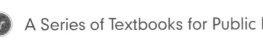

A Series of Textbooks for Public Health

U0596036

MEDICAL STATISTICS

医学统计学

主　编／赵进顺　倪春辉　毛广运

副主编／廖　奇　吴思英　易洪刚　施红英

秘　书／廖　奇

ZHEJIANG UNIVERSITY PRESS
浙江大学出版社

图书在版编目(CIP)数据

医学统计学＝Medical Statistics:英文 / 赵进顺,倪春辉,毛广运主编. —杭州:浙江大学出版社,2020.7

ISBN 978-7-308-20298-5

Ⅰ.①医… Ⅱ.①赵… ②倪… ③毛… Ⅲ.①医学统计-统计学-医学院校-教材-英文 Ⅳ.①R195.1

中国版本图书馆 CIP 数据核字(2020)第 103976 号

Medical Statistics(医学统计学)

赵进顺　倪春辉　毛广运　主编

丛书策划	朱　玲
责任编辑	陈丽勋
责任校对	李　晨
封面设计	春天书装
出版发行	浙江大学出版社
	(杭州市天目山路 148 号　邮政编码 310007)
	(网址:http://www.zjupress.com)
排　版	浙江时代出版服务有限公司
印　刷	杭州高腾印务有限公司
开　本	787mm×1092mm　1/16
印　张	25
字　数	835 千
版 印 次	2020 年 7 月第 1 版　2020 年 7 月第 1 次印刷
书　号	ISBN 978-7-308-20298-5
定　价	75.00 元

Contributors

叶海亚·阿布卡里亚/Abqariyah，Yahya（马来亚大学医学院社会和预防医学系/Department of Social and Preventive Medicine，Faculty of Medicine，University of Malaya）

艾自胜/Ai，Zisheng（同济大学医学院医学统计学教研室/Department of Medical Statistics，School of Medicine，Tongji University）

柏建岭/Bai，Jianling（南京医科大学公共卫生学院生物统计学系/Department of Biostatistics，School of Public Health，Nanjing Medical University）

珍妮·鲍曼/Bowman，Jenny（自由撰稿人和编者 freelance writer and editor）

岑晗/Cen，Han（宁波大学医学院公共卫生学院/School of Public Health，Medical School of Ningbo University）

戴悦/Dai，Yue（福建医科大学公共卫生学院卫生管理学系/Department of Health Management，Public Health School，Fujian Medical University）

黄民耀/Derry，Minyao Ng（宁波大学医学院/Medical School of Ningbo University）

丁玉松/Ding，Yusong（石河子大学医学院预防医学系/Department of Preventive Medicine，School of Medicine，Shihezi University）.

董长征/Dong，Changzheng（宁波大学医学院公共卫生学院/School of Public Health，Medical School of Ningbo University）

范引光/Fan，Yinguang（安徽医科大学公共卫生学院流行病与卫生统计学系/Department of Epidemiology and Health Statistics，School of Public Health，Anhui Medical University）

冯丹/Feng，Dan（中山大学公共卫生学院营养学系/Department of Nutrition，School of Public Health，Sun Yat-sen University）

冯晴/Feng，Qing（南京医科大学公共卫生学院营养与食品卫生学系/Department of Nutrition and Food Hygiene，School of Public Health，Nanjing Medical University）

凤志慧/Feng，Zhihui（山东大学公共卫生学院职业与环境健康学系/Department of Occupational and Environmental Health，School of Public Health，Shandong University）

郭欣/Guo，Xin（山东大学公共卫生学院卫生毒理与营养学系/Department of Toxicology and Nutrition，School of Public Health，Shandong University）

玛丽亚·哈莱姆/Haleem，Maria（宁波大学医学院/Medical School of Ningbo University）

韩丽媛/Han，Liyuan（中国科学院大学华美医院，中国科学院大学宁波生命与健康产业研究院/Hwa Mei Hospital，Ningbo Institute of Life and Health Industry，University of Chinese Academy of Sciences）

何灿霞/He，Canxia（宁波大学医学院公共卫生学院/School of Public Health，Medical School of Ningbo University）

何斐/He, Fei（福建医科大学公共卫生学院流行病与卫生统计学系/Department of Epidemiology and Health Statistics, Public Health School, Fujian Medical University）

胡付兰/Hu, Fulan（深圳大学医学部公共卫生学院流行病与卫生统计学教研室/Department of Epidemiology and Biostatistics, School of Public Health, Health Science Center, Shenzhen University）

华启航/Hua, Qihang（宁波大学医学院公共卫生学院/School of Public Health, Medical School of Ningbo University）

荆春霞/Jing, Chunxia（暨南大学基础医学院公共卫生与预防医学系/Department of Public Health and Preventive Medicine, School of Medicine, Jinan University）

敬媛媛/Jing, Yuanyuan（川北医学院预防医学系/Department of Preventive Medicine, North Sichuan Medical College）

孔璐/Kong, Lu（东南大学公共卫生学院劳动卫生与环境卫生学系/Department of Occupational and Environmental Health, School of Public Health, Southeast University）

冷瑞雪/Leng, Ruixue（安徽医科大学公共卫生学院流行病与卫生统计学系/Department of Epidemiology and Health Statistics, School of Public Health, Anhui Medical University）

李煌元/Li, Huangyuan（福建医科大学公共卫生学院预防医学系/Department of Preventive Medicine, Public Health School, Fujian Medical University）

李京/Li, Jing（潍坊医学院公共卫生学院预防医学系环境卫生教研室/Division of Environmental Health, Department of Preventive Medicine, School of Public Health, Weifang Medical University）

李静/Li, Jing（徐州医科大学公共卫生学院卫生学系/Department of Hygiene, School of Public Health, Xuzhou Medical University）

李举双/Li, Jushuang（温州医科大学公共卫生与管理学院预防医学系/Department of Preventive Medicine, School of Public Health and Management, Wenzhou Medical University）

李晓枫/Li, Xiaofeng（大连医科大学公共卫生学院流行病学教研室/Department of Epidemiology, School of Public Health, Dalian Medical University）

李永华/Li, Yonghua（济宁医学院公共卫生学院食品安全与健康教研室/Department of Food Safety and Health, School of Public Health, Jining Medical University）

李育平/Li, Yuping（扬州大学临床医学院，江苏省苏北人民医院/Clinical Medical School of Yangzhou University, Northern Jiangsu People's Hospital）

李真/Li, Zhen（宁波大学医学院公共卫生学院/School of Public Health, Medical School of Ningbo University）

廖奇/Liao, Qi（宁波大学医学院公共卫生学院/School of Public Health, Medical School of Ningbo University）

林玉兰/Lin, Yulan（福建医科大学公共卫生学院流行病与卫生统计学系/Department of Epidemiology and Health Statistics, Public Health School, Fujian Medical University）

刘丽亚/Liu, Liya（宁波大学医学院公共卫生学院/School of Public Health, Medical School of Ningbo University）

卢光玉/Lu, Guangyu（扬州大学医学院预防医学系/Department of Preventive Medicine, Medical College of Yangzhou University）

马俊香/Ma, Junxiang（首都医科大学公卫学院劳动卫生与环境卫生学系/Department of Occupational and Environmental Health, School of Public Health, Capital Medical University）

马儒林/Ma, Rulin（石河子大学医学院预防医学系/Department of Preventive Medicine, School of Medicine, Shihezi University）

安妮·马穆沙什维利/Mamuchashvili, Anny（宁波大学医学院/Medical School of Ningbo University）

毛广运/Mao, Guangyun（温州医科大学公共卫生与管理学院预防医学系,温州医科大学附属眼视光医院临床研究中心/Department of Preventive Medicine, School of Public Health and Management, and Center on Clinical Research of the Eye Hospital, Wenzhou Medical University）

毛盈颖/Mao, Yingying（浙江中医药大学公共卫生学院流行病与卫生统计学教研室/Department of Epidemiology and Health Statistics, School of Public Health, Zhejiang Chinese Medical University）

孟琼/Meng, Qiong（昆明医科大学公共卫生学院流行病与卫生统计学系/Department of Epidemiology and Health Statistics, School of Public Health, Kunming Medical University）

孟晓静/Meng, Xiaojing（南方医科大学公共卫生学院职业卫生与职业医学系/Department of Occupational Health and Occupational Medicine, School of Public Health, Southern Medical University）

倪春辉/Ni, Chunhui（南京医科大学公共卫生学院实验教学中心/Experimental Teaching Center, School of Public Health, Nanjing Medical University）

潘红梅/Pan, Hongmei（昆明医科大学公共卫生学院营养与食品科学系/Department of Nutrition and Food Science, School of Public Health, Kunming Medical University）

庞道华/Pang, Daohua（济宁医学院公共卫生学院营养与食品卫生学教研室/Department of Nutrition and Food Hygiene, School of Public Health, Jining Medical University）

培尔顿·米吉提/Peierdun, Mijiti（新疆医科大学公共卫生学院流行病学教研室/Department of Epidemiology, School of Public Health, Xinjiang Medical University）

仇梁林/Qiu, Lianglin（南通大学公共卫生学院营养与食品卫生学系/Department of Nutrition and Food Hygiene, School of Public Health, Nantong University）

曲泉颖/Qu, Quanying（锦州医科大学公共卫生学院流行病学教研室/Department of Epidemiology, School of Public Health, Jinzhou Medical University）

邵方/Shao, Fang（南京医科大学公共卫生学院生物统计学系/Department of Biostatistics, School of Public Health, Nanjing Medical University）

沈冲/Shen, Chong（南京医科大学公共卫生学院流行病学系/Department of Epidemiology,

School of Public Health，Nanjing Medical University)

施红英/Shi，Hongying（温州医科大学公共卫生与管理学院预防医学系/Department of Preventive Medicine，School of Public Health and Management，Wenzhou Medical University)

孙桂菊/Sun，Guiju（东南大学公共卫生学院营养与食品卫生学系/Department of Nutrition and Food Hygiene，School of Public Health，Southeast University)

孙桂香/Sun，Guixiang（徐州医科大学公共卫生学院流行病与卫生统计学系/Department of Epidemiology and Health Statistics，School of Public Health，Xuzhou Medical University)

孙宏鹏/Sun，Hongpeng（苏州大学医学部公共卫生学院少儿卫生与社会医学系/Department of Child Health and Social Medicine，School of Public Health，Medical College of Soochow University)

孙鲜策/Sun，Xiance（大连医科大学公共卫生学院劳动卫生与环境卫生教研室/Department of Occupational and Environmental Health，School of Public Health，Dalian Medical University)

唐春兰/Tang，Chunlan（宁波大学医学院公共卫生学院/School of Public Health，Medical School of Ningbo University)

唐少文/Tang，Shaowen（南京医科大学公共卫生学院流行病学系/Department of Epidemiology，School of Public Health，Nanjing Medical University)

童智敏/Tong，Zhimin（昆山疾病预防控制中心/Kunshan Municipal Center for Disease Control and Prevention)

王春平/Wang，Chunping（潍坊医学院公共卫生学院预防医学系/Department of Preventive Medicine，School of Public Health，Weifang Medical University)

王辉/Wang，Hui（北京大学医学部公共卫生学院妇幼卫生系/Department of Maternal and Children Health，School of Public Health，Peking University Health Science Center)

王建明/Wang，Jianming（南京医科大学公共卫生学院流行病学系/Department of Epidemiology，School of Public Health，Nanjing Medical University)

王津涛/Wang，Jintao（四川大学华西公共卫生学院环境卫生与职业医学系/Department of Environmental Health and Occupational Medicine，West China School of Public Health，Sichuan University)

王乐三/Wang，Lesan（中南大学湘雅公共卫生学院流行病与卫生统计学系/Department of Epidemiology and Health Statistics，Xiangya School of Public Health，Central South University)

王丽君/Wang，Lijun（暨南大学医学院公共卫生与预防医学系/Department of Public Health and Preventive Medicine，School of Medicine，Jinan University)

王强/Wang，Qiang（江苏大学医学院预防医学与卫生检验系/Department of Preventive Medicine and Public Health Laboratory Science，School of Medicine，Jiangsu University)

王少康/Wang，Shaokang（东南大学公共卫生学院营养与食品卫生学系/Department of

Nutrition and Food Hygiene, School of Public Health, Southeast University)

王涛/Wang, Tao (温州医科大学公共卫生与管理学院预防医学系/Department of Preventive Medicine, School of Public Health and Management, Wenzhou Medical University)

王晓珂/Wang, Xiaoke (南通大学公共卫生学院职业医学与环境毒理学系/Department of Occupational Medicine and Environmental Toxicology, School of Public Health, Nantong University)

王子云/Wang, Ziyun (贵州医科大学公共卫生学院流行病与卫生统计学系/Department of Epidemiology and Health Statistics, School of Public Health, Guizhou Medical University)

黄丽冰/Wong, Li Ping (马来亚大学医学院社会和预防医学系/Department of Social and Preventive Medicine, Faculty of Medicine, University of Malaya)

吴冬梅/Wu, Dongmei (南京医科大学公共卫生学院职业医学与环境卫生学系/Department of Occupational Medicine and Environmental Health, School of Public Health, Nanjing Medical University)

吴继国/Wu, Jiguo (南方医科大学公共卫生学院环境卫生学系/Department of Environmental Health, School of Public Health, Southern Medical University)

吴秋云/Wu, Qiuyun (徐州医科大学公共卫生学院卫生学系/Department of Hygiene, School of Public Health, Xuzhou Medical University)

吴思英/Wu, Siying (福建医科大学公共卫生学院流行病与卫生统计学系/Department of Epidemiology and Health Statistics, School of Public Health, Fujian Medical University)

吴莹/Wu, Ying (南方医科大学生物统计教研室/Department of Biostatistics, Southern Medical University)

肖艳杰/Xiao, Yanjie (锦州医科大学公共卫生学院流行病学系/Department of Epidemiology, School of Public Health, Jinzhou Medical University)

徐进/Xu, Jin (宁波大学医学院公共卫生学院/School of Public Health, Medical School of Ningbo University)

许望东/Xu, Wangdong (西南医科大学公共卫生学院循证医学中心/Department of Evidence-Based Medicine, School of Public Health, Southwest Medical University)

严玮文/Yan, Weiwen (南京医科大学公共卫生学院预防医学实验教学中心/Experimental Teaching Center of Preventive Medicine, School of Public Health, Nanjing Medical University)

杨丹婷/Yang, Danting (宁波大学医学院公共卫生学院/School of Public Health, Medical School of Ningbo University)

杨艳/Yang, Yan (西南医科大学公共卫生学院营养与食品卫生教研室/Department of Nutrition and Food Hygiene, School of Public Health, Southwest Medical University)

姚美雪/Yao, Meixue (徐州医科大学公共卫生学院流行病与卫生统计学系/Department of Epidemiology and Health Statistics, School of Public Health, Xuzhou Medical University)

叶洋/Ye, Yang（江苏大学医学院预防医学与卫生检验系/Department of Preventive Medicine and Public Health Laboratory Science, School of Medicine, Jiangsu University）

易洪刚/Yi, Honggang（南京医科大学公共卫生学院生物统计学系/Department of Biostatistics, School of Public Health, Nanjing Medical University）

尹洁云/Yin, Jieyun（苏州大学医学部公共卫生学院流行病与卫生统计学教研室/Department of Epidemiology and Health Statistics, School of Public Health, Medical College of Soochow University）

于广霞/Yu, Guangxia（福建医科大学公共卫生学院预防医学系/Department of Preventive Medicine, School of Public Health, Fujian Medical University）

俞琼/Yu, Qiong,（吉林大学公共卫生学院流行病与卫生统计学教研室/Department of Epidemiology and Health Statistics, School of Public Health, Jilin University）

袁芝琼/Yuan, Zhiqiong（大理大学公共卫生学院营养与食品卫生学教研室/Department of Nutrition and Food Hygiene, School of Public Health, Dali University）

曾芳芳/Zeng, Fangfang（暨南大学医学院公共卫生与预防医学系/Department of Public Health and Preventive Medicine, School of Medicine, Jinan University）

查龙应/Zha, Longying（南方医科大学公共卫生学院营养与食品卫生学系/Department of Nutrition and Food Hygiene, School of Public Health, Southern Medical University）

张丹丹/Zhang, Dandan（浙江大学基础医学院病理学与病理生理学系/Department of Pathology and Pathophysiology, School of Basic Medical Sciences, Zhejiang University）

张俊辉/Zhang, Junhui（西南医科大学公共卫生学院流行病与卫生统计学教研室/Department of Epidemiology and Health Statistics, School of Public Health, Southwest Medical University）

张莉娜/Zhang, Lina（宁波大学医学院公共卫生学院/School of Public Health, Medical School of Ningbo University）

张利平/Zhang, Liping（潍坊医学院公共卫生学院预防医学系环境卫生教研室/Division of Environmental Health, Department of Preventive Medicine, School of Public Health, Weifang Medical University）

张巧/Zhang, Qiao（郑州大学公共卫生学院卫生毒理学教研室/Department of Toxicology, School of Public Health, Zhengzhou University）

张思懋/Zhang, Simin（南京医科大学公共卫生学院社会医学和健康教育系/Department of Social Medicine and Health Education, School of Public Health, Nanjing Medical University）

张晓宏/Zhang, Xiaohong(宁波大学医学院公共卫生学院/School of Public Health, Medical School of Ningbo University）

赵进顺/Zhao, Jinshun（宁波大学医学院公共卫生学院/School of Public Health, Medical School of Ningbo University）

赵苒/Zhao, Ran（厦门大学公共卫生学院预防医学系/Department of Preventive Medicine, School of Public Health, Xiamen University）

赵秀兰/Zhao，Xiulan（山东大学公共卫生学院营养与毒理学系/Department of Nutrition and Toxicology，School of Public Health，Shandong University）

赵研/Zhao，Yan（匹兹堡大学医学中心/University of Pittsburgh Medical Center）

郑馥荔/Zheng，Fuli（福建医科大学公共卫生学院预防医学系/Department of Preventive Medicine，School of Public Health，Fujian Medical University）

仲崇科/Zhong，Chongke（苏州大学医学部公共卫生学院流行病与卫生统计学教研室/Department of Epidemiology and Health Statistics，School of Public Health，Medical College of Soochow University）

周舫/Zhou，Fang（郑州大学公共卫生学院劳动卫生教研室/Department of Occupational Health，School of Public Health，Zhengzhou University）

周志衡/Zhou，Zhiheng（广州市华立科技职业学院健康学院/Health College of Guangzhou Huali Science and Technology Vocational College；深圳市福田区第二人民医院/ The Second People's Hospital of Futian District，Shenzhen）

邹祖全/Zou，Zuquan（宁波大学医学院公共卫生学院/School of Public Health，Medical School of Ningbo University）

Preface

Public health is the science and art of disease prevention. It targets many facets necessary to the well-being of society, including prolonging life, the promotion of physical health through organized community efforts directed at environmental sanitation, the control of community infections, the education of the individual in the principles of personal hygiene, the development of the social machinery to ensure that every individual in the community has an adequate standard of living for the maintenance of health, and the organization of medical and nursing services to aid early diagnosis and enable preventive treatment of diseases. Public health includes many sub-branches, among which the most important ones are preventive medicine, medical statistics, epidemiology, and health services. Preventive medicine is an important part of medical science, which, when integrated with basic medicine and clinical medicine, forms the entire frame of modern medicine. Because preventive medicine, medical statistics, and epidemiology are three important compulsory subjects for international students majoring in clinical medicine, Zhejiang University Press organized public health experts from five universities in China and the University of Texas in the United States of America to compile an English textbook entitled *Preventive Medicine*, *Medical Statistics and Epidemiology*, which was published in 2014. In recent years, this textbook has played an important role in teaching preventive medicine, medical statistics, and epidemiology to international students majoring in clinical medicine in China.

With the continuous expansion and internationalization of higher education in China and many developments in preventive medicine, medical statistics, and epidemiology, a revised edition of this important textbook was required. In 2018, Zhejiang University Press organized experts to reprint the textbook. For the revised edition, the quality was raised significantly to meet global demands. The authors endeavor to improve the quality of this textbook and reflect the latest developments in the fields of preventive medicine, medical statistics, and epidemiology. In addition, the authors present a resource to standardize and unify the quality of teaching and materials for international students majoring in clinical medicine in China.

The new edition is a series of textbooks for public health including *Preventive Medicine*, *Medical Statistics*, and *Epidemiology*.

This book, *Medical Statistics*, describes the basic concepts of medical statistics and the common methods applied in practice. It includes 17 chapters. Chapters 1, 2, and 3 introduce the basic statistical terminologies and descriptive statistics for quantitative data and categorical data. Chapter 4 introduces how to make statistical tables and graphs. Chapter 5 is about parameter estimation and introduces point and interval estimation, confidence interval (CI), and 95% CI. Chapter 6 introduces the basic idea, key steps, and the major considerations of a hypothesis test. Chapters 7, 8, 9, and 10 introduce the most commonly used hypothesis testing methods, including t-test, analysis of variance (ANOVA), chi-square test, and non-parametric tests. Chapter 11 is about linear correlation and regression, focusing on linear correlation analysis as well as the fitting and evaluation of a linear regression model. Chapters 12, 13, and 14 illustrate how to develop an appropriate model, specifically the multiple linear regression model, multiple logistic regression model, and multiple Cox proportional hazards model. Because the impact due to other potential confounders can be properly adjusted, compared to a simple linear regression model, the multiple regression models are now widely accepted as a better approach to assess the independent effect or influence of a predictor on a quantitative response variable or dichotomous response variables in a cross-sectional, case-control, or cohort study. Chapter 15 explains the foundations of the study design. Chapter 16 briefly introduces the principles and techniques of sample size and power estimates. Chapter 17 provides a basic introduction and guidance on the proper application of commonly used statistical methods by using SPSS software, which readers can follow to learn how to perform simple analyses. This book aims to provide a basic introduction and guidance on the proper application of commonly used statistical methods, with sufficient background information and details that readers might carry out similar analyses themselves. This book provides a good starting point, both for students who want to systematically grasp the concepts of medical statistics and for researchers who want to increase their knowledge of medical statistics relating to their field.

In addition to this textbook, a concise bilingual manual with *pinyin* has been compiled. The authors envision this manual to be useful in bridging the language barrier faced by international students studying clinical medicine in China, especially those starting internships in Chinese hospitals, or by Chinese doctors who intend to practice in a foreign country and hope to have a convenient guide to refer to while practicing. This manual consists of the following parts: Part 1 includes a translation of all laboratory reports used in Chinese hospitals, which are categorized by department for ease of use, how to interpret each report, and the normal values; Part 2 consists of questions to ask during history taking in both English and Chinese with *pinyin*, to allow a doctor or an intern to obtain information despite the language barrier; Part 3 includes various tips and checklists of the most common physical examination; Part 4 lists the common communication skills necessary for various patient scenarios, including but not limited to "Breaking Bad News" and "Explaining Medication"; Part 5 consists of case report forms (discharge summary for hospitalized patients and medical records for outpatient department); Part 6 is a guide on the use of the basic Chinese hospital software; Part 7 shows clinical formulae needed in the clinical practice. This manual will be easy and convenient to use and ensures that any student or doctor have quick and easy access to topics of interest.

In addition, courseware presented in MS PowerPoint is available to supplement this book. And a question bank can be accessed by scanning the QR code at the end of each chapter. Institutions that use this book as teaching material can contact Zhejiang University Press.

More than 40 institutions of higher education both in China and abroad participated in the compilation of this series of textbooks, which is the crystallization of the knowledge and experience of experts in the field of public health from countries such as China, the United States of America, and Malaysia. All editorial committees pooled their best efforts together to ensure that this series of textbooks is not only innovative but also practical and reflects the latest developments in the related fields.

Finally, a special thanks goes to Mrs. Linda Bowman for her wonderful help in the process of reviewing the manuscript.

However, due to limited time, mistakes and omissions in the books are inevitable; therefore we sincerely seek the readers' feedback. For comments and suggestions, please email us at zhaojinshun@nbu. edu. cn.

Zhao Jinshun, Ni Chunhui, Mao Guangyun

Contents

Chapter 1   Introduction and Basic Concepts

1.1   General Overview

1.1.1   What Is Medical Statistics?

Statistics is a branch of applied mathematics that focuses on the collection, organization, analysis, interpretation, and presentation of data. It contains a series of powerful and vital methods that help with our researches and studies and has become one of the most commonly applied disciplines in the past several decades.

In general, statistics can be classified into two categories: **mathematical statistics** and **applied statistics**. The former is mainly interested in developing novel strategies and measures of statistics based on probability theory (a major component of mathematics) and others. The latter, applied statistics, guides the performance of statistical practices containing data collection, organization, analysis, and interpretation precisely and efficiently in fields such as science, economics, psychology, industry, and society. **Medical statistics** is a branch of applied statistics, applying statistics to medical practices, such as the investigation of disease burden, screening of influential factors associated with the initiation and development of disease, assessment of the efficacy and safety of a medication, effective prevention, and control of the disease, and so on.

Medical statistics has been widely accepted as a profound applied natural science and a series of vital methods dealing with the study design, data collection, data management, data mining, and data analysis. Among these methods, most routine medical statistics focus on **descriptive statistics** and **inferential statistics**. Descriptive statistics describes and summarizes the features or characteristics of data using a sample that has been randomly selected from the studied population. While inferential statistics focuses on the estimations of population characteristics or relationships between two or among several features based on a randomly selected sample. To summarize, descriptive statistics serve as a basis for inferential statistics, which extracts useful knowledge about a population from samples collected—the final objective of medical statistics.

Descriptive statistics is often related to two types of the sample or population distribution properties: the **central tendency** (or location) which seeks to characterize the distribution's central or typical value, and the **tendency of dispersion** (or variability) which characterizes the extent to which members of the distribution depart from its center and each other. Descriptive statistics uses statistical indices such as the mean, standard deviation, rate, ratio, graphs such as histograms and bar graphs, and tables to make the information easier to view and interpret.

Unlike descriptive statistics which is solely related to the observed data's properties, the inferential statistics aims to apply the conclusions that have been obtained from a sample to a population—the properties of a population from a randomly selected sample. There are two main categories of inferential statistics: estimating parameters, which aims to estimate the value of a population parameter (i. e. the population mean) based on the statistics derived from the sample data (i. e. the sample mean), and hypothesis tests, of which the sample is used to estimate whether there are significant differences among several corresponding populations or the predictors are significantly associated with the response variable. For example, you might be interested in knowing if a medication is effective for breast cancer or whether physical exercise helps children grow faster and healthier. The contents of statistical analysis can be summarized in brief as follows (Figure 1.1).

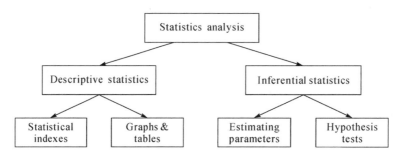

Figure 1. 1   Content Structure of Statistics Analysis

1.1.2   Procedures of Statistics Research

It is the culmination of a long process to achieve findings in a study using medical statistics. Carrying out a study includes constructing the study design (features determination and measurements), devising the sampling technique and sample size, collecting and cleaning the data, determining proper analysis methods, drawing a reasonable conclusion, and presenting the results effectively. The overall quality of the outcome depends on the entire chain of events. A single weak link would produce unreliable results. The basic procedures of medical statistics are summarized as follows.

1.1.2.1   Study Design

During the study design phase, researchers need to formulate a research question that can be answered with statistical analysis, allowing them to carry out projects precisely and efficiently. It requires the researchers to have a medical background to avoid missing any important factors that may affect the conclusions and to be proficient with statistical methods to define the problem and the objective of the study. The group to be studied is determined during this phase.

1.1.2.2 Data Collection

The objective of data collection is to collect and evaluate data from the sample that is required in the study. In this step, the samples should be selected from the study populations using appropriate sampling plans and determining sample size. Then, the features of the participants in the sample should be properly measured using a questionnaire or other instruments. The investigators must check and evaluate the quality of collected data to avoid missing data, outlier, or logical errors to improve the data reliability.

1.1.2.3 Data Management and Analysis

The saying, "garbage in, garbage out," indicates the importance of high-quality data to your study. The process of designing, reviewing and cleaning data is called data management which concerns the data set creation, data entry, check and correction of missing values, outliers, and logical errors, and standardization and transformation of data. Then, statistical methods including descriptive statistics and statistical inferences are applied to sample data to extract reasonable conclusions.

Although important information extracted from your data is usually consistent based on your sample, the data should be comprehensively analyzed with appropriate statistical approaches since different methods will lead to (slightly) different conclusions even based on the same sample. Only proper methods will produce reasonable conclusions using high-quality data. As a result, the requirements of each statistical method should be considered and evaluated before application to obtain more robust and reliable findings.

1.1.2.4 Making decisions

This stage is to draw reasonable conclusions and answer your questions properly based on the results obtained in step 3. Many tools such as statistical tables and graphs (STG) can help better organize the output and present findings. The concept of STG will be introduced in Chapter 4.

1.2   Basic Conceptions in Statistics

1.2.1 Population and Sample

A **population** is a set of similar individuals or objects to the interest of a specific study. A statistical population can consist of people, animals, or schools—anything that an investigator concerns. For example, when studying the height of adult men, the population is the heights of all the adult men in the world. If we are studying the intelligence quotient (IQ) of students at a university, the population is the set of IQs for all the students in the university. The size of the population can vary from very large to small, depending on what the investigator intends to study. Sometimes, the size of the population is too large, making it impractical to investigate each member of the population. Such a population is called an

infinite population such as the stars in the sky or the germs in a body. Contrarily, the population with a limited number of individuals is called a **finite population** such as the number of students in a high school or the number of residents in a small town.

There are two types of population in research: the **target population** and the **study population**. The target population, also known as the theoretical population, refers to the entire group of individuals for which survey data are used to generalize the conclusions. The study population, also known as the accessible population, is a subset of the target population where researchers have access to and draw samples from. The study population is the population that investigators can measure and apply their conclusion, sometimes limiting to a region, state, city, county, or institution of a target population. Therefore, the study population is usually much smaller than the target population. As an example, if a doctor wants to study the mortality of institutionalized elderly with Alzheimer's, the target population is all the institutionalized elderly with Alzheimer's, and the study population may only contain all institutionalized elderly with Alzheimer's in some hospitals in a city.

Regardless of the type of study, populations are typically extremely large in practice, especially on the national or international level. Suppose we want to know the average birth weight of premature infants in a city. The best way to achieve the objective, in theory, is to perform a census or general investigation, collecting and examining all birth weights of these premature infants in the city, which is too large and impractical to collect. Another good option is to randomly select a subset of premature infants in the city, obtain the values of birth weight of each participant and estimate the average birth weight of all premature infants in this city. The latter is easier to apply and more commonly performed than the former. In statistics, the process of selecting a subset of individuals from a population in a random manner is called **sampling** and the subset of individuals drawn from a population is called **sample**. The number of individuals within a sample is called **sample size**.

Only the sample as representative of the population can be used for further statistical inferences. Therefore, a sample must be selected in an appropriate way, such as through a process of random selection in which everyone in a population has an equal chance to be selected. This is called **random sampling**, and the sample size should be large enough for further statistical inference. If each participant in the population is not selected randomly, called **non-random sampling**, further statistical inferences cannot be performed using this sample. Finally, careful exploration of a random sample instead of the population can greatly reduce the labor and cost involved, and highly increase the feasibility of a well-conducted study. In some conditions, it might be the only way to apply a study.

1.2.2 Homogeneity and Heterogeneity

In statistics, **homogeneity** means that the variables (i.e. people, cells, or traits) within a data set share the same or very similar traits or characteristics. In a homogeneous sampling, all items in the sample are selected with similar or identical traits, which means that participants in a homogeneous sample might share the same age, location, or employment. For example, a data set made up of 20-year-old college students who obtained the scholarship is a homogeneous sample because all individuals in the sample are 20-year-old college students. A homogeneous sample is chosen when the trait or characteristic of a population is the interest of the study.

In statistics, **heterogeneity**, the opposite of homogeneity, also called variability, means the subjects in a population are slightly different though they have good homogeneity. A heterogeneous population or sample is one in which each participant has a different value for the characteristic you are interested in. For example, if everyone in your group varies from 40 to 70 kg, they would be heterogeneous in weight. In practice, heterogeneity is extremely common as patients will be different in many factors including demographics, clinical manifestations, and medical histories.

1.2.3   Parameter and Statistic

Statistical indices such as mean, median, variance, standard deviation, and rate are commonly used to describe the features or characteristics of a sample or population. In statistics, the index used to describe the features of a population is defined as a **parameter**, whereas the measurement derived from sample data is called a **statistic**, which is often used to estimate the parameter of a corresponding population (Figure 1.2). Suppose we have all premature infants' birth weights in a population and calculate its average birth weight, which is a parameter. If we select a random sample from the population and calculate the average, it is a statistic.

As a subset of a population, a sample is not equal to the population. Usually, the difference between a sample statistic and the parameter of the corresponding population exists when the sample does not represent the entire population of data. This is called

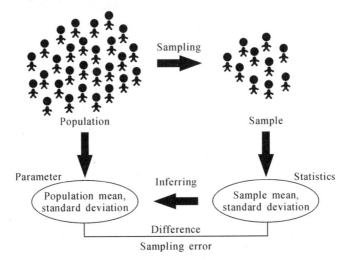

Figure 1.2   Relationship between Population and Sample

sampling error, which will be introduced in detail in Chapter 5. In practice, sampling error cannot be completely avoided using randomizing sample selection. Fortunately, it can be reduced by increasing the sample size to some extent, which will be introduced in detail in Chapter 5 too.

1.2.4 Variable and Data

Data analysis mainly focuses on the study of the features of a population, inferring the differences among populations or estimating the relationships between predictors and response variable, using randomly selected samples. The first task you complete before any statistical analysis is to identify the type of each feature in your data as a specific statistical method is only suitable for a particular type of feature, which is also called variable. In statistics, a **variable** is defined as a characteristic of the participant. We can record information about a feature with a variable in a study. The associated information on a specific variable is defined as the value of a variable. Finally, the accumulation of the values is called **data**.

In general, the variables can be classified into two major types: numerical and categorical variables (Figure 1.3). **Numerical variables**, also known as **quantitative variables**, consist of numbers representing counts or measurements with specific units, such as kilograms, hours, meters. A numerical variable can be further classified into either a continuous or a discrete variable. A **continuous** variable can take any value within a range, such as a person's height and weight. A **discrete** variable contains values that are countable without decimals. For example, the number of books in a bag and the number of children in a family are both considered discrete variables. Other examples are shown in Figure 1.3.

Categorical variables, also known as **qualitative variables**, contain values that are selected from a limited number of possible values. A categorical variable can be further separated into either a nominal or ordinal variable. **Nominal variables** contain two or more categories such as male/female, alive/dead, and blood type (O, A, B, AB). **Ordinal variables** contain values that can be naturally ordered. For example, exam grades (i. e. fail, pass, good, excellent) can be ranked with excellent better than good and good better than pass. Other examples include cancer degree (I, II, III, IV) or therapeutic effect (ineffective, improved, effective, cured), where intrinsic order exists among the categories within these variables. More examples can be found in Figure 1.3.

Different types of variables can be transformed from one to another as needed. Although an ordinal variable can be transformed into a continuous variable in some conditions, most of these transformations are unidirectional—from numerical to ordinal and to nominal. In Figure 1.4, the numerical variable (age) can be transformed into an ordinal variable (young, middle-aged, old), and then be transformed into a nominal variable (young or old).

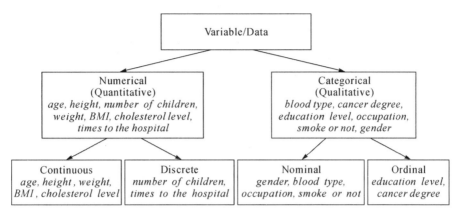

Figure 1. 3   Types of Variable/Data

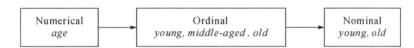

Figure 1. 4   Transformation of Different Variable Types

1.2.5 Error

In statistics, an **error**, which can be classified into sampling or non-sampling error, indicates the difference between the observed value and the "true" value. The greater the error, the less the data are representative of the sample or population.

In many conditions, a **sampling error** refers to differences between the statistics of a sample and the parameter (true values) of the population because of the heterogeneity. It occurs when we use sample statistics as an estimate of the desired population. Sometimes, a sampling error also represents the differences among the same statistics of several samples randomly selected from the same population. No sampling error occurs if the conclusions are depending on a census which means that each participant in a population will be investigated, but it is expensive and impractical. The only way sampling errors can be reduced is to increase the sample size.

Non-sampling error is caused by factors outside of the sample selection process. A non-sampling error can occur at any stage of a census or sampling study, which mainly includes the systematic error, missing data error, and personal error. **Systematic error** is caused by inaccuracies, mainly during the measurement process that is inherent to the system instead of the chance. It can be caused by things like defective instruments and misuse of instruments. Systematic error is the most common non-sampling error, which can be reduced by better study design, proper instrument calibration, standard data collection, and appropriate statistical approaches. **Missing data error** represents the errors induced by too much missing data that decreases the power of statistical inference. This error can be reduced by designing more adequate methods of data collection during the investigation.

Personal error is caused by faulty procedures conducted by the observers, such as writing a wrong record or performing a wrong procedure. Providing more training and supervision during the investigation will reduce personal error. Unlike sampling error, non-sampling error tends to increase with bigger sample sizes as more efforts are needed to collect and process data.

1.2.6 Probability and Relative Frequency

In statistics, events that are influenced by chance are called **random events**. For example, flipping a coin generates an outcome, a head or a tail, with a 50% probability of each occurs. Each possible result of a random experiment is called an **outcome**. In this experiment, the outcomes are either heads or tails. The collection of all the possible distinct outcomes of a random experiment is called **sample space**.

Although the random event is unpredictable, we can use **probability** to measure the chances that we will observe it at a certain time. Suppose A is an outcome of a random experiment, the probability of A can be denoted by $P(A)$ or $Pr(A)$. For example, "H" is used to represent as head in a coin-flipping experiment, the probability of the head is 0.5 (or 50%) and can be recorded as $P(H)=0.5$ or $Pr(H)=0.5$. The probability of an event E, expressed as $P(E)$, is always between 0 and 1. The cumulative probability, which is calculated by the sum of all the probabilities, of the sample space (the collection of all possible outcomes) is always equal to 1. In statistical analysis, a random event with probability $\leqslant=0.05$ or 0.01 is defined as a **small probability event**, which has been widely accepted as the criteria in almost all statistical inferences.

A classical approach to estimate probability is the calculation of **relative frequency**, which is a measure of the number of times that an event occurs divided the number of total events. The relative frequency is an experimental quantity rather than a theoretical one. This is a very common and useful way that is used after the data collection. Suppose in a 100-times coin flipping experiment, we observed 48 heads and 52 tails. The relative frequency of head is 0.48 $\left(\dfrac{48}{100}\right)$ using Formula (1.1).

$$\text{Relative frequency}=\frac{\text{The number of the event occurrence}}{\text{The total number of the experiment conducted}} \qquad (1.1)$$

(Liao Qi, Mao Guangyun, Zhao Yan, Zhao Jinshun)

Question Bank

Chapter 2   Descriptive Statistics for Quantitative Data

After the data collection of a study, the long-waited, exciting data management and analysis are awaiting. Descriptive statistics that describe features or characteristics from a sample, serve as the basis of further data analysis. This will be introduced in this chapter, including frequency distribution, measures of the central tendency and variation, normal distribution, and others.

2.1   Frequency Distribution

2.1.1   Frequency Distribution

One way for organizing the quantitative data is to classify observed values of a specific quantitative variable into ordinal categories, and then to calculate the frequency for each category. A list containing the frequency by category is called a frequency distribution table. In statistics, a frequency distribution is defined as the correspondence of a set of frequencies with the set of categories, intervals, or values into which a population is classified. Nowadays, a frequency distribution has been widely used as the first step to investigate the features of a variable in a sample. It can be displayed as a frequency distribution table or histogram, a statistical graph with a set of bars (or smoothed lines) to show the frequency of each related group.

2.1.2   Frequency Distribution Table

A frequency distribution table is a statistical table to display the frequency distribution of your data. It contains three major components: the group, frequency, and associated relative frequency of each group. A frequency distribution table can be used for both categorical and numeric variables.

2.1.2.1   Frequency Distribution Table of Discrete Variables

As can be found in Chapter 1, a quantitative variable can be either a continuous or discrete variable. In statistics, a continuous variable can take any value within a given range with decimals, while a discrete variable is countable, such as negative and non-negative integers, in a finite amount. For example, the number of decayed teeth in an experiment is a discrete variable, within the set $\{0, 1, 2, \cdots\}$.

Since the frequency distribution of a discrete variable is easier to understand than that of a continuous variable, we would like to show readers the techniques of preparing a frequency distribution table for discrete data. The method involves classifying the data into groups based on values, calculating the frequencies and relative frequencies for each group and displaying the distribution with a statistical table. The following example illustrates the theory behind the frequency distribution table and procedures to construct the table for a discrete variable.

Example 2. 1　Previous studies suggest delayed treatment is a leading risk factor of coronary artery lesions in patients with Kawasaki disease (KD). The treatment time, defined as the number of days before the treatment, of 100 KD patients was collected in a KD study and displayed in Table 2. 1. How can we obtain the treatment time distribution of this study?

Table 2. 1　The Time (d) before the Treatment of KD

7	4	7	4	11	5	7	9	7	3	8	8	6	6	8	7	6	4	4	6
10	9	7	7	4	5	8	5	8	5	3	5	8	5	9	7	6	9	2	6
2	6	3	8	8	5	7	6	9	5	10	6	6	6	6	6	5	8	5	7
4	7	6	9	2	6	6	6	10	8	7	7	6	6	8	9	7	5	5	6
4	6	5	7	2	5	4	5	6	6	5	4	10	4	11	9	4	8	3	1

The preparation of the frequency distribution table starts with identifying the maximum and minimum values from your sample—in this case, 11 and 1 respectively. Since there are 11 distinct values of treatment time from the study, the table should contain 11 groups (rows), one for each distinct treatment time, ranging from 1 to 11. If fewer groups are required, discrete values can be converted into ordinal ones, grouping different treatment times into ranges. The number of cases per group and associated relative frequency for each category is calculated and listed in Table 2. 2.

Table 2. 2　Distribution of Number of Days before the Treatment of KD

Days before treatment	Frequency	Relative frequency /%	Cumulative frequency	Cumulative relative frequency /%
1	1	1. 0	1	1. 0
2	4	4. 0	5	5. 0
3	4	4. 0	9	9. 0
4	11	11. 0	20	20. 0
5	16	16. 0	36	36. 0
6	23	23. 0	59	59. 0
7	15	15. 0	74	74. 0
8	12	12. 0	86	86. 0

| | | | **Continued** |
Days before treatment	Frequency	Relative frequency /%	Cumulative frequency	Cumulative relative frequency /%
9	8	8. 0	94	94. 0
10	4	4. 0	98	98. 0
11	2	2. 0	100	100. 0
Total	100	100. 0	—	—

Although neither the cumulative frequency nor cumulative relative frequency are needed, they are usually listed in a frequency distribution table to help readers better understand the data. The cumulative frequency (or cumulative relative frequency) is the sum of the frequency (or relative frequency) for that class and all previous classes in a frequency distribution table.

Using the above frequency distribution table, we observed that the majority (77. 0%) of KD patients received treatment between 4 and 8 days after the onset of the disease. Fewer patients obtain the treatment within 3 days or after 8 days after disease onset, and the most common treatment time is the 6th day.

2. 1. 2. 2   Frequency Distribution Table of Continuous Variables

Since a continuous variable contains an infinite amount of numbers, it is impractical to list all the values as what we have done for the discrete data. It makes the generation of the frequency distribution table for continuous data more complicated than that of discrete data. Example 2. 2 provides the strategy and procedures for developing a frequency distribution table for continuous data.

Example 2. 2   To investigate the condition of central obesity among male adults in a city, a researcher selected 105 male adults from his city in a random manner and obtained their waist circumference presented in Table 2. 3.

Table 2. 3   The Waist Circumference (cm) of 105 Male Adults

68. 4	85. 8	96. 5	96. 2	97. 0	109. 1	123. 8
82. 5	97. 6	102. 4	98. 1	106. 1	110. 4	116. 0
73. 7	95. 8	101. 2	102. 0	98. 3	98. 9	109. 0
81. 3	97. 5	86. 3	97. 2	104. 6	99. 8	116. 1
84. 5	89. 9	89. 9	98. 6	110. 2	113. 1	127. 5
83. 1	95. 7	100. 7	101. 5	106. 8	97. 9	122. 9
80. 0	96. 8	92. 2	95. 0	97. 0	105. 1	111. 7
79. 4	80. 5	95. 0	93. 9	104. 4	117. 1	133. 0
86. 5	90. 2	89. 5	98. 6	101. 2	109. 0	128. 0

Continued

80. 9	97. 2	88. 5	79. 5	108. 8	105. 6	93. 3
91. 5	93. 3	92. 7	89. 0	101. 2	116. 4	93. 0
78. 2	88. 9	100. 0	100. 0	95. 5	109. 2	92. 2
80. 9	85. 5	92. 2	91. 5	104. 5	113. 0	112. 0
102. 1	88. 4	95. 7	88. 1	106. 3	109. 3	94. 5
83. 7	80. 1	98. 2	98. 1	103. 7	115. 0	113. 6

We can construct a frequency distribution table for continuous data following the procedures below.

Step 1: Calculate the range of the data.

Range=maximum value (133. 0 cm)−minimum value (68. 4 cm)=64. 6 cm

Step 2: Decide the number of classes and calculate the class width. The number of classes usually ranges from 8 to 15 with 10 as the most popular choice. In addition, we can use more classes for larger data sets. The width of each class is determined using the following formula.

$$\text{Class width}=\frac{\text{Range}}{\text{Number of classes}}$$

If the number of class is defined as 8, 10, and 15, the width of each class will be 8. 075, 6. 46, and 4. 31 cm, respectively. We can round these numbers to 8, 7, or 5 cm. We'll pick 5 cm as the class width in this example.

Step 3: Divide the range of the data into classes with equal width.

Choose either the minimum value or a convenient value below the minimum for the lower limit of the first class. In our example, 65 cm is chosen as the lower bound of the first class, containing the count of men with waist circumference between 65. 0 and 70. 0 cm. The first class is labelled as "65. 0~," where the upper bound can be omitted. The second class contains the count of men with waist circumference between 70. 0 and 75. 0 cm, one class width higher than the first class. Unlike other classes, the upper bound of the last class needs to be included in the interval. The rationale for this classification is to make sure that all the observed data will be included in the frequency distribution table with no overlap. The class groups of this example are illustrated in the first column of Table 2. 4. Sometimes, illogical class groupings(e. g. 1~5, 5~10, 11~15) can also be detected in some published papers, in which the boundaries of the categories are ambiguous.

Step 4: Count the number of cases (frequency) and relative frequency for each class, shown in the second column in Table 2. 4. Similar to Example 2. 1, the cumulative frequency and cumulative relative frequency of each group are also reported in the last two columns in Table 2. 4.

Table 2. 4 shows an overall picture of what the data look like by representing a distribution of the waist circumference of these 105 male adults. As can be seen in Table

2. 4, the waist circumference is from 65. 0 to 135. 0 cm with 85. 72% of participants with waist circumference over 80. 0 cm and under 115. 0 cm. The class of 95. 0 to 99. 9 cm contains the largest number of observations. Although a little information about the raw data is lost in a frequency distribution table, more important and concise information will be extracted from the data. It is of great value to fully understand the features of the 105 male adults' waist circumference.

Table 2. 4   Frequency Distribution of Waist Circumference for 105 Male Adults

Grouping intervals /cm	Frequency	Relative frequency /%	Cumulative frequency	Cumulative relative frequency /%
65. 0~	1	0. 95	1	0. 95
70. 0~	1	0. 95	2	1. 90
75. 0~	3	2. 86	5	4. 76
80. 0~	10	9. 52	15	14. 29
85. 0~	12	11. 43	27	25. 71
90. 0~	12	11. 43	39	37. 14
95. 0~	24	22. 86	63	60. 00
100. 0~	14	13. 33	77	73. 33
105. 0~	11	10. 48	88	83. 81
110. 0~	7	6. 67	95	90. 48
115. 0~	5	4. 76	100	95. 24
120. 0~	2	1. 90	102	97. 14
125. 0~	2	1. 90	104	99. 05
130. 0~135. 0	1	0. 95	105	100. 00
Total	105	100. 0	—	—

2.1.3   Histogram and Bar Charts

As compared to a frequency distribution table, a more concise and intuitive way to display the frequency distribution is the utilization of statistical graphs such as a bar chart or histogram. Histogram is a collection of non-overlapping bars representing the frequency distribution of one continuous variable. The horizontal axis of a histogram usually displays the consecutive, non-overlapping intervals of equal size, while its vertical axis depicts either the frequency (usually in a data set with small sample size) or the relative frequency (often in a sample with a large number of participants) of observations within each interval. The histogram representing the distribution of the treatment time in 100 KD patients is illustrated in Figure 2. 1.

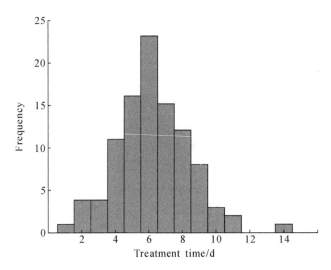

Figure 2. 1   Number of Days before the Treatment in 100 KD Patients

Unlike the histogram, bar charts are mainly used to display the frequency distribution of nominal or ordinal data. In a specific bar chart, bars should have equal width and a space between each bar is permitted.

Histogram and bar chart should be clearly labelled with an informative title and the relevant variables specified along each axis. If the units of measurement are involved, these should also be specified. Additionally, the vertical scale of the histogram or bar chart should always begin at zero as frequency scales start at zero.

2.1.4   Uses of a Frequency Distribution

The most important usage of a frequency distribution is to reveal its shape, center tendency, and variation of the associated data. One property of a distribution is its skewness, which is usually used to determine whether the distribution is symmetric or asymmetric. A symmetric distribution has its right or left side approximately a mirror image of another. As shown in Figure 2. 2, the waist circumference of 100 individuals is symmetrically distributed, ranging from 65.0 to 135.0 cm, with gradually decreased frequency of each subgroup from the center to the end of each side. Furthermore, symmetric distributions can also be detected in many other biological measurements such as systolic pressure, diastolic pressure, and heart rate of healthy adults. Among all symmetric distributions, the normal distribution is particularly more important than others because many statistical theories and principles are derived from the normal distribution. The normal distribution is characterized by a single peak, bell-shaped curve, and the symmetric around the highest value.

Asymmetric distributions can be classified into two categories: positively or negatively skewed distributions. A positively skewed distribution is determined if the area under the curve (AUC) of the right tail is much larger than that of the left tail. Figure 2. 3 shows the

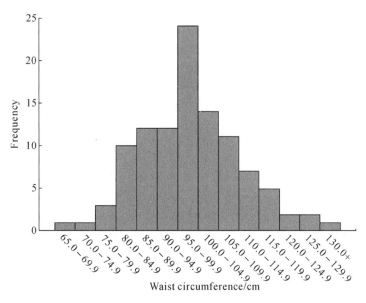

Figure 2. 2   Waist Circumferences for 100 Male Adults

distribution of insulin levels (μIU/mL) among 3,811 individuals and an example of classical positively skewed distribution in which most individuals have insulin levels less than 20 μIU/mL. Meanwhile, if the AUC of the right tail is much smaller than that of the left part, it will be defined as a negatively skewed distribution.

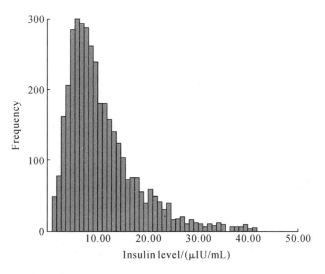

Figure 2. 3   Insulin Levels among 3,811 Individuals

A further property of a distribution curve is its kurtosis, which refers to the degree of peaking. If a curve is more peaked than the normal distribution, it is said to be leptokurtic. Otherwise, it is platykurtic. In general, kurtosis is not as important as the skewness when assessing a distribution's type.

Another feature of a distribution is the number of peaks. If a single peak or mode is observed, the distribution is a unimodal distribution (Figures 2.1, 2.2, and 2.3). The normal distribution is an example of unimodal distributions. In some conditions, if a distribution has two or more peaks, it is called a multimodal distribution. Figure 2.4 is an example of a multimodal (double-peaked) distribution in which the heights of the boys are taller than those of the girls.

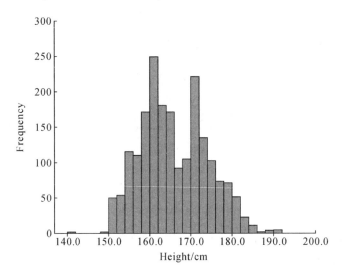

Figure 2.4 Heights of 2,009 College Students in a City in China

2.2 Normal Distribution

2.2.1 Skewness Coefficient

As can be seen above, a histogram is a good option to display the distribution of quantitative data, with which we can concisely understand the features. Any quantitative data can be described using a histogram. Histograms can be further classified into two major categories: symmetric distribution and asymmetric distribution depending on their associated skewness coefficient, which is a characteristic of a distribution to describe the degree of deviation from symmetry and usually represented with α. Here, symmetry means the area under the curve (AUC) on one side of a point is equal to the AUC on the opposite side (Figure 2.5a). In general, α will be equal to or very close to 0 in a symmetric distribution, and α will be greater than or less than 0 when the distribution is positively (Figure 2.5b) or negatively (Figure 2.5c) skewed, respectively. In many conditions, we can also concisely describe the distribution using the density curves (Figure 2.6). **Skewness coefficient** is a characteristic to describe the degree of distribution deviation from symmetry. When the distribution is symmetrical, the skewness coefficient is 0. When the heavy tail of a distribution is on the left side, the skewness coefficient will be greater than 0 and the distribution is positively skewed (Figure 2.6b). While the heavy tail of the distribution is on the right side, the skewness coefficient will be less than 0 and the distribution is negatively skewed (Figure 2.6c).

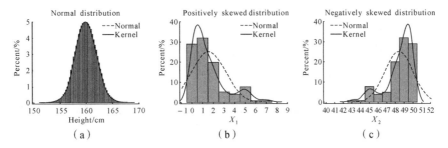

Figure 2. 5   Types of Distribution for Quantitative Data

Solid lines refer to the actual distribution, while dashed lines indicate the normal distribution

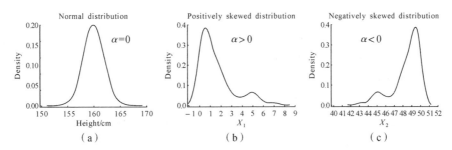

Figure 2. 6   Types of Distribution

2.2.2   Coefficient of Kurtosis

Although a skewness coefficient is important and useful to examine the type of the distribution of interest, it is insufficient to fully assess the characteristics of a symmetric distribution. As can be seen in Figure 2.7, the three distributions with different heights of

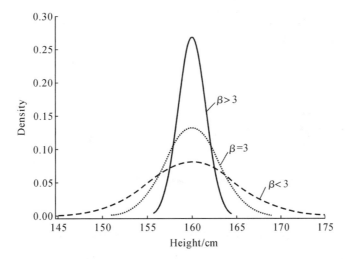

Figure 2. 7   Kurtosis of a Distribution

the peak all have the same skewness coefficient. As a result, we need another measure to further describe the shape of a probability distribution. The coefficient of kurtosis is a commonly used measure to reflect the flatness or kurtosis of the height of a distribution curve, and it is usually represented with β. A kurtosis greater than, equal, or less than 3 leads to a sharp peak, normal peak, or platy peak, respectively.

2.2.3 Normal Distribution

In statistics, a symmetric distribution with a skewness coefficient (α) of 0 and the kurtosis coefficient (β) of 3 is defined as a normal distribution, which is considered as a special symmetric distribution. The AUC associated with a specific value (X) can be calculated using the following equation (density function).

$$f(X) = \frac{1}{\sigma\sqrt{2\pi}}e^{\frac{-(X-\mu)^2}{2\sigma^2}}, \quad -\infty < X < +\infty$$

The normal distribution is the most widely used continuous distribution and is the basis of other statistical approaches. It is also frequently called the Gaussian distribution to commemorate the well-known mathematician Karl Friedrich Gauss.

The features of a normal distribution can be summarized as follows:

(a) A bell-shaped curve is presented above the horizontal axis with the two ends never touching the horizontal axis.

(b) It is symmetric at the point μ, which is also the mean, mode, and median of the normal distribution. AUC to the left (highlighted with brighter shade) and right (highlighted with darker shade) of the point μ is completely symmetrical (Figure 2.8a).

(c) The maximal value of $f(X)$ is at the point of $X = \mu$, and $f(x)$ decreases quickly when X leaves the μ.

(d) The population mean (μ) is also called the location parameter since it determines the location of a normal distribution. If the μ varies, the location of a normal distribution will be changed accordingly (Figure 2.8b). The population standard deviation (σ) is called the shape parameter. If the μ is fixed and the σ is changed, the shape of a normal distribution will be also varied (Figure 2.8c).

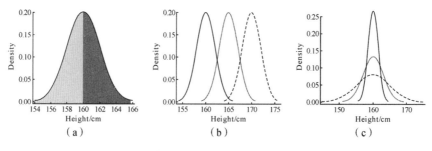

Figure 2.8   Characteristic of a Normal Distribution

(e) The total AUC of a normal distribution is equal to 1. The AUC value of the band that is 1.96σ around the mean ($\mu-1.96\sigma$ to $\mu+1.96\sigma$) or 2.576σ around the mean is 95% and 99%, respectively (Figure 2.9a and 2.9b). If $\mu=0$ and $\sigma=1$, the band for AUC=0.95 or 0.99 is from -1.96 to 1.96 or from -2.576 to 2.576, respectively (Figure 2.9c and 2.9d).

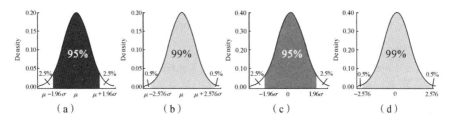

Figure 2.9 The AUC of a Normal Distribution

2.2.4 Standard Normal Distribution

If a continuous variable (X) follows the normal distribution $[X \sim N\ (\mu,\ \sigma^2)]$ and is transformed into a new variable (Z) with the equation: $Z=\dfrac{X-\mu}{\sigma}$, the new variable Z will follow the standard normal distribution with $\mu=0$ and $\sigma=1$ (Figure 2.9c and 2.9d). The standard normal distribution is a special case of the normal distribution. In practice, a lot of statistical approaches have been developed based on the standard normal distribution, which is recognized as the most important distribution in statistics.

2.2.5 Reference Value

In practice, we usually need a widely accepted criteria to judge whether a specific value is in the normal range or not, especially in a specific disease diagnosis. This criterion in medicine is called a reference value (RV) or medical reference value. The RV is defined as the constants of various physiological and biochemical indices, such as human morphology, function and metabolites, in most general people. If the data meet the normal or close to normal distribution, the RV of two-sided probability can be calculated by the equation: $\overline{X} \pm Z_{\frac{\alpha}{2}} S$. It means that the RV will be ($\overline{X} - Z_{\frac{\alpha}{2}} S, \overline{X} + Z_{\frac{\alpha}{2}} S$). While the RV of one-sided probability may be $RV > \overline{X} - Z_{\frac{\alpha}{2}} S$ or $RV < \overline{X} + Z_{\frac{\alpha}{2}} S$. However, if the data are obviously skewed, it can be estimated using the percentile approach. Therefore, the RV of two-sided probability can be calculated using $P_{\frac{\alpha}{2}} \sim P_{1-\frac{\alpha}{2}}$. Meanwhile, the RV of one-sided probability may be $RV > P_{\alpha}$ or $RV < P_{1-\alpha}$. Among all potential RVs, the most commonly used one is 95% RV which refers to the constants of various indices in 95% general people.

2.3 Measures of Central Tendency

Though a frequency table or histogram can generally provide an overview of the features of continuous data, it is insufficient for someone using these tools to comprehensively understand the characteristics of data in detail. To achieve this goal, we need to describe the central tendency and dispersion of the data.

As can be seen in Figure 2. 10a, the subgroup at the center of the distribution has the largest percent, and the closer to the center, the higher of the percent. This phenomenon is called a central tendency. A **measurement of central tendency** is defined as the assessment of the average or typical value of a set of scores using several indices. They are also useful for making comparisons between groups. Because different variables have different distributions, there is no single standard procedure for determining the central tendency for all variables. In this section, we will briefly introduce four commonly used indicators for the central tendency measurement: mean, geometric mean, median, and mode.

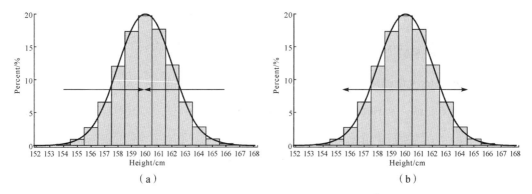

Figure 2. 10   Central Tendency (a) and Dispersion (b) of a Normal Distribution

2.3.1   Mean

In statistics, the most commonly used measure of central tendency is the **arithmetic mean**, which is also called the mean. It is calculated by the sum of all the values in a set of data divided by the number of values:

$$\overline{X} = \frac{\sum X}{n} \tag{2.1}$$

where $\overline{X}$ stands for the sample mean; $\sum$ refers to the sum of the values, and n is the total number of records in the data set. In general, the sample statistics are represented by English letters, and the population parameters are represented by Greek letters. For instance, the mean for a population is usually denoted by μ.

Example 2. 3   Calculate the mean treatment time for KD patients in Example 2. 1.

$$\overline{X} = \frac{\sum X}{n} = \frac{7 + 4 + 7 + \cdots + 3 + 1}{100} = 6.2$$

Thus, the mean number of days before treatment of this sample is 6. 2 d.

If a constant value is individually added to the value of each observation, the sample mean will increase by the value of that constant. The same rule applies when a constant is subtracted from the value of each observation, in which the sample mean will decrease by that amount. In this example, if each patient receives treatment one day earlier, the mean treatment time will be 5. 2 d.

In statistics, the calculation of the mean involves all actual scores of a variable, producing a good representative of the sample. Mean is generally used to indicate the central tendency for data that is normally distributed. Mean is heavily influenced by outliers, extremely large or small values that are far from the sample mean. The mean of skewed distributions may not coincide with the median. Furthermore, the mean measurement can only be applied for numerical data rather than ordinal and nominal data including dichotomous data.

2.3.2 Geometric Mean

Even as the mean has been the most commonly used indicator to represent the central tendency of a normal distributed continuous variable, the measure poorly represents the skewed data in certain conditions. For instance, we have a positively skewed variable, which follows either the exponential (1, 2, 4, 8, 16, etc.) or logarithmic distribution ($\frac{1}{2}, \frac{1}{4}, \frac{1}{8}$, $\frac{1}{16}$, etc.). The arithmetic mean is an inappropriate indicator for its central tendency due to outliers, but the logarithm-transformed data, in which the raw data are transformed by the log-algorithm, e. g. $y = \log10(x)$ or $y = \log(x)$, meet the criteria of normal distribution.

To calculate the geometric mean, we first calculate the arithmetic mean of the logarithm-transformed values of x, denoted as y, using $\bar{y} = \dfrac{\sum y}{n}$. Then the $\bar{y}$ is returned to its original form by using the anti-log-transformation of the $\bar{y}$ with either the equation $\bar{x} = \exp10(\bar{y})$ or $\bar{x} = \exp(\bar{y})$. This log-transformation based mean is called a geometric mean and abbreviated as G. Another way to calculate G is the nth square root of the product of n numbers, which is also shown in Formula (2. 2).

$$G = \sqrt[n]{x_1 x_2 \cdots x_n} = \lg^{-1}\left[\frac{\sum \lg x}{n}\right] \tag{2.2}$$

Example 2. 4   The Center for Disease Control and Prevention (CDC) of W city vaccinated 50 children using influenza vaccine. One month later, the antibody titers were measured, and the results were presented in Table 2. 5. Please calculate the average level of the antibody in these 50 children.

Table 2. 5   The Antibody Concentration of Influenza in 50 Children of W City

8	32	64	128	128
8	32	64	128	128
16	32	64	128	128

Continued

16	32	64	128	128
16	32	64	128	128
16	64	64	128	128
32	64	128	128	128
32	64	128	128	128
32	64	128	128	128
32	64	128	128	128

The data follow an exponential distribution, making routine arithmetic mean inaccurate to represent the central tendency. The geometric mean is the proper measure for the data.

$$G = \lg^{-1}\left[\frac{\sum(\lg 8 + \lg 8 + \lg 16 + \cdots + \lg 128)}{50}\right] = 64.9$$

The geometric mean is generally used when the data meet a log-normal distribution, which means the raw data do not follow a normal distribution but the log-transformed data do. Many variables in medicine including serum antibodies follow a log-normal distribution. A geometric mean is used extensively in microbiological and serological research, in which distributions are often skewed positively. In general, geometric mean is usually smaller than the arithmetic mean of the raw data since the data are positively skewed in this condition and some outlier will greatly magnify the arithmetic mean.

2.3.3 Median

Although data transformation can effectively improve the normality of some data, it is not omnipotent in any condition. The **median** is another measure that is resistant to outliers and is the middle value when data are sorted in an ascending order as half values will be smaller than the median and the other half larger than the median. Median is abbreviated as M.

The median can be obtained according to the following steps.

(a) Sort the data from smallest to largest.

(b) If the number of observations (n) is odd, the median is the middle value as shown in Formula (2.3). If n is even, the median is the mean of the two values at the nearest position to the middle location in the ordered list as shown in Formula (2.4).

$$n \text{ is odd, } M = X_{\frac{n+1}{2}} \tag{2.3}$$

$$n \text{ is even, } M = \frac{1}{2}\left(X_{\frac{n}{2}} + X_{\frac{n}{2}+1}\right) \tag{2.4}$$

Example 2.5 The number of days before treatment among 9 randomly selected KD patients in a hospital is given below.

Table 2.6 The Number of Days before Treatment of 9 KD Patients

2	5	4	5	7	6	5	4	10

The data are sorted in an ascending order: 2, 4, 4, 5, **5**, 5, 6, 7, 10. Since n is odd, the median of the days before treatment is 5.

Unlike the mean, a median is only a location measurement and is not sensitive to outliers. Even if the minimum or maximum value of the data from Table 2.6 is changed to extreme values—e. g. the largest value is revised to 2,000, or 500,000—the median will remain at 5. Median can also be used to describe the central tendency of any distributed continuous data as well as ordinal data. However, since it takes no account of the influence due to majority of values in your sample on the central tendency, it has much poorer representativeness of the data as compared to the mean. Median is suggested to be applied to examine the average level of a very skewed continuous data when both the routine mean and transform-based mean cannot be used.

Finally, if the distribution is exactly symmetric, the mean and median are very close to each other or the same. If the distribution is positively skewed, the median will be less than the mean. In contrast, if the distribution is negatively skewed, the median will be greater than the mean.

2.3.4 Mode

As stated above, the mean, geometric mean, and median can all be used to assess the central tendency of continuous data with unimodal distribution. However, they cannot be used for categorical data and multimodal distributed continuous data. To solve this problem, statisticians have developed other indicators such as the mode. The **mode** is the single value or multiple values with the largest frequency in a data set. Please note that the mode only can be the raw data value (s) with the largest frequency rather than the associated frequency. For example, two modes, both 4 and 5, are observed in the data presented in Table 2.7 since these two numbers appear most frequent in these 10 KD patients.

Table 2.7 Number of Days before the Treatment of KD

2	4	4	5	5	5	6	4	10

As compared to both mean and median, the mode is the simplest indicator for the measurement of a central tendency, and it has no mathematical properties. In other words, the mode cannot be added, subtracted, multiplied, or divided. This may be the largest limitation of the mode. Although it can be applied as a summarized measurement for all types of data including nominal and ordinal data, the mode is never suggested when either the mean or median can be used because of its limitation mentioned above.

2.3.5　Choice of Measures of Central Tendency

We must know that the best indicator for the central tendency measurement of continuous data often depends on the associated distribution. This is the reason the frequency table or histogram is first applied to investigate the distribution type. If a distribution is symmetric and unimodal, the mean, median, and mode should be nearly the same. In this case, the mean is usually used as the measure of central tendency because it takes each value of the data into account and has the best representativeness of the sample.

When the data follow the unimodal distribution, but are not symmetric and cannot be transformed into a normal or similar distribution, the median instead of mean is the first option for the central tendency description. This is because the mean is quite sensitive to extreme values, causing it to overestimate or underestimate the actual average level of the data due to some outliers.

When your data follow bimodal or multimodal distributions or you have ordinal or categorical data, the mode should be considered since both mean and median are not suitable for the types of data.

2.4　Measures of Variation

A measure of central tendency alone is insufficient to fully describe the features of continuous data. Different data with the same central tendency may also be quite different (Figure 2.8c) because they may have different variations. As can be seen in Figure 2.10b, from the center to both sides, the percentage of each subgroup decreases when the heights leave the center. This phenomenon is defined as dispersion which refers to the variation of continuous data. Therefore, to comprehensively describe a quantitative variable, both a measure of center and a measure of variation should be employed. In practice, several indices including range, inter-quartile range, variance, standard deviation, and coefficient of variance are usually applied to comprehensively assess the dispersion of numerical data.

2.4.1　Range

The **range** of a set of data is defined as the difference between the largest value and the smallest value.

$$R = X_{max} - X_{min} \tag{2.5}$$

Although the range is easy to compute, its usefulness is limited since it only considers the minimum and maximum values of your data and is highly affected by outliers. Therefore, a range cannot be used to properly reveal the actual dispersion as compared to other indices and is seldom to be a routine indicator of variation nowadays.

2.4.2　Inter-quartile Range

Inter-quartile range (IQR) is developed to overcome the limitation of the range. To fully understand the IQR, readers must understand the definition of percentile. Suppose we have obtained the marks of medical statistics in an ascending order (from low to high). Then we averagely split the sequence into 100 parts. If a mark falls into the ith part, it is defined as the ith percentile. If a mark is in the 90th percentile, then 90% of observations can be found below this mark. In a word, a percentile is an accumulative percentage, and the median is a special percentile (50th percentile). If the sorted data sequence is averagely split into four parts, the 25th, 50th (median), and 75th percentile are defined as the first, second, and third quartiles (Figure 2.11).

The **IQR** is calculated by subtracting the 25th percentile (the first quartile, denoted by Q_1) from the 75th percentile (the third quartile, denoted by Q_3) of your data:

$$IQR = P_{75} - P_{25} = Q_3 - Q_1 \qquad (2.6)$$

As the IQR is the difference between Q_1 and Q_3, it only represents the middle 50% of the data and completely disregards the other half. Although the IQR will not be affected by outliers and is more resistant to variation than the range, it is not a perfect indicator for the variation assessment since it does not take each value into account by excluding 50% of your sample. Therefore, the IQR is only applied to a very skewed distribution in which data cannot be transformed to a normal or similar distribution. The IQR is generally used to describe the dispersion only when the mean cannot be used, in which a median can also be used as the measure of central tendency.

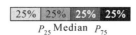

P_{25} Median P_{75}

Figure 2.11   Quartiles and IQR

2.4.3   Variance

To detect the appropriate index to display the dispersion of numerical data, many statisticians have performed a lot of exploratory researches. In a paper titled " The Correlation Between Relatives on the Supposition of Mendelian Inheritance," Dr. Ronald Fisher suggests that variance can be used to properly disclose the variation of numerical data. He defined the variance of a population (σ^2) as the mean squared distance from the mean, which can be expressed as $\dfrac{\sum (X - \mu)^2}{N}$ (see details in Formula (2.7)). While the variance of a sample (S^2) is calculated by the sum of squared distance from the mean divided by $n-1$ instead of by the sample size (n) (Formula (2.8)) because he observed that the difference between σ^2 and S^2 would be smaller by using $n-1$ rather than n in the calculation of S^2.

Dr. Fisher defined $n-1$ as the degrees of freedom (df), which is a very important concept and commonly used in a lot of statistical approaches. In statistics, the degree of freedom refers to the number of variables whose values are unrestricted when fitting a multiple variable model. For example, a researcher has obtained two multiple-variable models: $y_1 = 3a + 2b - 4c$ and $y_2 = 5a + 4b + 2c + 6d$. In the first equation, we observed 3 variables (a, b, and c) included in the model. We know that the number of variables to be varied restrictively is equal to $3 - 1 = 2$. While in the second formula, it has 4 variables (a, b, c, and d) and the number of variables that varies freely is $4 - 1 = 3$.

$$\text{Population variance: } \sigma^2 = \frac{\sum_{i=1}^{N} (X_i - \mu)^2}{N} \tag{2.7}$$

where X_i represents the raw data; μ indicates the population mean; and N is the number of participants in a population.

$$\text{Sample variance: } S^2 = \frac{\sum_{i=1}^{n} (X_i - \overline{X})^2}{n - 1} \tag{2.8}$$

where X_i represents the raw data; $\overline{X}$ indicates the sample mean; n is the sample size; and $n - 1$ refers to the degree of freedom.

As the variance involves squaring the deviations, its unit will be different from the original unit of your data; e. g. if the variable is systolic pressure measured in mmHg, the unit of the variance is $mmHg^2$, which causes inconvenience when using mean and variance to describe the features of numeric data.

2.4.4 Standard Deviation

To resolve the inconvenience due to different units between the variance and raw data, a German statistician named Carl Friedrich Gauss developed the standard deviation to replace the variance. The **standard deviation** (SD) also known as the mean square deviation (MSD) is the square root of the variance. SD is zero only when all the data values are the same. The SDs of a population and sample are represented by σ and S, respectively.

$$\text{Population standard deviation: } \sigma = \sqrt{\frac{\sum_{i=1}^{N} (X_i - \mu)^2}{N}} \tag{2.9}$$

$$\text{Sample standard deviation: } S = \sqrt{\frac{\sum_{i=1}^{n} (X_i - \overline{X})^2}{n - 1}} \tag{2.10}$$

Example 2. 6 The body mass index (BMI) of 20 college students randomly selected from a population are presented in the following table. Question: Does there appear to be a difference in the variation between the male and female students? (Suppose the data meet a normal distribution, respectively)

Table 2. 8 The BMI of 20 College Students of W City Stratified by Gender

Female	18.59	19.23	19.74	18.95	18.73	21.76	17.15	23.62	20.57	21.48
Male	19.05	20.76	22.49	18.75	23.32	24.22	19.00	18.34	21.30	17.96

Compared to range and IQR, the SD is the best option to describe the variations of the BMI as the data are normally distributed. Formula (2.10) can be used to calculate the SD of the BMI of both genders.

$$S_{\text{female}} = \sqrt{\frac{\sum(X - \overline{X})^2}{n-1}} = 1.89 \text{ kg/m}^2$$

$$S_{\text{male}} = \sqrt{\frac{\sum(X - \overline{X})^2}{n-1}} = 2.24 \text{ kg/m}^2$$

As S_{male} is greater than S_{female}, we may think that male students appear to have greater variability in BMI than females. Unlike the variance, both SDs calculated above have the same unit as the unit of the original BMI data. Nowadays, the SD has been widely accepted as the most important and commonly used index of the dispersion measurement since it takes the variation of each value in your data into account and maintains consistency of the units between SD and original data.

The SD has limitations: Suppose we have obtained heights and weights from 100 college students. Although we can calculate the two SDs as $S_{\text{height}} = 3$ cm and $S_{\text{weight}} = 2.5$ kg, we do not know which variation is larger since they have different units and cannot be compared directly. Another limitation of the SD is that it will be strongly affected by the sample mean. Suppose we have collected data on the weights of 50 rats and 50 pigs ($X_{\text{rat}} = 150.01$ g and $S_{\text{rat}} = 3.95$ g; and $\overline{X}_{\text{pig}} = 199,433.23$ g and $S_{\text{pig}} = 3,326.60$ g). As S_{pig} is much larger than S_{rat}, we may think that the variation of weights of pigs is much larger than that of the rats. However, depending on Figure 2.12, S_{pig} is much lower than S_{rat} relative to the associated sample mean. In addition, the value of SD can be dramatically affected by outliers.

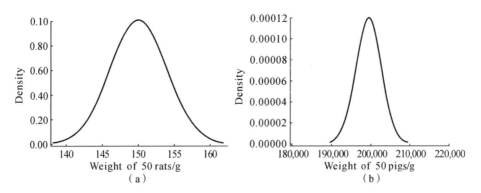

Figure 2.12　Distributions of the Weights for 50 Rats (a) and 50 Pigs (b)

2.4.5　Coefficient of Variation

Although the SD has been widely accepted as the best indicator for assessing the variation of normally distributed quantitative data, it also has limitations. First, it cannot be used to compare variations with different units. For example, you have collected the data of height and weight in 100 boys and want to know whether the heights have larger variations than that of the weights (suppose the heights and weights are normally distributed). To answer this question, you may calculate and compare the SDs for these two variables— suppose $S_{height} = 3.5$ cm and $S_{weight} = 2.1$ kg. With different units, it is not logical to compare these two SDs directly. Second, the SD cannot be used to compare the variations of data with tremendously different means. Suppose you have a data set including 50 elephants and 50 rats— $\overline{X}_{elephant} = 2,000,000$ g, $\overline{X}_{rat} = 100$ g, $S_{elephant} = 5,000$ g, and $S_{rat} = 20$ g. Although the two SDs have the same unit and $S_{elephant}$ is much larger than S_{rat}, we cannot conclude that the variation of the 50 elephants is greater than that of the 50 rats because the dispersion relative to mean tells a different story.

To fill this gap, statisticians have developed another measure: coefficient of variation (CV). In statistics, CV is a measure of dispersion relative to the mean. It is calculated as the ratio of SD to the mean. It is often expressed as a percentage.

$$CV = \frac{S}{\overline{X}} \times 100\% \qquad (2.11)$$

CV is very convenient and useful in comparing two or more variations that follow normal or similar to normal distributions. The following example will help you fully understand the definition and usage of CV.

Example 2.7　With the following sample data for 20 adolescents, find the CVs for heights and weights and compare the results.

Table 2.9　Heights and Weights of 20 Adolescents

ID	Height/cm	Weight/kg
1	164.0	50.0
2	158.0	48.0
3	151.0	45.0
4	160.0	48.5
5	155.0	45.0
6	159.0	55.0
7	162.0	45.0
8	155.0	39.0
9	165.0	49.0
10	162.0	62.0
11	160.0	55.0
12	173.0	57.0
13	170.0	60.0
14	170.0	65.0
15	160.0	48.0
16	172.0	69.0

		Continued
ID	Height/cm	Weight/kg
17	170. 0	70. 0
18	167. 0	53. 0
19	170. 0	53. 0
20	180. 0	69. 0

Sample mean and SD are calculated first.

Height: $\overline{X}=160.82$ cm, $S=7.16$ cm

Weight: $\overline{X}=50.05$ kg, $S=6.07$ kg

CVs are calculated using Formula (2.11).

Heights: $CV=\dfrac{S}{\overline{X}}\times100\%=\dfrac{7.16}{160.82}\times100\%=4.45\%$

Weights: $CV=\dfrac{S}{\overline{X}}\times100\%=\dfrac{6.07}{50.05}\times100\%=12.13\%$

Therefore, we may conclude that the height is less dispersed than the weight.

2.4.6　Choice of Measures of Variation

In this section, we have introduced five indicators for the variation assessment. Identifying the best indicator under different scenarios needs careful consideration. In general, a more appropriate measure of variation for a given data set often depends on the distribution of the data. If a distribution is symmetric and unimodal, the SD is the best one since it takes all scores into account. If two or more variables have different units or tremendously different central tendency, the CV that measures the dispersion using the same relative scale outperforms SD. When the data are asymmetrically distributed and cannot be transformed into a normal distribution, the IQR is often a better choice than the SD or the CV. The range, in comparison, is seldom used.

(Shi Hongying, Shao Fang, Mao Guangyun, Zhao Yan, Zhao Jinshun)

Question Bank

Chapter 3 Descriptive Statistics for Categorical Data

In Chapter 2, readers have learned the description and summary of continuous data. This chapter will focus on the descriptive statistics for categorical data. A categorical variable consists usually a fixed number of outcomes such as a person's gender, country of origin, and city of birth.

3.1 Absolute Number

Data are a collection of different values of one or more different variables, with many values represented as either absolute numbers or relative numbers. An **absolute number** is an actual/observed value. For example, there are 30 patients and 450 healthy controls in a data set, in which the heights of the first two participants are 175.3 cm and 169.8 cm, respectively. All these values including 30, 450, 175.3, and 169.8 are absolute numbers. The absolute number is commonly used in statistics since almost all the original data are presented by absolute numbers.

Although they are common, simple, intuitive, and meaningful, absolute numbers may provide incorrect impressions in some conditions. For example, in a cross-sectional survey, researchers found 48 and 56 boys with metabolic syndrome in urban and rural regions. Can we conclude that metabolic syndrome is more prevalent in rural boys than those in the urban areas just because the numbers of patients in the former is larger than that of the latter? The evidence is insufficient for us to make the conclusion since the number of patients is insufficient and the sizes of two populations are unknown. To answer this question, we need to use relative numbers.

3.2 Relative Number

The **relative number** is the ratio of two values, which can be both absolute and other relative numbers. In statistics, relative numbers consist of proportion, rate, and ratio, and are widely used in the descriptive statistics for categorical data.

3.2.1 Proportion

A **proportion** is defined as a comparative relation of a part to the whole. It is usually a ratio of counts in which the numerator (the top number) is a subset of the denominator (the bottom number). The proportion can be calculated by the following equation.

$$\text{Proportion} = \frac{\text{The number of individules in the part within a whole}}{\text{The sum of individules in all parts within a whole}} \times 100\% \quad (3.1)$$

A proportion can be used to describe the structure (constitution) of a group of people with categorical characteristics (such as gender and blood type). It can be also denoted as a percentage.

Example 3.1   Suppose a total of 2,761 adolescents (1,478 boys and 1,283 girls) have participated in a survey. The proportions of boys and girls who participated are calculated in Table 3.1.

Table 3.1   The Number and Proportion (Percentage) of Boys and Girls Participated in the Survey

Sex	No. of adolescents	Proportions
Boys	1,478	$\frac{1,478}{2,761} = 53.5\%$
Girls	1,283	$\frac{1,283}{2,761} = 46.5\%$
Pooled	2,761	100.0%

3.2.2   Rate

A **rate** refers to the frequency of a specific event by the numbers of all **possible events** during a certain period of time. Similar to the proportion, a rate is also a ratio of two counts in which the numerator is a subset of the denominator. However, a rate is usually applied as a measure to reveal the epidemic intensity of a disease of interest in medical statistics. If the rate of a specific disease is much higher than that of another disease, the specific disease may present a major health problem during the study period. Unlike proportions that sum up to 100%, rates are usually independent of each other and the sum of them can be over, under or equal to 100.0%.

A series of rates are used in practices. Among them, incidence rate, prevalence rate, and mortality rate are the commonly used ones. An incidence rate is defined as the number of **new cases**, which have occurred in a study population over a specified period of time, divided by the total number of participants of the same population. It is mainly performed to assess the effectiveness of some specific preventive measures. If the preventive strategies and measures of a disease of interest are satisfied, this disease's incidence rate will be dramatically decreased.

A prevalence rate is determined as the number of **all cases** (both new and old cases) divided by the total number of possible cases in a population within a specific time period (Formula (3.2)). Like incidence, a prevalence rate can be applied to assess the efficacy of both preventive and therapeutic measures. If the prevalence of a disease is quite high, the preventive strategies and clinical medications are unsatisfied, and this disease might soon become a major health concern.

$$\text{Prevalence} = \frac{\text{The number of persons with a given disease at the time of investigation}}{\text{The total number of persons investigated}} \quad (3.2)$$

A mortality rate (or death rate) is the ratio of the number of deaths by the whole number of subjects during the period in a population. It is strongly related to clinical techniques. If the therapeutic skills are high enough, many diagnosed patients would be cured, and the mortality rate will decrease. In practice, several death rates can be applied to different conditions. Among them, a crude death rate is defined as a ratio of the number of **all deaths** by the total number of participants in a population over the period of time. For example, the child mortality rate is one of the most commonly reported death rates for a given population. To investigate which disease is the most dangerous one causing child mortality, the disease-specific mortality rate is a good option. In general, a disease-specific mortality rate is defined as a ratio of the number of deaths due to a specific disease by the whole number of diagnosed patients with this disease. Based on the rank of different disease-specific mortality rates, you can identify the leading causes of death in your population and prioritize interventions accordingly. Besides, if we want to know the death rates at different ages or genders, you can calculate the age-specific or gender-specific mortality rate. All mortality rates mentioned above will help you understand the major health concerns and associated spectrum in your population, which will guide the discovery of high-risk people, develop proper strategies of disease prevention and control, and provide precise prevention and efficient medications as early as possible.

Let's take an example to better understand the definitions and applications of rates.

Example 3.2   In a cross-sectional study, researchers found that a total of 48 boys of 833 residents from the urban area and 56 boys of 1,928 villagers in the rural counterparts were metabolic syndrome patients. Please calculate the prevalence of the disease for each area.

In the urban area, 48 patients were detected in 833 boys, and the prevalence of boys with metabolic syndrome in the urban region is:

$$\text{Prevalence in the city} = \frac{48}{833} \times 100\% = 5.8\%$$

Meanwhile, 56 patients were identified in 1,928 boys from the rural area, and the prevalence of boys with metabolic syndrome in the rural region is 2.9%, less common (or serious) than that in the rural region.

$$\text{Prevalence in the village} = \frac{56}{1,928} \times 100\% = 2.9\%$$

3.2.3 Ratio

A **ratio** is the computation of one number divided by another, in which the numerator may be a subset of the denominator or completely independent of the denominator. It indicates a relationship between two numbers representing how many times of the numerator containing the denominator. It is simply expressed by the following equation.

$$\text{Ratio} = \frac{A}{B} \tag{3.3}$$

As can be seen from the previous sections, the numerators in both the rate and proportion calculations are a subset of the denominators, restricting the values of both to between 0 and 1. The numerator (A) for ratio, however, can be correlated to or independent of the denominator (B), and A can be larger or smaller than or equal to B. It means that the values of a ratio will not be limited to a small range. In addition, a ratio can be of both two absolute numbers and two relative numbers. As usual, we use fold to represent the result if A is larger than B. Otherwise, it will be commonly represented using a percentage.

Example 3.3   The mortality rate of infants from the city in a specific time period is 4.68‰, while the mortality rate of infants in country is 15.34‰. Please calculate the ratio of the mortality rates of infants from the country and city.

As the rates in the city and country are 4.68‰ and 15.34‰, respectively, the relative ratio of rates in country to the city is equal to $\frac{15.34‰}{4.68‰} = 3.28$, indicating that the mortality rate of infants in the country is 3.28 times of that in the city, much more serious than that in the city. More efforts and resources should be provided in the country to promote infants' health and to reduce the higher mortality rate of infants in the country.

3.3   Considerations of the Application of Relative Number

(a) The denominator cannot be too small, requiring the total number of observations to be large enough when applying for a relative number. Insufficient observations will increase the impact of random error and decrease the representativeness of the sample, causing the relative number to be extremely unstable and biased to reflect the real situation. For example, if the denominator is 2 in a survey of smoking rate, the result contains only four different scenarios: both participants are smokers, or both are non-smokers, or one is a smoker and the other is a non-smoker. In a view of statistics, this result is significantly affected by chance with large sampling error. In this scenario, it is suggested to present the results using absolute numbers instead of relative numbers. Alternatively, the researcher should provide a CI of the rate accompanied by the relative number. The information on the CI will be discussed later.

(b) The difference between the rate and the proportion cannot be ignored. Although the numerator is a subset of the denominator in both rate and proportion, they have a different meaning. In general, a rate is usually applied as a measure to disclose the epidemic intensity of a specific disease and associated within a period, while a proportion is a time-independent indicator and mainly used to represent the composition of each part in an object. In statistics, a rate is much more commonly used than a proportion. A proportion cannot be used to disclose the intensity of a specific disease or phenomenon, whereas a rate can. If a proportion is misused as a rate, a false conclusion will be made.

(c) The average rate cannot be calculated with the same formula in continuous data. Suppose we have two rates as $p_1 = \frac{17}{50} = 0.34$ and $p_2 = \frac{15}{30} = 0.5$. According to the equation of mean for continuous data, the average rate in this example is $\frac{0.34 + 0.50}{2} = 0.42$. However, according to the definition of rate, the average rate is $\frac{17 + 15}{30 + 50} = 0.40$. The latter is correct because it recognizes the difference between sample sizes when calculating the mean. The former is only suitable for the mean calculation for numerical data, while a rate is a relative number belonging to categorical data rather.

(d) Comparability of the data from different periods should be considered. For example, a researcher wants to know whether the exposure $A(E_a)$ is more dangerous than the exposure $B(E_b)$. He carefully designed and conducted an investigation and compared the data he collected with data collected 50 years ago. Based on the data analysis, he concluded that the exposure A was much more dangerous than the exposure B since the prevalence of a specific disease in the data collected 50 years ago was significantly higher than that of the most recent data. The conclusion can be incorrect as the two data may be incomparable—such as the differences in nutritional status and physical fitness, largely affecting the prevalence of the disease when being exposed to either exposure A or B.

(e) A proper hypothesis test is needed to compare among rates. Suppose you obtained two or more rates after an investigation, with all these statistics calculated based on samples. These statistics cannot be used as the criteria of the comparison because they only display the features of a sample. Since the final objective of any researches is to disclose the characteristics of a population, comparisons of several populations or the relationship between features in the population depend on the proper application of statistical inferences that is derived from statistics.

3.4　Standardized Rate

Before the introduction of the standardized rate, let's look at an example first.

Example 3.4　A clinician wanted to know which medication (A and B) is better for the disease X. He collected data from several hospitals and presented the results in the following table.

Table 3. 2   Efficacy Comparison of Medication *A* and *B*

Patient category	Medication *A*			Medication *B*		
	Enrolled	Effective	Rate/%	Enrolled	Effective	Rate/%
Children	60	42	70. 0	120	78	65. 0
Adult	180	78	43. 0	40	2	5. 0
Pooled	240	120	50. 0	160	80	50. 0

As we can see clearly in the above table, the effective rates of both medications are 50.0%, but can we conclude that the two medications have the same efficacy for disease X? The effective rates of either the children or adults in medication A are higher than those in medication B (70.0% vs. 65.0%, 43.0% vs. 5.0%). It can be inferred that medication A is better than medication B. Further analysis reveals that the patients' compositions for the two medications are extremely different. To address the problem, statisticians have developed standardized rates to account for crucial differences in features of difficult populations.

In statistics, a standardized rate refers to an adjusted rate in which the different compositions among several populations are corrected based on a standard population. Age, gender, and severity of disease are three most common confounding factors in many studies. In this example, the proportions of children received medication A and B are 25% and 75%, respectively. Meanwhile, we observed that the effective rates for children and adults in both medications are also quite different. The possible cause of the "equal" efficacy is due to that more children, whose efficacy is much higher than that of adults, are enrolled in medication B. The potential impact due to the inconsistency of the compositions of the two medications can be mitigated using the standardized rate instead of the crude rates, which are calculated routinely without adjusting for confounding factors. In statistics, a standardized rate can be calculated in two ways: direct or indirect method. In this chapter, we only introduce the principles and steps of direct standardized rate estimation. Readers can teach themselves for the indirect method of standardized rate.

Regarding the direct method, all the populations are compared with the standard population, a widely accepted, stable, and representative population or sample with an extremely large sample size. If no optimal standard population can be used, the combination of all observations in your study can be considered as the surrogate.

The procedures of the calculation of the standardized rate are as follows.

(a) Combine the samples by the same age groups as a standard population.

(b) The expected number of effective cases for each stratum can be calculated with the following equations:

$$\text{Expected number } (N_e) = \text{Standard population } (P_s) \times \text{Effective rate } (p) \qquad (3.4)$$

$$\text{Standardized rate } (R_s) = \frac{\sum_{i=1}^{k} N_{ei}}{\sum_{i=1}^{k} P_{si}} \times 100\% \qquad (3.5)$$

The steps of standardized rate calculation in this example are as follows.

Step 1: Calculate the standard population of each stratum.

Children: $60+120=180$

Adults: $180+40=220$

The standard population consists of 180 children and 220 adults.

Step 2: Calculate the expected number for each stratum in different medications.

The expected number of effective cases in children for medication A:

    $180 \times 0.7 = 126$

The expected number of effective cases in adults for medication A:

    $220 \times 0.43 = 94.6 \approx 95$

The standardized rate of medication A:

    $\frac{126+95}{180+220} \times 100\% = 55.25\%$

The expected number of effective cases in children for medication B:

    $180 \times 0.65 = 117$

The expected number of effective cases in adults for medication B:

    $220 \times 0.05 = 11$

The standardized rate of medication B:

    $\frac{117+11}{180+220} \times 100\% = 32\%$

Step 3: Make a conclusion.

Since the standard rate for medication A is higher than that of medication B, we conclude that medication A is better than medication B.

3.5 Binomial and Poisson Distribution

3.5.1 Overview of Binomial Distribution

Before the introduction of the binomial distribution, readers should understand the discrete variable and Bernoulli experiment first. As can be seen in Chapter 1, a discrete variable contains values that are discrete, such as gender and education levels. If a random variable (x) has two mutually exclusive outcomes such as female or male, disease or non-disease, and passed or failed, it is generally referred to as a "success" or "failure" variable, also defined as a Bernoulli random variable, which is proposed by a Swiss scientist named Jacob Bernoulli. A trial associated with a Bernoulli random variable is called a Bernoulli experiment, which refers to a trial that was conducted repeatedly in the same condition and the results are independent of each other.

The Bernoulli distribution, also known as the binomial distribution or two-point distribution, is a discrete probability distribution developed by Dr. Jacob Bernoulli to describe the feature of the results of a Bernoulli experiment. If a new random variable x is utilized to represent the number of patients cured, x will meet a binomial distribution. In statistics, a binomial distribution usually has three assumptions:

(a) The number (n) of the Bernoulli trial is very huge or countless and each trial has two possible outcomes;

(b) Each outcome in the n-times trial is independent, which means that a specific outcome will not be affected by any previous outcome;

(c) The condition for each experiment and its associated probability of success (p) remains the same.

The probability of k-time success in an n-times Bernoulli trial can be computed using the function below:

$$P(x=k) = C_n^k \pi^k (1-\pi)^{n-k} \qquad k=1,2,3,\cdots,n \qquad (3.5)$$

where π represents the population rate and k indicates the times of success.

Suppose we want to randomly select 10 infants from a population of 100. If the probability of getting a girl is 0.5, what is the probability of getting exactly 4, 5, or 6 girls from the random selection of 10 infants? As each outcome is independent, the results of the sampling meet a binomial distribution. The probability of obtaining exactly 4, 5, or 6 girls is:

$$P(x=4) = C_{10}^4 \times 0.5^4 (1-0.5)^6 = 0.2051$$
$$P(x=5) = C_{10}^5 \times 0.5^5 (1-0.5)^5 = 0.2461$$
$$P(x=6) = C_{10}^6 \times 0.5^6 (1-0.5)^4 = 0.2051$$

Example 3.5　Please calculate the probability that a family with 5 kids consists of 2 boys and 3 girls, with the probability of getting a boy at 0.51 at each birth.

$$P(x=2) = C_5^2 \times 0.51^2 (1-0.51)^3 = 0.306$$

As the outcome of each birth is either a boy or a girl, it meets a binomial distribution. The probability, 30.6%, can be calculated using Formula 3.5 or statistical software.

3.5.2　Characteristics of a Binomial Distribution

As can be seen in Figure 3.1, the binomial distribution is a typical discrete distribution and determined by two parameters: sample size and the population rate (π). When the sample size is stable, a positively skewed distribution will be changed to a negatively skewed one with the increase of π (Figure 3.1(a) to 3.1(d)), in which the distribution will be positive, symmetric, or negative as π is less than, equal to, or greater than 0.5. While when π is stable, the binomial distribution will be close to a normal distribution with the increase of sample size (Figure 3.1(e) to 3.1(h)).

In general, the binomial distribution can be considered as a normal or close to normal

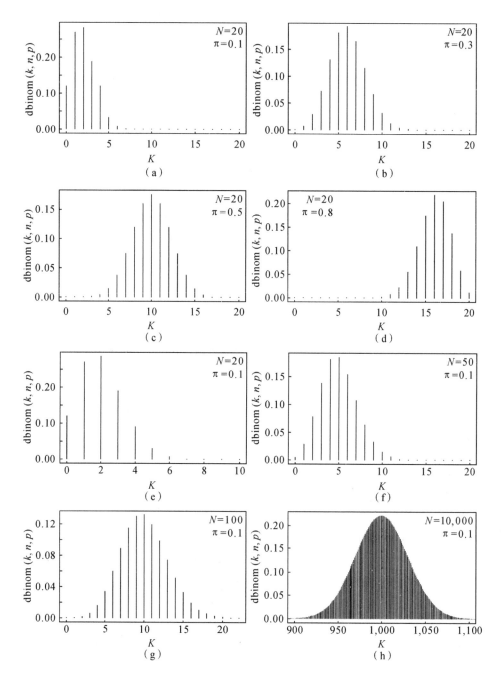

Figure 3. 1   Binomial Distribution

distribution when both $n \times \pi$ and $n \times (1-\pi)$ are greater than 5 (Figure 3.1(h)). If we do not know the value of π, it can be replaced by the sample rate (p). In this condition, we also can examine its central tendency and dispersion of the binomial distribution. The mean and variance of the binomial distribution can be calculated by the following equations:

$$\mu = np \tag{3.6}$$

$$\sigma = np\ (1-p) = npq \tag{3.7}$$

where n is the number of trials or the sample size; p represents the probability of success; and q indicates the probability of failure.

Example 3.6　It is known that the probability to develop cancer in mice carrying a specific mutation is 0.6. What's the probability that at least 6 mice develop cancer in 15 mutant mice? How many mice are expected to develop cancer in 15 mutant mice? What's the variance?

(a) The number of mice that develops cancer follows the binomial distribution. In this example, $p=0.6$, $q=0.4$, $n=15$, and $k=6$.

$$P(x{\geqslant}6)=1-P(x{<}6)=1-[P(x{=}5)+P(x{=}4)+P(x{=}3)+P(x{=}2)+$$
$$P(x{=}1)+P(x{=}0)]$$
$$=1-(0.0245+0.0074+0.0016+0.0003+0+0)$$
$$=0.9662$$

(b) $n{\times}p=15{\times}0.6=9$ and $n{\times}(1-p)=15{\times}0.4=6$. As both are greater than 5, this binomial distribution is approximately normally distributed.

The mean is:

$$\mu=np=15{\times}0.6=9$$

The variance is:

$$\sigma=np(1-p)=15{\times}0.6{\times}0.4=3.6$$

The probability that at least 6 mice will develop cancer in 15 mutant mice is 0.9662. Nine mice are expected to develop cancer within the sample, and the variance is equal to 3.6.

3.5.3　Poisson Distribution

In statistics, the binomial distribution is usually applied to describe the features of a Bernoulli experiment, in which the rate of a random event will not be too small. If the rate of a Bernoulli experiment is too small, the event will follow a Poisson distribution rather than a binomial distribution. The Poisson distribution is a special case of the binomial distribution, in which the event is rare.

The **Poisson distribution** is a discrete probability distribution commonly seen in statistics and was published in 1838 by a French mathematician named Simeon Denis Poisson (Figure 3.2). It is usually applied to represent the distribution of rare events in a large population when:

(a) a rare event can be counted in a huge population and independently occurs in a random manner in a given interval, which can be a period of time or space i.e. during a week or per mile;

(b) the mean number of occurrences, represented by lambda (λ), in the interval or the rate of occurrences is known and finite.

The probability of k events occurring in a time period t for a random variable can be estimated using the following equation:

$$P(x=k) = \frac{u^k e^{-\mu}}{k!} \qquad (3.8)$$

where $\mu = \lambda t$, representing the expected number of events over the time period t.

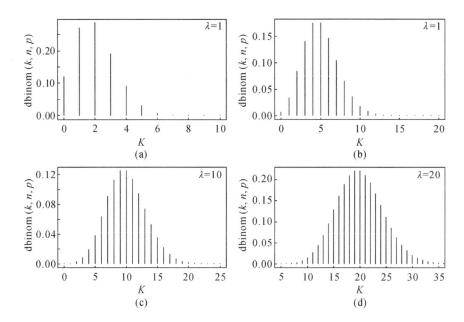

Figure 3. 2　Poisson Distribution

As can be seen in Figure 3.2, the Poisson distribution is mainly determined by the parameter (λ). Although it is a discrete distribution, it becomes similar to a normal distribution as the λ increases. It is widely accepted that when the λ is greater than 20, the Poisson distribution can be considered as a normal or close to normal distribution, which we can investigate its associated central tendency and dispersion. Unlike the binomial distribution, the mean of the Poisson distribution is equal to the variance, which can be used to check whether a random variable follows a Poisson distribution. In the health care field, the Poisson distribution is often used to investigate the number of occurrences of an event per time unit or space. For example, we can use the Poisson distribution to examine the number of insects in a unit of space.

$$\mu = \sigma^2 = \lambda t \qquad (3.9)$$

Example 3. 7　Eight particles per ml air are detected in a classroom. Assume that the number of particles in the air follows the Poisson distribution, what is the probability that 5 particles are in 1 ml air in a random sampling from the classroom?

Equation (3.8) is used to calculate the probability:

$$P(x = k) = \frac{8^5 e^{-8}}{5!} = 0.0916$$

We conclude that the probability of 1 ml air containing 5 particles is 0.0916 or 9.16%.

3.5.4   Why Is the Poisson Distribution a Special Case of the Binomial Distribution?

If a random variable follows the Binomial distribution, its associated mean and variance are equal to np and $np(1-p)$, respectively. When the p is small ($p \approx 0$), $1-p$ will be very close to 1, and $np(1-p)$ will be approximately equal to np. Therefore, the mean and variance are almost identical when p is small, and the Binomial distribution becomes the Poisson distribution. When the number of trials (n) is large, the calculation of the probability of a Binomial distribution will become very cumbersome and time consuming and can be approximated with Poisson distribution formulae.

(**Zhang Dandan**, **Mao Guangyun**, **Zhao Yan**)

Question Bank

Chapter 4　Statistical Tables and Graphs

4.1　Introduction

After obtaining a series of results when the data analysis has been performed, we need to organize and show results to audiences. In general, results can be presented in three ways: text, statistical tables, and graphs, with statistical tables and graphs most commonly used to summarize and present the features of data. A statistical table can be used to briefly arrange your data in several rows and columns, or in a more complex structure, while a statistical graph is an aesthetically-pleasing diagrammatical illustration of a set of data.

The main guideline of creating a statistical table or graph (STG) is that the results should be self-explanatory and understandable without the need for reading the text. The terms used in an STG should be well-defined, and all attributes should be accompanied by required meaningful labels. Besides, too many or too few groups are not recommended in an STG. A proper STG will transport your findings more efficiently.

4.2　Statistical Tables

Statistical tables can present concise numerical information, such as the number of observations and features of the central tendency and variations, which vary depending on the study objective. In general, a statistical table is presented in numbered and captioned blocks.

4.2.1　Principles of Making Statistical Tables

(a) Display and expression of one central idea.

(b) Clear and ordered: grouping should be logical and easy to compare.

(c) Canonical expression of data.

4.2.2　Structures of Statistical Tables

As can be seen in Table 4.1, a statistical table consistently includes a title, headings (row and column captions), lines, numbers, and a footnote or other ancillary features.

(a) Title. The title is the main heading to summarize the major contents of the statistical table. It is usually placed at the top of the table and labelled with the word "Table," followed by numbers, such as Table 1 or Table 2. The remaining portion of table titles should contain a brief overview of the contents of the data.

(b) Headings: row and column captions. The horizontal headings or subheadings of the row in a statistical table are called row captions. They are usually the variables to illustrate the meaning of each row and must be placed at the left of the data. While a column caption is also called the box head of a statistical table. It is the vertical heading and subheading of the column, usually represented as several groups and must be placed on the top of the data. Only the first letter of the box head is in capital letters and the remaining words must be written in lowercase. If the column captions are grouped by only one variable, it is classified into a simple table. However, if the column captions are stratified by two or more variables, it will be called a composite table. As compared to the column captions, row captions are more important in a typical statistical table.

(c) Lines. In the statistical table, only horizon lines are permitted with fewer lines the better. The general adopted format is "three-line table," which includes a top line, a bottom line and a line separating the heading from the data.

(d) Numbers. The body of the statistical table consists of numbers, numerical information classified into row and column captions. In Arabic numerals, the digits are aligned, and the number of decimals is consistent. The symbol "—" is used if there is no number for that cell, and the symbol "..." is used to represent the missing number.

(e) Footnote. If necessary, the footnote is a statement below the table to provide additional explanation. It can be used to explain any codes, abbreviations or symbols in the table. We can also explain all nonstandard abbreviations using symbols as follows: * , † , ‡ , § , || , ¶ , * * , †† , ‡‡ , § § , |||| , ¶¶ , etc.

Table 4. 1   Characteristics of the Study Participants by Gender

Variables	Men ($n=4,050$)	Women ($n=4,316$)
Age/years	46.55 ± 19.48	44.07 ± 18.80
BMI/(kg/m^2)	27.46 ± 4.99	28.17 ± 6.02
Waist circumference/cm	97.89 ± 14.31	93.37 ± 14.33

Data are presented as mean $\pm$ standard deviation (SD)

4.2.3   Types of Statistical Tables

(a) Simple table. A simple table as shown in Table 4.1, the most common statistical table, usually has one level of heading.

(b) Composite table. In some conditions, the column captions may be stratified by another categorical variable, in which the statistical table may have two or more levels of headings. This is called a composite table. As shown in Table 4.2, the total number of people screened, the number of patients diagnosed with hypertension and the prevalence rates are stratified by gender.

Table 4. 2   Prevalence of Hypertension in an Elderly Population with Different Ages and Genders

Age group /years	Men			Women		
	Total number	Hypertension	Rate /%	Total number	Hypertension	Rate /%
60~	329	107	32. 52	314	88	28. 03
65~	231	66	28. 57	239	85	35. 56
70~	258	79	30. 62	201	86	42. 79
75~	165	57	34. 55	125	52	41. 60
80~85	231	94	40. 69	193	97	50. 26

4.2.4   General Rules of the Statistical Table

(a) A table should be simple and understandable, requiring no further explanations.

(b) Proper and clear headings for columns and rows help audiences understand the contents of the table.

(c) Suitable approximation may be adopted, and figures may be rounded off.

(d) The units of measurements should be labelled.

(e) If the numbers of features are large, two or more statistical tables may be required.

(f) Thick lines are used to separate the data under big classes, and thin lines are used to separate the sub-classes of data.

(g) The number of lines should not exceed 3 or 4.

4.3   Graphs

Although a statistical table has strength to efficiently disclose your results, graphical representation of data usually helps the audience understand large and complex data. A statistical graph (visualization) illustrates descriptive statistics diagrammatically, conveys information extracted from your data efficiently, and eases the burden of understanding large data.

Like a statistical table, a statistical graph also has common features. For instance, scales should be labelled clearly with appropriate dimensions added. The plotting symbols are also important. As a graph is used to give an impression of pattern in the data, bold and relatively large plotting symbols are desirable. With currently available statistical software, one can perform extensive exploration of the data, not only to determine more carefully their structures but also to find the best means of summary and presentation.

This chapter introduces several types of frequently used statistical graphs including histogram, stem-and-leaf plot, bar chart, box plot, pie chart, percentage bar chart, scatter plot, and line chart. Their applications, strengths, and limitations are introduced next.

4.3.1 Histogram

A **histogram** is a commonly used statistical graph to show the distribution of one numerical variable. It consists of equal-width bars with heights proportional to the frequency of the range of values these bars represent. To generate a histogram, we generally divide the range of values of a numeric variable into a series of equidistant groups (or "bins") and calculate the frequency or percentage of observations that fall into each group. The horizon labels of a histogram show the midpoint value of each group. While the vertical axis shows the relative frequency. As can be seen in Figure 4.1, which is drawn according to the data in Table 4.3, the waist circumference (WC) of 8,366 residents in an area ranges from 60 to 143 cm and the distribution is symmetric around WC of 92 cm with more than half (56.94%) of residents have the WC between 80 and 100 cm.

Table 4. 3 Frequency Distribution Table of Waist Circumference (cm) in 8,366 Residents

Waist circumference /cm	Frequency	Cumulative frequency	Percentage /%	Cumulative percentage/%
60. 0∼	84	84	1. 00	1. 00
68. 0∼	632	716	7. 55	8. 55
76. 0∼	1,230	1,946	14. 70	23. 25
84. 0∼	1,566	3,512	18. 72	41. 97
92. 0∼	1,735	5,247	20. 74	62. 71
100. 0∼	1,462	6,709	17. 48	80. 19
108. 0∼	914	7,623	10. 93	91. 12
116. 0∼	454	8,077	5. 43	96. 55
124. 0∼	242	8,319	2. 89	99. 44
135. 0∼143. 0	47	8,366	0. 56	100. 00
Total	8,366	8,366	100. 00	100. 00

Advantages:

(a) Histograms show the type of distribution of continuous data.

(b) Histograms can be used to estimate the central tendency and dispersion of numerical data.

(c) Histograms help find outliers, which affect the accuracy of further data analysis.

Limitation:

Histograms only provide an overview of the data, and we cannot obtain more detailed information as a typical frequency distribution table since no actual values can be obtained from it.

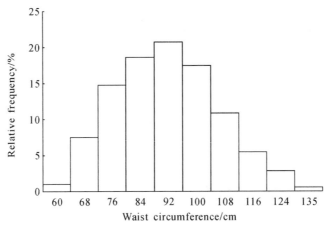

Figure 4. 1 Histogram of Waist Circumference Distribution

4.3.2 Stem-and-Leaf Plot

Another way to visually disclose the distribution of continuous data is a **stem-and-leaf plot**. It is simpler to construct and more informative than a histogram, which does not show any actual observed values. A stem-and-leaf plot is commonly applied when dealing with numerical data with small sample sizes. For example, a researcher has collected the blood urea nitrogen (g/L) of 40 study subjects as follows:

5.7	3.2	3.6	4.6	7.1	5.0	4.3	3.6	4.3	3.6
5.0	3.9	5.4	6.8	3.9	3.6	3.6	2.5	3.9	8.6
3.2	4.6	4.6	3.6	3.9	5.4	7.5	3.2	2.9	4.6
5.4	2.5	6.8	5.4	3.9	2.9	6.4	5.7	2.9	5.4

Readers can use any statistical software such as SPSS, R, STATA, SAS, or Python to construct a stem-and-leaf plot. The procedures of the construction of a stem-and-leaf plot using SPSS can be found at https://jingyan. baidu. com/article/0964eca2434e9f8285f536cd. html.

```
2 | 5 5 9 9 9
3 | 2 2 2 6 6 6 6 6 6 9 9 9 9 9
4 | 3 3 6 6 6 6
5 | 0 0 4 4 4 4 4 7 7
6 | 4 8 8
7 | 1 5
8 | 6
```

Figure 4. 2 Stem-and-Leaf Plot of Blood Urea Nitrogen (g/L) in 40 Study Subjects

Figure 4. 2 is an example of the stem-and-leaf plot consisting of stems and leaves. The stems and leaves are separated by a vertical line, with the stems to the left and leaves to the right. Typically, the leaf represents the last digit of the number, and the stem contains the remaining digits. Leaves are subgroups of stems. For example, the first group in Figure 4. 2 is 2 | 5 5 9 9 9, where 2 is the stem and 5, 5, 9, 9, 9 are the leaves, containing five values 2.5, 2.5, 2.9, 2.9, and 2.9 in this group.

Advantages:

(a) All of the data are shown in the stem-and-leaf plot.

(b) Data can be organized at any time for dynamic modification.

(c) It is useful to identify the mode and find outliers.

Limitation:

The plot is only useful for smaller sized data sets (<100 data points).

4.3.3 Bar Chart

A **bar chart** is one of the most widely used approaches for visually displaying the features of either continuous or categorical data when being stratified by another variable. In a bar chart, various groups are represented along the horizontal axis, usually arranged either alphabetically or by the size of their proportions. The height of each bar usually represents the average level of a continuous variable or the frequency of a categorical variable. Similar to a statistical table, your data can be presented with a simple bar (Figure 4.3) or a composite bar (Figure 4.4).

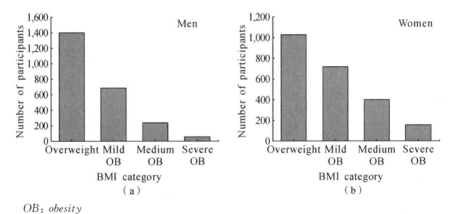

OB: *obesity*

Figure 4.3   Number of Participants Determined as Overweight or Obesity

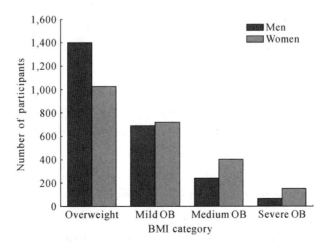

OB: *obesity*

Figure 4.4   Number of Participants Determined as Overweight or Obesity by Gender

Considerations of a bar plot construction:

(a) Several rectangles (also called bars) are applied to construct a bar plot, in which the number of the bars must be equal to the number of groups.

(b) The height of each bar represents the average level of a continuous variable or the proportion of a categorical variable for each group.

(c) A constant space exists between any consecutive bars and the width of bars should be equal.

(d) The vertical axis should start at 0, which is the same in a histogram.

Table 4.4   Number of the Study Participants Determined as Overweight or Obesity by Gender

Category	Men		Women	
	Cases	Percentage/%	Cases	Percentage/%
Overweight	1,398	58.67	1,026	44.55
Mild obesity	687	28.83	719	31.22
Medium obesity	237	9.95	402	17.46
Severe obesity	61	2.55	156	6.77
Pooled	2,383	100.00	2,303	100.00

Advantages:

(a) Bar charts display the average level or proportion of a variable among several groups.

(b) Bar charts make comparison of a variable easier among several groups.

Limitation:

A bar plot may provide insufficient information compared to a statistical table.

4.3.4 Box Plot

A **box plot** is a method to compare the distributions of groups of numerical data. Neither a histogram or a bar plot is competent for this job. A box plot can be applied not only to display the central tendency and dispersion for one or more continuous variables but also to examine whether they are comparable (Figures 4.5 and 4.6). As can be seen in Figure 4.5, a box plot consists of a box, a top line, a bottom line, and outliers plotted as individual points. The height of the box represents the IQR of the data, which is the distance between the 25th percentile (P_{25}) and 75th percentile (P_{75}). While the bottom and top lines usually indicate the minimum and maximum of the data without outliers. The range of the bottom line to top line is 1.5 times as much as the IQR (height of the box). The horizon line within the box is the median of the data. The dots below the bottom line or above the top line are outliers. Based on a box plot, we can examine both the central tendency through the median and the degree of variation. Furthermore, the distribution type of the data can be detected, such as the case in Figures 4.5 and 4.6, where the spread of the fasting plasma glucose of both men and women follow the normal distribution, and the level of fasting plasma glucose in men is higher than that in women.

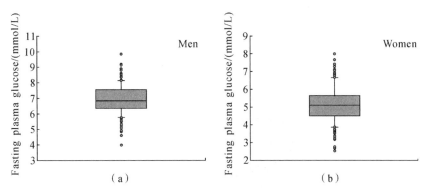

Figure 4.5   Levels of the Fasting Plasma Glucose in 150 Men (a) and 150 Women (b) Respectively

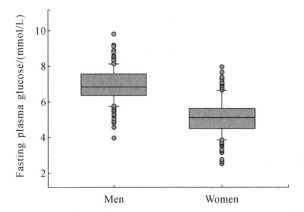

Figure 4.6   Levels of the Fasting Plasma Glucose in 150 Men and 150 Women by Gender

Advantages:

(a) Box plots graphically represent the features of continuous data, depicting both the median and spread in a glance.

(b) Box plots are useful to detect extreme values.

(c) Box plots can be applied to describe the distributions of several discrete data.

(d) Box plots are useful for intuitive analysis and the side-by-side comparison of different data sets.

Limitation:

Outliers detected by a box plot might not be actual outliers, which means that whether a value is an outlier cannot be determined only by means of a box plot.

4.3.5   Pie Chart

A **pie chart** is a very commonly used statistical graph for relative numbers to display the construction of an object, which is generally split into several slices to illustrate the associated proportions. In a pie chart, the area of each slice indicates its quantitative proportion. In many conditions, each slice will be arranged in a sequence by the descending order of proportions when creating a pie chart. Slices may also be arranged alphabetically or on other rational bases. Besides, colors, textures, or arrows can be used to help readers better understand a pie chart (Figure 4. 7).

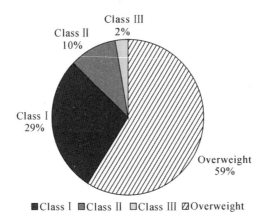

Figure 4. 7 The Composition of Overweight and Different Levels of Obesity in Men

Notes:

Different categories can be distinguished by different colors, text, and percentages. The sum of the percentages for all categories should be 100%.

Advantage:

Pie charts display relative numbers in an easy-to-understand format.

Limitation:

Pie charts are not suitable for large amounts of data with many groups.

4.3.6 Percentage Bar Chart

Like the pie chart, a **percentage bar chart** is another way to disclose the compositions of relative numbers as well as comparisons of several relative numbers. It consists of a few bars in which each bar displays a proportion of multiple categories stacked in a single row or column. Internal stacked colors are used to indicate the percentage participation of a sub-type of data. Figure 4. 8 is a percentage bar chart based on Table 4. 5.

Table 4. 5 Blood Pressure Levels of Study Participants Based on the Monitoring Results

Gender	Normotension	Hypertension		
		Class I	Class II	Class III
Male	2,736 (79. 26)	546 (15. 82)	145 (4. 20)	25 (0. 72)
Female	2,813 (81. 23)	424 (12. 24)	148 (5. 72)	28 (0. 81)

Data were presented as cases (%)

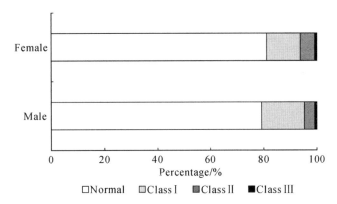

Figure 4.8   Construction of Blood Pressure Levels in Male and Female Participants

Advantage:

The percentage of each part can be easily seen.

Limitation:

It is difficult to apply to categorical data with too many groups.

4.3.7   Scatter Plot

The statistical graphs mentioned so far are mainly used for assessing features of data or investigating differences in the central tendency or dispersion among different groups. These graphs cannot estimate the relationship between or among two or more variables. To answer this question, statisticians have developed the scatter plot, which is used to display the relationship between two numerical variables. Figure 4.9 is an example of a typical scatter plot, which visually discloses the relationship between the Body Mass Index (BMI) and the waist circumference (WC) of 30 subjects. To examine the relationships among three or more variables at the same time, a scatter plot matrix (Figure 4.10) can efficiently reveal the correlation between multiple variables.

Figure 4.9 is the scatter plot using data from Table 4.6, where each circle represents a pair of the WC and the BMI of a subject, with the value of WC determining the position on the horizontal axis and BMI determining the position on the vertical axis. The plot clearly illustrates a pattern where both variables move in the same direction, indicating a positive correlation between two variables.

Table 4.6   BMI and WC of 30 Subjects

ID	BMI /(kg/m²)	WC/cm	ID	BMI /(kg/m²)	WC/cm
1	29.10	99.9	16	27.47	87.7
2	22.56	81.6	17	20.98	71.7
3	29.39	90.7	18	27.96	86.5

Continued

ID	BMI /(kg/m²)	WC/cm	ID	BMI /(kg/m²)	WC/cm
4	30.94	108.0	19	23.2	91.0
5	30.62	112.8	20	29.74	110.4
6	27.33	100.3	21	24.05	81.0
7	26.68	86.7	22	29.28	107.5
8	23.68	81.0	23	20.48	73.9
9	39.76	125.7	24	30.38	95.1
10	25.93	90.6	25	23.93	79.0
11	37.60	114.5	26	25.85	93.0
12	19.44	73.4	27	32.14	111.4
13	36.16	116.1	28	29.14	93.7
14	30.23	99.3	29	20.84	73.8
15	31.42	99.8	30	22.85	83.5

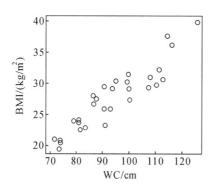

Figure 4. 9   Scatter Plot of WC and BMI in 30 Subjects

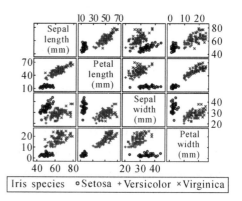

Figure 4. 10   Scatter Plot Matrix for Iris Data

In statistics, a scatter plot or scatter-plot matrix is a very useful approach to examine the relationship between or among two or more continuous variables. It is usually the first step of the investigation of the relationships among several numerical variables, with the potential explanatory variable arranged on the horizontal axis (the X-axis) of a scatter plot and the potential response variable on the vertical axis. Unlike a histogram or bar plot, the value of horizontal or vertical axes of a scatter plot does not necessarily starts from 0. Categorical variables can be represented using different colors or symbols in a scatter plot (Figure 4. 10).

Advantages:

(a) Scatter plots can be used to identify outliers.

(b) Scatter plots can visually describe the direction and the degree of the correlation.

(c) Each observation is graphically displayed, leaving no information behind.

Limitation:

Scatter plots may be difficult to read (and to construct) if values are close to each other.

4.3.8 Line Chart

A **line chart** is another commonly used statistical graph. It is suitable to describe the trend of the variations of a specific variable accompanied by another variable value, especially to display the trend of a variable changing over time. For example, a researcher wanted to investigate the trend of the variation between age and the serum folate level. He collected the associated data in 10 adults (Table 4.7) and created a line chart (Figure 4.11)

Table 4.7 Serum Folate Levels at Different Ages

Age	Folate/(nmol/L)	Age	Folate/(nmol/L)
18	25.31	23	27.18
19	26.5	24	26.85
20	25.73	25	27.67
21	26.38	26	27.63
22	26.25	27	28.14

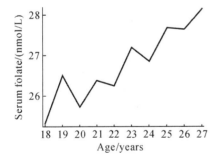 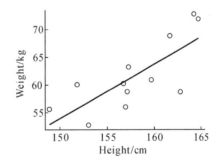

Figure 4.11   Line Chart of the Variation of Serum Folate Concentration with Age

Figure 4.12   Relationship between Height and Weight in 12 Boys

Unlike a scatter plot or scatter-plot matrix that is mainly applied to estimate the correlation between variables, a line chart is used to reveal variation and trend among variables, with data points joined by a straight line in a line chart. Although we may find a trend line in a scatter plot in some condition (Figure 4.12), it is a straight rather than polygonal line. In a line chart, both the horizontal and vertical axis does not have to start from 0. If there is only one polyline in a line chart, it is called a single line diagram, while a composite line chart is defined as a line chart with two or more polylines.

Advantage:

Line charts visually reflect the trend of the variations between one variable and another, usually over intervals of time.

Limitation:

Line charts are less intuitive when the sample size is small.

(**Mao Yingying, Mao Guangyun, Zhao Yan**)

Question Bank

Chapter 5   Parameter Estimation

The objective of a research is to understand the features of a population, but the number of entire participants in a population is usually huge or innumerable, making it expensive, time consuming, or impossible to collect and evaluate. An example is a census, in which data are collected directly from each individual participant enrolled in the population, thus producing summary statistics about the population. To overcome this problem, statisticians would selectively sample a subset of the population, to efficiently estimate the characteristics of the population. As compared to a census, a sampling study not only provides a less expensive, faster way to collect data but also produces quite accurate estimates about the population characteristics if it is designed carefully and properly.

5.1   Statistical Inference

Nowadays, a sampling study has become one of the most commonly used approaches to understand an unknown population. Figure 5.1 illustrates the principle and process of a sampling study. Firstly, we randomly select a number of participants from a population to obtain a representative sample. Then we summarize the sample data characteristics by descriptive statistics (descriptive statistics have been introduced in detail in Chapters 2 and 3 of this book). Finally, we use sample statistics to make inferences about unknown population parameters.

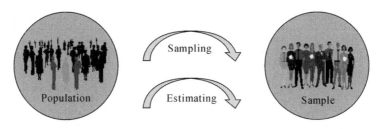

Figure 5.1   The Principle and Process of a Statistical Inference

In statistics, the practice of making statements about the parameters of a population based on random sampling is called **statistical inference**, also known as inferential statistics. Statistical inference is the leading way to understand a population and generally includes two parts: **parameter estimation** and **hypothesis testing**. In general, parameter estimation is the process of estimating unknown population parameters based on a random sample extracted from the same population; while hypothesis testing mainly focuses on providing evidence about the parameters describing a population. This chapter will introduce the parameter estimation in detail. The principle, steps, and considerations of hypothesis testing will be introduced in detail in Chapter 6.

5.2 Random Sampling and Sampling Error

5.2.1 Random Sampling

Randomly chosen samples play an irreplaceable role in statistical inference as any inferential statistics starts with random sampling. In statistics, each participant in a random sample should be selected from the population in a random manner, in which each participant has the same chance to be selected. Detailed introduction of random sampling can be found in the section of 15.3.2.2 of this book.

5.2.2 Sampling Error

Suppose your university has 20,000 male students, and their heights follow a normal distribution ($\mu = 174.96$ cm, $\sigma = 4.00$ cm, see Figure 5.2(a)). One hundred male college students (the sample) from your university (the population) are randomly selected, and the sample mean is 175.07 cm ($\bar{x}$, a statistic). In this sampling study, the sampling error equals 0.11 cm which is the difference between the statistic and parameter: $\bar{x}$ (175.07 cm) $- \mu$ (174.96 cm) = 0.11 cm. In another case, suppose you take 200 samples, each consisting of 100 randomly selected male college students, and calculate the mean and standard deviation of the height for each sample (Summary data are presented in Table 5.1). A histogram is constructed to show the distribution of these sample means (Figure 5.2(b)).

Table 5.1 The Sample Mean and Standard Deviation of the 200 Randomly Selected Samples

ID	Height_Mean	Height_StdDev	ID	Height_Mean	Height_StdDev
1	173.2	4.8	101	175.6	4.8
2	175.7	4.5	102	174.1	4.9
3	173.8	2.4	103	175.1	4.0
4	175.3	4.3	104	175.4	5.6
5	174.5	2.8	105	175.1	2.7
6	175.0	2.7	106	175.1	5.1
7	175.0	3.5	107	175.2	4.0
8	175.6	5.1	108	174.5	4.1
⋮	⋮	⋮	⋮	⋮	⋮
100	174.9	3.5	200	174.2	3.4

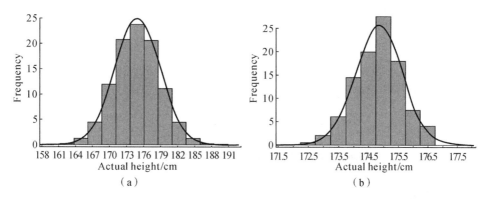

Figure 5. 2 Distributions of 20,000 Heights (a) and 200 Sample Means (b)

As can be seen in Table 5. 1, each sample mean of height is close to population mean of height (μ), thus differences among all of these 200 sample means and to the population mean height exist (see both Table 5. 1 and Figure 5. 2(b)). In statistics, the difference between a statistic and a parameter among different samples is defined as **sampling error**.

Sampling error arises primarily due to the following reasons.

In a typical sampling study, the sample is randomly selected from a population, thus the value of a specific variable will be quite different because of the variations among enrolled participants. Since only a subset of participants is selected, the difference between a statistic and parameter is completely induced by the sampling randomness. If many random samples of same size are drawn, the statistic of interest from each sample will also be different even though all samples are randomly selected from a single population (Table 5. 1). Such a difference among the samples is common and should be included in the sampling error, too.

(a) Sampling. In a classic sampling study, the sample is randomly selected from a population. Since only a small part of participants is selected, such a sample cannot give the complete picture of the properties of the whole population. However, if more participants from a population are included in the sample, the difference, sampling error, can be reduced. This is common as the sampling error decreases with the increase of the sample size of your sample.

To illustrate, in Figure 5. 3 (a Venn diagram), the rectangle represents a specific population, and each circle refers to a sample of the same sample size. As the samples can be different, the sample means can also be quite different. We denote the mean of the ith sample by $\overline{X}_i$. Therefore, the sampling distribution of these sample means include $\overline{X}_1$, $\overline{X}_2$, $\overline{X}_3$, and so on. If the samples are chosen with replacement, an infinite number of samples can be drawn from the population.

(b) Individual variation. The most fundamental cause of the sampling error may be due to the heterogeneity of a population in which participants are different from each other. If all individuals are completely the same, no sampling error will exist. In general, the greater the individual variation, the larger the sampling error.

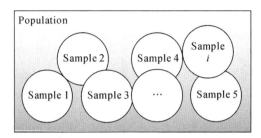

Figure 5. 3   A Population Mean and Sample Mean

5.2.3   Standard Error

As stated in Chapter 2, the central tendency and variation of the $\overline{X}_i$ should also be assessed using a mean and standard deviation. In statistics, the mean of the sample means $(\overline{\overline{X}})$ is called an expectation. In this example, it equals 174. 94 cm and is very close to the population mean, μ (174. 96 cm). The mean of sampling distribution of the sampling means, the expectation, is generated by repeated sampling and taking the average of these sample means. It is usually used to estimate the population mean disregard the population distributions.

In statistics, the standard deviation of a statistic (e. g. sample mean, sample rate) is defined as a **standard error of the mean**, which is also called a standard error (SE) in short, and can be calculated using Formula (5. 1),

$$\sigma_{\overline{X}} = \frac{\sigma}{\sqrt{N}} \tag{5. 1}$$

where $\sigma_{\overline{X}}$ is the population-based standard error (also called theoretical standard error); σ is the population standard deviation; N is the number of participants in a population.

In practice, σ and N are usually unknown in a population, especially an infinite population. They are replaced with the sample standard deviation (s) and the sample size (n) of a sample randomly selected from the population. Therefore, the estimate of $\sigma_{\overline{X}}$ is

$$s_{\overline{X}} = \frac{s}{\sqrt{n}} \tag{5. 2}$$

where $s_{\overline{X}}$ is the sample standard error (estimation of a population standard error); s is the sample standard deviation; n is the sample size of a sample.

As each sample comes from the same population, a dispersion of the statistic only can be due to the different sampling (Figure 5. 3). So, an SE is completely induced by the sampling and has been widely accepted as the indicator of sampling error. SE is positively associated with the standard deviation and negatively related to the square root of the number of participants in your data. That said, if the variability of a population has been determined, then the population standard deviation will be fixed. Thus, if a sample has been selected from this population, then increasing the sample size will largely reduce the standard error so as to make your data more robust.

For example, if $n=25$, the standard error of the sample mean is $\dfrac{\sigma}{\sqrt{25}}=\dfrac{\sigma}{5}$. However,

if the sample size is enlarged to $n=100$, the standard error is reduced to $\dfrac{\sigma}{\sqrt{100}}=\dfrac{\sigma}{10}$. This

implies that the larger sample size of the random sample, the less variation in the sample means (Figure 5.4). Since the expectation (mean of the sample means) is very close to the population mean, this further implies that larger sample size will not only decrease the sampling error to make your findings more robust and credible, but also to improve the representation of your sample to a population so that the expectation is much closer to the actual population mean.

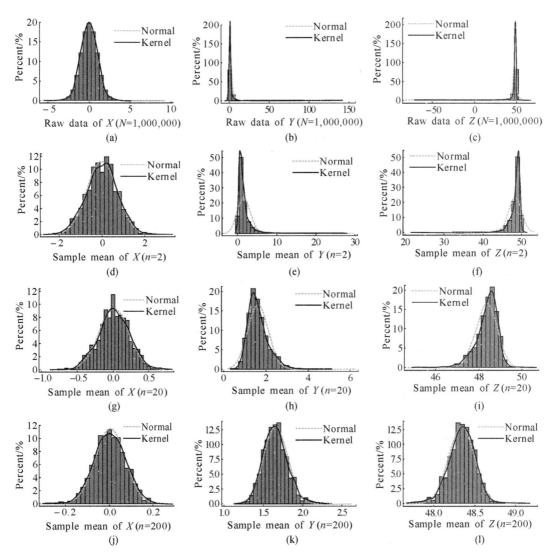

Figure 5.4   Central Limit Theorem

Comparisons between the standard deviation and standard error are as follows.

(a) Both the standard deviation and standard error are indices to assess the dispersion of numerical data.

(b) The standard deviation is mainly used to reveal the dispersion of numerical data that follows the normal or is approximately close to normal distribution. It is also applied to assess the representative of means to data. The larger the standard deviation, the worse the representative of the mean to the data.

(c) The standard error refers to the difference between a statistic and a parameter or the dispersion of the values of a specific statistic among samples randomly selected from a population. It is usually applied to assess the sampling error and the representative of your sample to the population. The larger the standard error, the worse robustness of your sample and the poorer representative of your sample to the population, making your final findings less credible.

(d) The standard error is typically less than the standard deviation as the sample size is usually greater than 1.

5.3　Central Limit Theorem

In most conditions, the sampling error refers to the numerical difference between a sample statistic and the corresponding population parameter. Since the latter is typically unknown, the exact sampling error is also unrecognized. If sample data are used to make inferences about the population, the central limit theorem lays a basis for determining the probability of various levels of sampling error.

Central Limit Theorem 1: If a population is normally distributed, the sampling distribution of $\overline{X}$ is also normally distributed, in which the mean equals the population mean ($\overline{X}=\mu$) and a standard error equals the population standard deviation divided by the square root of the sample size ($\sigma_{\overline{X}}=\dfrac{\sigma}{\sqrt{n}}$).

Central Limit Theorem 2: Suppose you have random samples of a population. Regardless of the population's actual distribution, if the sample size is large enough, the distribution of the sample means ($\overline{X}$) will be normal or approximately normal in which $\mu_{\overline{X}}=\mu$ and $\sigma_{\overline{X}}=\dfrac{\sigma}{\sqrt{n}}$. The larger the sample size, the closer it is to a normal distribution (Figure 5.4).

Figure 5.4 discloses the characteristics of the distributions of based on a normal, a positively and a negatively skewed population (the shapes of populations are displayed in the first column). The other three columns reveal the shape of the sample mean distribution with elevated sample sizes. As can be seen in Figure 5.4, as sample size increases, the distribution of the sample mean gets closer to a normal distribution.

Simulation studies indicate that:

(a) a statistic is always different from its associated parameter;

(b) the values of statistics calculated from each sample differ from each other though these samples are randomly selected from the same population;

(c) the mean of a statistic is nearly equal to its associated parameter;

(d) the dispersion of a statistic is less than that of the raw data;

(e) the statistic will be close to a normal distribution if the sample size is sufficient, regardless of the distribution type of the associated population.

This tells us that the distribution of a statistic has the same center as its population and a smaller dispersion. This phenomenon becomes more obvious with the increasing sample size.

5.4　*t*-Distribution

As stated above, the standard normal distribution is a special normal distribution, in which the mean (μ) is 0 and standard deviation (σ) equals 1. It is very useful in many fields and widely accepted as the basis of many statistical approaches. The standard normal distribution is based on the equation: $Z = \dfrac{X-\mu}{\sigma}$ or $Z = \dfrac{\overline{X}-\mu}{\sigma_{\overline{X}}}$. In general, μ and σ are unknown. Although we can obtain a very similar μ from the expectation ($\overline{\overline{X}}$) based on multiple random selection from the population, the value of σ is still unknown. This severely restricts the wide application of standard normal distribution in practice.

5.4.1　Definition of *t*-Distribution

To solve this problem, statisticians have done many studies. In 1908, a British statistician named William Sealy Gosset suggested that a sample standard deviation (d) could be used to replace the σ in the above-mentioned equations because he believed that s is very close to σ if the sample is randomly selected from a population, and published the result under the pseudonym "Student" using the notation. As Dr. Gosset's finding makes the universal application of this special normal distribution a reality, it is named as *t*-distribution (also called Student's *t*-distribution) to commemorate his great contributions in statistics:

$$t = \frac{\overline{X}-\mu}{s_{\overline{X}}} = \frac{\overline{X}-\mu}{\dfrac{s}{\sqrt{n}}} \tag{5.3}$$

As we can see in Figure 5.5, a series of *t*-distributions with the same mean ($\mu=0$) but with slightly varying spreads are displayed, which are determined by their degrees of freedom (df, representing as $v = n - 1$). With the increase of v, the shape of the *t*-distribution will look more like the Gaussian distribution which is called the standard normal distribution. In fact, the standard normal distribution is a special *t*-distribution when the sample size is sufficiently large.

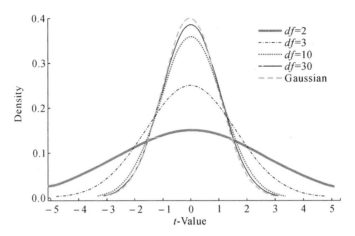

Figure 5. 5   t-Distributions

5.4.2   Properties of t-Distribution

(a) t-Distribution is a family of density curves, each determined by the degrees of freedom (υ).

(b) t-Distribution is bell shaped and symmetric around 0.

(c) With the increase of υ, the t-distribution will converge to the standard normal distribution, a special t-Distribution with $\upsilon = \infty$.

(d) The total AUC of a distribution is equal to 1. It is clearly observed in Figure 5. 6 that t_2 is greater than t_1, while the tailed AUC associated with t_1 (the sum of the highlighted with bright and dark shades) is obviously greater than that of t_2 (highlighted with dark shade). In summary, the tailed AUC of a specific t-distribution is negatively associated with the absolute value of t-score.

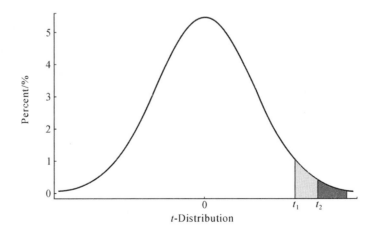

Figure 5. 6   AUC of t-Distribution

In practice, a tailed AUC is usually applied to represent a specific p-value, which is widely used in statistical inference, especially in hypothesis testing which will be introduced in Chapter 6. To help readers perform statistical inference based on calculated t-statistics, statisticians have provided the t-critical-value table based on t-distribution (Appendix 2), which consists of rows (degrees of freedom, υ) and columns (p-values for one-sided or two-sided). The body of the t-critical-value table is the collection of associated t-values. Suppose we have a random sample with sample size 7. Here, the degree of freedom is 6 ($\upsilon = n - 1 = 6$). If the significant level is set up as $\alpha = 0.05$ and we select the two-sided test, the associated critical t-value ($t_{\frac{0.05}{2}, 6}$) is 2.447, located at the intersection of the 6th row and 6th column. This means, 2.5% of the t-values fall into the right tail above 2.447 and another 2.5% of t-values fall into the left tail below -2.447. Further usage of t-distribution will be illustrated in Chapter 6 when we discuss hypothesis testing.

5.5   Parameter Estimation

The parameter estimation is the process of using sample data to understand the characteristics of the population. There are two primary estimation methods: point estimation and interval estimation.

5.5.1   Point Estimation

Suppose we want to know a parameter in a population but the number of participants contained in this population is very large. The parameter cannot be obtained directly but can be estimated through a sampling study, in which we randomly select a sample from the population, calculate the statistical sample mean, and use this statistic to estimate the unknown parameter. This process is called point estimation because the specific statistic is a single numerical value compared to a range of numbers when making inference about the population. In statistics, the **point estimation** is the estimation of a population parameter using a single statistic. Let's see a typical example of point estimation. Suppose the president of a university wants to know the average triglyceride (TG) of 30,000 students in his university. He asked his secretary to select a random sample of 100 students in his university, measured the TG concentration from these 100 students and calculated the average TG, say $\overline{TG} = 1.32$ mmol/L. Based on sample statistics, he then concludes that the average TG concentration of all 30,000 students in his university is 1.32 mmol/L.

The point estimation is used to infer the possible value of a parameter without considering the potential impact on the results due to sampling error. Although it can be reduced by either random sampling or increased sample size, sampling error is inevitable and should be well considered during the study design phase. In fact, the point estimation does not express the uncertainty in the estimation, therefore, it is rarely reported without the corresponding standard deviation values.

5.5.2   Interval Estimation

To make up for the lack of sampling error consideration in the point estimation, statisticians have developed the interval estimation method, in which the parameter estimate incorporates the level of confidence (e. g. 95%) that the true parameter value falls into the range of two numbers. The estimated interval is also called the confidence interval (CI), which is an interval that the parameter of interest will probably be contained in the interval with certain confidence. If the probability of producing an interval containing the true value of the parameter is 95% or 99%, the associated interval will be called the 95% or 99% CI. In practice, 95% is the most commonly used reliability in the interval estimation.

5.5.3 Calculation of a CI for Population Mean

In practice, we may use interval estimation to calculate a CI for population mean. A very commonly used approach to estimate a parameter is using the interval estimation to obtain a CI using a specific confidence level, such as the 95% CI. Given the fact that the sample mean follows the t-distribution, the two critical values of two-sided probability with a confidence level of $1-\alpha$ will be $-t_{\frac{\alpha}{2},v}$ and $t_{\frac{\alpha}{2},v}$, respectively. While the critical value of one-sided probability with a confidence level of $1-\alpha$ will be $-t_{\alpha,v}$ or $t_{\alpha,v}$.

(a) CI for population mean with two-sided probability

$t=\dfrac{\overline{X}-\mu}{S_{\overline{X}}}$, so $P(-t_{\frac{\alpha}{2},v}<\dfrac{\overline{X}-\mu}{S_{\overline{X}}}<t_{\frac{\alpha}{2},v})=1-\alpha$. In other word, if the confidence level equals to $1-\alpha$, we may find that $-t_{\frac{\alpha}{2},v}<\dfrac{\overline{X}-\mu}{S_{\overline{X}}}<t_{\frac{\alpha}{2},v}$. Then we can obtain an expression as $-t_{\frac{\alpha}{2},v}S_{\overline{X}}<\overline{X}-\mu<t_{\frac{\alpha}{2},v}S_{\overline{X}}$ when performing appropriate transformation. Thus, we can obtain another formula as follows:

$$\overline{X}-t_{\frac{\alpha}{2},v}S_{\overline{X}}<\mu<\overline{X}+t_{\frac{\alpha}{2},v}S_{\overline{X}} \tag{5.4}$$

Therefore, a population mean (μ) will generally be included in an interval as: $(\overline{X}-t_{\frac{\alpha}{2},v}S_{\overline{X}},\overline{X}+t_{\frac{\alpha}{2},v}S_{\overline{X}})$. So, the 95% CI with two-sided probability can be expressed by $(\overline{X}-t_{\frac{0.05}{2},v}S_{\overline{X}},\overline{X}+t_{\frac{0.05}{2},v}S_{\overline{X}})$.

Example 5.1 A college admissions director wished to estimate the average age of all students in his college. He selected a sample of 25 students in a random manner from all students and obtained the results as follows: $\overline{age}$ is 22.9 years, S is 1.5 years, and the ages of all students in his college are normally distributed. Question: What is the average age of all students in the college, with the confidence level at 95%?

Answer:

$$S_{\overline{X}}=\frac{S}{\sqrt{n}}=\frac{1.5}{\sqrt{25}}=0.3$$

Since the confidence level is 95% and the sample size is 25, α will be 0.05 and the degree of freedom (v) = 25 − 1 = 24. Based on the critical values table for t-distribution (Appendix 2), we know that the critical value of two-sided probability $t_{0.025,24}$ is 2.064. Therefore, the 95% CI of all students' average age in this college is:

$$(22.9-2.064\times0.3, 22.9+2.064\times0.3)=(22.3, 23.5)$$

The result means that we are 95% confident that the average age of all students is between 22. 3 and 23. 5 years, and there is a 5% chance that the true average falls outside of this range.

(b) CI for population mean with one-sided probability

If only one-sided probability is considered, the equation is as follows:

$$P\left(\frac{\overline{X}-\mu}{S_{\overline{X}}}<-t_{a,v}\right)=1-\alpha \text{ or } P\left(\frac{\overline{X}-\mu}{S_{\overline{X}}}>t_{a,v}\right)=1-\alpha \tag{5.5}$$

After the appropriate transformation, we obtain the equation for the CI:

$$\mu>\overline{X}-t_{a,v}S_{\overline{X}} \text{ or } \mu<\overline{X}+t_{a,v}S_{\overline{X}} \tag{5.6}$$

Example 5. 2　A researcher obtained data on the vital capacity (vital capacity is the maximum amount of air a person can expel from the lungs after a maximum inhalation) of 100 male adults in a city. The mean and standard deviations of this sample were 4,500 and 200 mL, respectively. Please estimate the 95% CI of the vital capacity of all male adults in this city.

Since the researcher only concerns whether the vital capacity is too low for all male adults in the city, the one-sided probability is appropriate. In this example, we know that $\overline{X}=4,500$ mL, $S=200$ mL, and $v=100-1=99$. With this information, we can calculate both the $S_{\overline{X}}$ and $t_{0.05,99}$ ($S_{\overline{X}}=\dfrac{S}{\sqrt{n}}=\dfrac{200}{\sqrt{100}}=20$ and $t_{0.05,99}=1.66$). Therefore, the 95% CI will be $\mu>\overline{X}-t_{a,v}S_{\overline{X}}=4,500-1.66\times20=4,466.8$ mL.

5.5.4　CI for the Difference between Two Population Means

Assume there are two normally distributed populations, defined as $N(\mu_1,\sigma_1^2)$ and $N(\mu_2,\sigma_2^2)$, where μ_1, μ_2, σ_1, σ_2 are all unknown. Now two samples are randomly drawn from the two populations. The sample sizes, means, and standard deviations of these two samples are denoted by (n_1, n_2), $(\overline{X}_1,\overline{X}_2)$, and (s_1^2,s_2^2). The CI for the difference between two population means $(\mu_1-\mu_2)$ with two-sided probability is estimated by the following expression:

$$(\overline{X}_1-\overline{X}_2)-t_{\frac{a}{2},v}S_{\overline{X}_1-\overline{X}_2}<(\mu_1-\mu_2)<(\overline{X}_1-\overline{X}_2)+t_{\frac{a}{2},v}S_{\overline{X}_1-\overline{X}_2}. \tag{5.7}$$

From here, the CI for the difference between two population means $(\mu_1-\mu_2)$ with one-sided probability can be calculated with the following formulae:

$$(\mu_1-\mu_2)>(\overline{X}_1-\overline{X}_2)-t_{a,v}S_{\overline{X}_1-\overline{X}_2} \text{ or } (\mu_1-\mu_2)<(\overline{X}_1-\overline{X}_2)+t_{a,v}S_{\overline{X}_1-\overline{X}_2} \tag{5.8}$$

Here $S_{\overline{X}_1-\overline{X}_2}$ is called the standard error of $(\overline{X}_1-\overline{X}_2)$ and can be obtained using the equation

$$S_{\overline{X}_1-\overline{X}_2}=\sqrt{S_c^2\times\left(\frac{1}{n_1}+\frac{1}{n_2}\right)} \tag{5.9}$$

S_c^2 is called the pooled variance or weighted average of S_1^2 and S_2^2 and can be calculated with the formula

$$S_c^2=\frac{(n_1-1)S_1^2+(n_2-1)S_2^2}{(n_1+n_2-2)} \tag{5.10}$$

If the sample sizes of the two samples are both large enough, say at least 60 or more, the standard error of $\overline{X}_1 - \overline{X}_2$ can also be estimated by the equation

$$S_{\overline{X}_1 - \overline{X}_2} = \sqrt{\frac{S_1^2}{n_1} + \frac{S_2^2}{n_2}} \tag{5.11}$$

Example 5.3 Assume that the population means of the red cell counts between healthy male and female residents in a city are different and the population standard deviations among them are equal. Two random samples are drawn from the respective population. The sample sizes, means, and standard deviations of these two samples are ($n_1 = 20$, $n_2 = 15$), ($\overline{X}_1 = 4.66 \ 10^{12}/L$, $\overline{X}_2 = 4.18 \ 10^{12}/L$), and ($S_1 = 0.47 \ 10^{12}/L$, $S_2 = 0.45 \ 10^{12}/L$). Please estimate the 95% CI for the difference of average red cell counts between healthy male and female residents.

Solution:

The pooled variance for the difference between healthy males and females, standard error of the difference, and pooled degrees of freedom are:

$$S_c^2 = \frac{(20-1) \times 0.47^2 + (15-1) \times 0.45^2}{20+15-2} = 0.2131$$

$$S_{\overline{X}_1 - \overline{X}_2} = \sqrt{S_c^2 \times \left(\frac{1}{n_1} + \frac{1}{n_2}\right)} = \sqrt{0.2131 \times \left(\frac{1}{20} + \frac{1}{15}\right)} = 0.1577$$

$$\nu = 20 + 15 - 2 = 33$$

At $\alpha = 0.05$, the critical value $t_{\frac{0.05}{2}, 23}$ for the two-sided test is 2.034 using the critical value table of t-distribution. Therefore, the 95% CI for the difference of average red cell counts between healthy male and female residents is $(4.66 - 4.18) \pm 2.034 \times 0.1577 =$ (0.16, 0.80) $10^{12}/L$.

5.5.5 Accuracy and Precision of CI

The first element of a CI is accuracy, which is defined as exactness or the quality of being true. In practice, accuracy is often determined by the research objective, the background of the real problem, sampling error and the associated confidence level. Accuracy refers to the ability to be depended on and freedom from error or defect (Figure 5.7). One of the major determinants of accuracy is the confidence level $1 - \alpha$. Generally, the closer the confidence level is to 1, the more reliable the estimation is. Among all potential reliability values, the most commonly used ones are 90%, 95%, and 99%.

The second element is precision, which is measured by the width of the CI ($C_U - C_L$). The narrower the CI, the more precise the estimation is. Factors affecting the precision include the variation, sample size, and reliability (also called the confidence level, $1 - \alpha$). When the reliability is fixed, the precision will be determined by the other two factors—the larger the individual variation or the smaller the sample size, the lower the precision is, and conversely, the higher the precision is.

In statistics, accuracy and precision are mutually restrained though they are both affected by the width of the CI. The broader the CI, the higher accuracy and lower precision

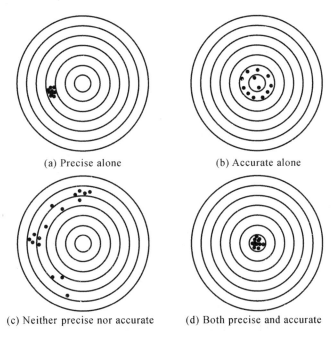

(a) Precise alone　　　　　　　　　　(b) Accurate alone

(c) Neither precise nor accurate　　　(d) Both precise and accurate

Figure 5. 7　Accuracy and Precision

are. On the contrary, the narrower the CI, the lower accuracy and higher precision are. As the width of a CI is mainly affected by the reliability $(1-\alpha)$ in a specific sampling study in which the sampling error and sample size are fixed, both accuracy and precision are affected by the reliability. To achieve higher accuracy, larger reliability (e. g. 99%) is needed. However, to obtain higher precision, smaller reliability (e. g. 90%) is preferred. Ninety-five percent is the most commonly used reliability scores since it better balances the accuracy and precision of a CI than others.

5.5.6　Interpretation of the 95% CI

Several considerations on the CI:

(a) Since μ is fixed when a population is determined, it is incorrect to conclude that the probability of μ in the CI is $1-\alpha$ once it is computed. As we know, the probability in a single experiment can only be either 0 or 1 when the outcome is negative or positive. In practice, the probability is equal to 1 when μ is in the interval. On the contrary, the probability will be 0 when μ is not included in the interval. A better way to interpret a level $(1-\alpha)$ CI is to say that such interval estimation method has probability $(1-\alpha)$ of producing an interval containing the μ.

(b) In a single experiment, we can increase the accuracy of the CI of μ by increasing $1-\alpha$, which will lead to increased $t_{\frac{\alpha}{2},v}$ and a wider CI.

(c) To improve the precision of a CI in a practical study, a smaller $1-\alpha$ should be applied, which will lead to decreased $t_{\frac{\alpha}{2},v}$ and a narrower CI.

(d) When $1-\alpha$ is fixed, both the accuracy and precision can be effectively reduced by increasing the sample size. The commonly used reliability of 95% is only a matter of convention with no strong theoretical reasons behind.

(e) It is tempting to interpret the 95% CI by saying that "there is a 95% probability that μ lies within the CI. " In fact, this interpretation is not completely correct. Though μ is a fixed parameter when the population is determined, the CI still varies among samples. For example, if we repeatedly draw 100 independent, random samples from the same population, we may obtain 100 different 95% CIs of μ. Theoretically, 95 out of 100 CIs will contain the μ, and 5 will not. As a result, we may say that this CI has 95% probability to contain the μ.

5.5.7　Comparison between the 95% RV and 95% CI

We have learned so far that the 95% RV is calculated using the formulae: $\overline{X} \pm t_{\frac{\alpha}{2}, \upsilon} S$, while the equation of 95% CI estimation is $\overline{X} \pm t_{\frac{\alpha}{2}, \upsilon} S_{\overline{X}}$. Though they are very similar, the RV and CI have different usages, requiring one to understand the distinction. A RV range is usually applied to assess whether a value is normal or not, mainly for a physiologic measurement in health-related measures. It also reflects the individual variation of your data to some extent, in which a narrow RV range means a small dispersion of your sample and better representative of the sample mean on your data. In contrast, the 95% CI is used to estimate a possible range of a specific parameter at 95% confidence. It usually reveals the sampling error of your study. If the reliability is fixed, narrower 95% CI often indicates smaller sampling error, better representative of your sample on the population and credibility of your findings.

(Bai Jianling, Mao Guangyun)

Question Bank

Chapter 6 Foundations of Hypothesis Test

6.1 Introduction

The final objective of a statistical analysis is to make inferences about the population of interest based on the information gained from a sample randomly selected from the population. Several approaches can be used to achieve our goals. Among them, parameter estimation, which has been introduced in Chapter 5, is a leading approach to well understand the features of a single population. However, if we want to know whether there is a significant difference among several populations, a parameter estimation will be insufficient and a series of statistical approaches called hypothesis tests can be applied to answer this question. In statistics, a hypothesis test mainly focuses on estimating whether a parameter is significantly different from others or a variable is undoubtedly linked to others. This chapter mainly covers the principle, steps, considerations, and others of a hypothesis test.

6.1.1 Objective of Hypothesis Test

A **hypothesis test** is a statistical approach to assess whether a specific hypothesis is true or not. In a hypothesis test, we usually aim to test whether a sample comes from a population, a parameter is significantly different from others, or a variable is really linked to others. The results of hypothesis tests are usually expressed in terms of a probability that measures how well the data and the hypothesis agree. In fact, a hypothesis test is also called a significant test, in which a specific test statistic is calculated on the assumption that the null hypothesis is valid and conclusions are made depending on whether the acquired p-value is less than the significant level or not.

Example 6.1 It is known that the μ of pulses for general male adults is 72 times/min. A doctor randomly selected 20 individuals in a mountainous area, measured their pulses, and obtained the sample mean of 76 times/min and standard deviation of 7 times/min. The doctor wanted to know whether the average pulse for male residents in the mountainous area is significantly faster than that for the general male adults? Can he conclude that the male residents in the mountainous area have faster pulse than general male adults because 76 is greater than 72?

Example 6.2 A clinician wanted to know whether medication A will have better efficacy than that of medication B.

To answer these questions, we can perform an appropriate hypothesis test.

6.1.2 Basic Idea of Hypothesis Test

In Example 6.1, we know that 76 is the sample mean, a point estimation of μ. As sampling error cannot be completely avoided in a sampling study, we cannot simply conclude that the pulse of male residents in the mountainous area (μ) is significantly higher than that of general male adults (μ_0) though 76 is greater than 72. As learned in Chapter 5, we will obtain different sample means though they are randomly selected from a same population. So, although μ is unknown, we may assume that two possible situations may be true. (a) No significant difference between μ and μ_0 exists. A higher sample mean (76) is mainly due to a sampling error. (b) μ is really different from μ_0. In other words, the sample comes from a population whose μ is not 72 at all. Although these two situations are both possible, only one will be true. To obtain the real answer to this question, hypothesis testing will give us a big hand.

Let's back to Example 6.1 again. Our objective is to answer whether the population mean of pulses for all general males in the mountainous area is equal to 72 or not. As we know, the relationship between 72 and μ maybe $\mu = 72$ or $\mu \neq 72$, and only one of them can be true. Among them, we really want to observe that $\mu \neq 72$ because in this condition we may conclude that people live in the mountainous area should receive additional health care as compared to a general population. Unfortunately, it is too difficult to obtain sufficient evidence to demonstrate that $\mu \neq 72$ directly. Inspired by data transformation, statisticians have solved this problem perfectly depending on the idea of counter-evidence. **The basic ideas of a hypothesis** are as follows: (a) We assume that $\mu = 72$ (null hypothesis, H_0) and the difference we observed is completely due to the sampling error. (b) To estimate a probability of obtaining a difference as large as or larger than what we have observed under this assumption. (c) If the probability equals to or less than 0.05 (a most commonly used significant level) or 0.01, we say that a small probability event has occurred. In accordance with what we have learned in Chapter 1, we have reason to doubt about the null hypothesis, reject it, and conclude that the population mean of pulse in male residents lived in a mountainous area is significantly different from general male adults. On the contrary, if the probability is greater than the significant level, we have no reason to doubt about the null hypothesis and have to conclude that no significant difference of pulse exists between the two populations. In this example, as the probability is 0.02 which is less than 0.05, we have reason to reject the null hypothesis ($\mu = 72$) and conclude that the population mean of pulse for male residents lived in a mountainous area is significantly higher than that of general male adults since the sample mean is larger than 72 (μ_0).

In fact, a hypothesis test is based on the thought of proof by contradiction and the principle of small probability event. As the latter has been carefully introduced in Chapter 1, here we would like to briefly illustrate the thought of proof by contradiction. First, we assume that there is no significant difference in the two population means ($\mu = \mu_0$). Then, we want to know whether sufficient evidence can be extracted from the data we obtained to support the assumption. If so, we may conclude that our assumption is true. Otherwise, we may believe that the assumption is false and its counterpart will be true and credible. In a word, the basic idea of a hypothesis test can be summarized in Figure 6.1.

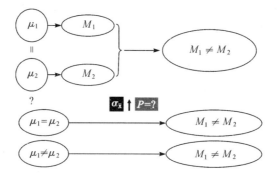

Figure 6.1   The Basic Idea of a Hypothesis Test (An Example of Two Independent Samples *t*-Test)

6.2   Key Steps in a Hypothesis Test

6.2.1   Set Up Your Hypothesis and Significant Level

The first step in a hypothesis test is to determine your hypothesis to be tested and the criteria we can use to make a conclusion, which is also called a significant level. In practice, we usually need to define two hypotheses containing a null hypothesis and an alternative hypothesis.

Null hypothesis is abbreviated as H_0 and usually defined as a statement to be tested in a hypothesis test. In statistics, a null hypothesis is often a statement of no difference among several parameters or no relationship among several variables and expected to be false. A hypothesis test is generally designed to assess whether H_0 is really false, in which we cannot conclude that the difference among parameters or relationships among variables is mainly attributable to sampling error. So, while setting up a null hypothesis we must take the following two aspects into account.

(a) The null hypothesis is usually set up as no difference among several parameters or no relationship among several variables though the associated statistics are different from each other or correlated.

(b) To test any statement about the population, we assume first that the null hypothesis is true. As Dr. R. A. Fisher remarked, "Null hypothesis is the hypothesis which is to be tested for possible rejection under the assumption it is true."

Notes:

Hypotheses always refer to some population parameters. For example, the null hypothesis for Example 6. 1 is:

H_0: $\mu = \mu_0 = 72$ times/min, which indicates that there is no significant difference between the population mean of pulse for males in the mountainous area and that for the general male adults.

Alternative hypothesis is the opposite of a null hypothesis and abbreviated as H_1. H_1 generally refers to a condition that there exists a significant difference among parameters or correlation among variables.

Although H_1 often represents a condition we hope to find, we mainly focus on collecting evidence to support the H_0 first. For Example, the alternative hypothesis for Example 6. 1 may be one of the followings:

(a) H_1: based on two-sided probability, which means that the two population means are significantly different.

(b) H_1: $\mu < \mu_0$ or $\mu > \mu_0$ when the one-sided probability is preferred.

In statistics, a **significant level** is a widely accepted criterion to be followed when making a conclusion in a hypothesis test. Whether H_0 to be rejected is mainly depending on its associated probability. In a typical hypothesis test, H_0 will be rejected when the probability is no more than the significant level, which is often abbreviated as α and the criteria of a small probability event. Otherwise, we cannot reject the H_0. Although α can be set up as 0. 05, 0. 01, or others, 0. 05 is the most commonly used one. If we choose $\alpha = 0. 05$, the probability of rejecting a correct null hypothesis is no more than 0. 05 or 5%. This means that we are 95% confident that the null hypothesis is false and should be rejected. Meanwhile, if α is set up as 0. 01, we may have 99% confidence to doubt about the H_0 and reject it.

6.2.2   Calculate the Test Statistic

As stated above, hypothesis test is a leading approach to achieve our goals in various researches. The key component of a hypothesis test is to decide whether H_0 will be rejected or not, which is mainly based on the associated p-value under the assumption of H_0. In a word, the calculation of the p-value is the core activity of a hypothesis test. Unfortunately, the calculation of a specific p-value is very difficult and complicated for many researchers, especially in the case of insufficient information. As is known to all, both the AUC of a distribution and a probability are from 0 to 1. So, statisticians suggest that the tailed AUC of a normal distribution can be used as the substitute probability. However, the precise calculation of the tailed AUC is also very difficult for the majority of investigators, especially for those lacking a strong advanced math background. In fact, we only care about whether the associated p-value is no more than the significant level rather than its specific value. As we learned in Chapter 5 (Figure 5. 6), the AUC is negatively associated with the t-value when the degree of freedom is fixed. So, we can calculate a t-value depending on the equation provided in Chapter 5, compare it with the critical t-value whose associated AUC equals to the significant level and make a decision in your hypothesis test. As the t-value is calculated based on your sample and plays a crucial role in the hypothesis test, it is also called a test statistic. In statistics, a test statistic is defined as a statistic based on a specific probability distribution and used to test whether the null hypothesis is true or not. In Example 6. 1, as the sampling distribution of the variable (pulse) meets t-distribution, we calculated the t-value using the equation $t = \dfrac{\overline{X} - \mu_0}{\dfrac{S}{\sqrt{n}}} = \dfrac{76 - 72}{\dfrac{7}{\sqrt{20}}} = 2. 56$, where t is the test statistic, $\overline{X}$ is the sample mean, μ_0 is the population mean, S is the standard deviation, n is sample size, υ is degree of freedom, and $\upsilon = n - 1 = 20 - 1 = 19$.

6.2.3 Determine the p-Value and Make Decision

As we know, H_0 will be rejected when the associated p-value is no more than the significant level in a hypothesis test. In fact, the p-value of a hypothesis test refers to the probability of obtaining another larger statistic from a population under the assumption of H_0 than the statistic of the current samples. The smaller the p-value, the stronger the evidence to against H_0. In a specific distribution, e. g. t-distribution, a p-value is a tailed AUC for one-sided probability or the sum of two-tailed AUC for two-sided probability (Figure 6. 2).

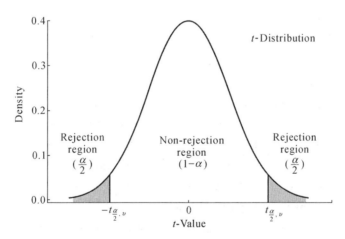

Figure 6. 2 The Rejection Area and Non-rejection Region

To make your decision in a hypothesis test, we can compare the test statistic (e. g. t-value) with the critical value which represents a special value, e. g. $t_{\frac{\alpha}{2}, \upsilon}$ (two-sided probability) or $t_{\alpha, \upsilon}$ (one-sided probability) whose associated AUC equals to the significant level (α). In a t-distribution with fixed degree of freedom, we can find that the p-value is inversely associated with the absolute value of the test statistic. The larger the absolute value of the test statistic, the smaller the p-value will be. So, if the absolute value of a test statistic is greater than that of the critical value, it is suggested that the associated p-value (the tailed AUC, highlighted with silver color) will be less than the significant level and a small probability event has occurred under the assumption of H_0. Therefore, we have reason to doubt about the H_0, reject it, and accept the alternative hypothesis (H_1) according to the significant level. Otherwise, we have no reason to doubt about the H_0 and have to accept it. In general, the critical values serve as the cutoff points of rejecting H_0 or not (Figure 6.2).

In summary, if $|t| \geqslant |t_{\frac{\alpha}{2},\nu}|$, it will be located in the rejection region and the p-value$\leqslant \alpha$ (Figure 6.2). So, according to the significant level, we have reason to doubt about the H_0, reject it, and accept that the H_1 is true. The conclusion will be that there exists a significant difference among several parameters or significant correlation among several variables. However, if $|t| < |t_{\frac{\alpha}{2},\nu}|$, it will be located in the non-rejection region and the p-value will be greater than α. So, according to the significant level, we have no reason to doubt about the H_0 and have to conclude that several parameters are not significantly different from each other or variables are not significantly correlated to each other.

In Example 6.1, t-value$=2.56$ (please see detail in section 6.2.2) and the critical value $t_{\frac{\alpha}{2},\nu}=t_{0.025,19}=2.093$ in a condition that the significant level is set up as $\alpha=0.05$ and $\nu=n-1=19$. As $2.56>2.093$, the p-value will be less than 0.05. So, according to the significant level $\alpha=0.05$, we can suspect that H_0 may be false, reject it, and conclude that the average pulse of male residents living in a mountainous area is significantly different from that of general male adults. Furthermore, as 76 (the point estimation of a population mean) is over 72, the final conclusion in this example will be that the male residents of a mountainous area have a significantly higher pulse than that of general male adults.

We can also obtain a more accurate range of p-value than only knowing whether it is no more than the significant level. Based on the Appendix 2, we may find that the two critical values for two-sided probability $t_{\frac{0.02}{2},19}=2.539$ and $t_{\frac{0.01}{2},19}=2.861$. As the test statistic ($t=2.56$) is between $t_{\frac{0.02}{2},19}$ and $t_{\frac{0.01}{2},19}$, the associated p-value will be located in the range of 0.01 to 0.02, which means that $0.01 < p\text{-value} < 0.02$. We also can get an accurate p-value by some specific statistical software including SAS, SPSS, STATA, R, and others. In Example 6.1, the accurate two-sided p-value based on SPSS is 0.0192.

Summary of the steps for a hypothesis test:

A hypothesis test is a process for assessing the significance of the evidence provided by the samples against a null hypothesis. The five common steps for all hypothesis tests are as follows.

Step 1: Set up H_0 and H_1. A hypothesis test is generally designed to assess the strength of the evidence against H_0, while H_1 is the alternative hypothesis that we will accept if the evidence enables us to reject H_0.

Step 2: Choose a significant level α. It refers to announce in advance how much evidence against H_0 you regard as decisive.

Step 3: Calculate the value of the **test statistic** on which the H_0 will be rejected. This statistic usually measures how far the data are from H_0.

Step 4: Determine the p-value based on the observed data. This is a specific probability assuming that H_0 is true, in which the test statistic will weigh against H_0 at least as strongly as it does for these data.

Step 5: Make a conclusion. One way to do this is to compare the p-value with α which is decided in Step 2. If the p-value is less than or equal to α, you can conclude that H_0 might be false and the alternative hypothesis can be accepted. While if it is greater than α, you can conclude that the data do not provide sufficient evidence to reject the null hypothesis. In general, your conclusion may be one or two sentences to summarize what you have found by a specific hypothesis test.

6.2.4 Cautions of a Hypothesis Test

(a) A proper study design is the basis of a hypothesis test. Potential confounding factors such as age, gender, and others among groups should be comparable. To achieve this goal, your sample should be randomly selected from the population in an observational study and participants enrolled in an experimental study should also be randomly assigned into different groups to receive different interventions. Otherwise, the conclusion of a hypothesis test will be incredible.

(b) Different types of data need a different hypothesis test. For example, paired t-test, paired chi-square test, and conditional logistic regression model should only be used for paired design study. A t-test cannot be used for the comparisons of three or more population means. Correlation and regression models are only performed to investigate the relationship between several variables. In a word, an appropriate hypothesis test should be applied strictly depending on the objective, the types of your data, different distributions, study designs, sample size, etc.

(c) Readers should correctly understand the meaning of significant difference or significantly correlated to each other. In general, "H_0 is rejected" does not mean that the difference is very big or obvious. It only indicates that the difference between the population means has reached the significant level α, while "H_0 is not rejected" represents that insufficient evidence is obtained to conclude that the H_0 is false. But it does not mean that H_0 is true. In other words, it only means that the difference among parameters based on the current samples has not reached a significant level. This is the reason why the expression of "significant difference or significantly correlated" is less and less used nowadays. Similar examples can be found in the principle of presumption of innocence in judicial practice: the defendant is presumed to be innocent before being proved guilty. If the defendant cannot be proved to be guilty under reasonable speculation based on sufficient evidence, he/she will be considered innocent. In this condition, that the defendant is innocent does not mean that he must be innocent. It just indicates that we cannot obtain sufficient evidence to prove that he is guilty at present. In fact, whether H_0 will be rejected is not only based on the real difference but also highly affected by the significant level, two-sided or one-sided probability you used, sample size, and others.

(d) The conclusion of a hypothesis test is probabilistic and cannot be absolutely correct or incorrect as it is obviously affected by the significant level (α), sample size, and others. It is believed that whether H_0 is rejected or not will inevitably induce two types of errors which will be introduced in detail in the following section of this chapter. So, you should provide the test statistic and specific p-value at the same time in your report. For example, if the p-value is 0. 019 in a hypothesis test, it should be that $P = 0. 019$ rather than only $P < 0. 05$.

(e) The difference and relation between statistical significance and professional significance should not be ignored. Statistical significance is generally a conclusion based on a statistical point of view and largely affected by the sample size and others. While a professional significance mainly focuses on the practical value of the conclusion. To draw a proper conclusion in research, both statistical significance and professional significance should be well considered.

6.3 Considerations of Hypothesis Test

In practice, carrying out a hypothesis test is not difficult, especially using some specific statistical softwares. However, performing a hypothesis test wisely is not so simple since each test is valid only when its requirements are met, which will be introduced in detail in the following chapters. This section only focuses on the two types of errors and power of a test.

6.3.1 Definitions of Two Types of Errors and the Power of a Hypothesis Test

As we know that the conclusion of a hypothesis test is probabilistic, which means it cannot be absolutely correct no matter whether the H_0 has been rejected or not. The errors due to a hypothesis test are called two types of errors containing type I error and type II error.

(a) **Type I error** is defined as the error due to rejecting a correct H_0. As we know that if the p-value of a hypothesis test is no more than the significant level (α), which usually equals to 0. 05, we will conclude that H_0 is false depending on the theories of small probability event. In general, only when $P = 0$ can we believe that H_0 will be completely false. However, $P \leqslant \alpha$ is not equal to $P = 0$. So, our conclusion cannot be true in some conditions. When the H_0 is true and rejected because of a quite small p-value, type I error will occur and equals to the p-value. The probability of type I error is generally denoted by α and equals to the p-value of a hypothesis test.

(b) **Type II error** is the error of failing to reject a false H_0. It occurs when the false H_0 has not been rejected due to a large p-value, e. g. $P > \alpha$ in a hypothesis test. In a specific hypothesis test, H_0 will not be rejected though it might be false when the p-value is greater than the significant level. In general, only when $P = 1$ can we believe that H_0 will be completely true. However, $P>\alpha$ is not equal to $P=0$. So, type II error will occur in this condition. In statistics, the probability of type II error is generally denoted by β and its range is from 0 to $1-\alpha$ in theory. The definitions of type I error and type II error, as well as the characteristics of them, are summarized in Table 6.1 and Figure 6.3.

Table 6.1   The Two Types of Error in the Acceptance Sampling Setting

Reality	Statistical decision based on sample	
	Reject H_0	Not reject H_0
H_0 is True	Type I error (α)	Correct decision ($1-\alpha$)
H_0 is False	Correct decision ($1-\beta$)	Type II error (β)

As shown in Table 6.1 and Figure 6.3, the probability of type I error is, in fact, α which is conventionally set at 0.05 and the probability of its logical complement is $1-\alpha$. Meanwhile, the probability of type II error is defined as β and the probability of its logical complement is $1-\beta$, which is called power. In statistics, the **power of a hypothesis test** refers to the ability to find an incorrect H_0 when it is really false. In fact, it is a probability that H_1 will be accepted when H_1 is really true. It is vitally important to obtain a proper power in a hypothesis test. In fact, insufficient power is one of the most common reasons for the negative findings when H_1 is true. It is widely accepted that the power of a hypothesis test should be over 0.8. Otherwise, your conclusion will be thought to be incredible. In summary, power should be well-considered and calculated in advance during your study design period.

6.3.2   The Source of Two Types of Errors

In statistics, census or general survey means that investigators can collect data from each participant of a specific population and calculate parameters directly. In a census, neither type I error nor type II error will occur anymore because both of them only come from a hypothesis test, in which type I error will occur when H_0 is rejected and type II error will appear when H_0 is not rejected. Furthermore, a hypothesis test will be performed only in a sampling study since no statistical inference will be needed in a census. In fact, in a sampling study, we must select a random sample from a specific population first, then collect data of the sample, perform the statistical description, and finish the statistical inference including a hypothesis test. So, we must know that both types of errors mainly come from the sampling error in a random sampling study.

6.3.3   Measures to Decrease Two Types of Error

It is of fundamental importance to take some effective measures to reduce type I error and type II error because both of them will decrease the credibility of our conclusion to some extent. As the two types of error mainly come from the sampling error, which is also called standard error and accurately assessed by the ratio of standard deviation by square root of the sample size ($\sigma_{\bar{x}} = \dfrac{\sigma}{\sqrt{n}}$). As we know that the standard deviation of a population is generally fixed when a population has been determined though we perhaps do not know its value. So, if we enlarge the sample size of our sample, the standard error will decrease and both types of error will also decrease at the same time. In a word, expanding sample size can effectively reduce both types of errors at the same time.

Unfortunately, a larger sample size will also greatly increase the cost of a study. This cannot be the first option in some conditions that we cannot afford the cost or obtain too many participants as we want. So, how can we do in a study that we cannot enroll as many participants as we can? As can be seen clearly in Figure 6.3, there is an intimate relationship between type I error and type II error, in which larger type I error will lead to smaller type II error (when the vertical line in the middle is moved to the left) or smaller type I error will be accompanied by larger type II error (when the vertical line in the middle is moved to the right). It means that techniques to minimize one error can unwittingly increase the chance of the other and we cannot reduce the two types of errors at the same time in a specific research when its sample size cannot be enlarged easily. In this condition, which will be the first consideration when we want to decrease the two types of error?

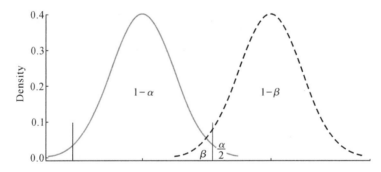

Figure 6.3   Relationship between Type I Error and Type II Error

As stated above, the range of type I error and type II error will be, in theory, from 0 to 0.05 and 0 to 0.95, respectively. So, as compared to type II error, it is suggested to decrease the type I error first because its interval is shorter than that of type II error when we cannot reduce them at the same time by expanding the sample size.

6.3.4   *p*-Value and the Significant Level

The **p-value** is the probability, computed assuming that H_0 is true, to represent that H_0 is true. In fact, a hypothesis test aims to give a clear statement to reject H_0 depending on the degree of evidence (*p*-value) based on the sample. A small *p*-value generally indicates that we have a strong evidence against H_0.

The significant level is a specific probability and widely accepted as the criterion of the occurrence of a small probability event. It is also the maximum probability of a type I error. Only when the p-value is no more than the significant level, can we conclude that the difference among parameters or correlation among variables are statistically significant. Otherwise, we may conclude that the difference or correlation is not statistically significant. In fact, no sharp border exists between "significant" and "not significant" as it is largely affected by the significant level. The smaller p-value we observed, the higher the probability to against H_0 and smaller probability to make mistakes when H_0 is rejected. To help readers better understand our findings, we frequently report the specific p-value such as $P=0.002$ rather than $P<0.05$ only. This expression clearly reveals that the probability of type I error will be 0.002 when we reject H_0. If we use $P<0.05$ instead of $P=0.002$, readers do not know what is the accurate probability of type I error ($P=0.049$? 0.01? 0.0001? or others) if we think H_0 is false and will be confused a lot.

6.3.5 Two-Tailed vs. One-Tailed Test

In any hypothesis test, the conclusion will mainly base on whether the p-value is no more than the statistical level (α). So, a key step of a hypothesis test is to calculate its associated p-value and compare it with α to make a decision. Unfortunately, the calculation of a specific p-value is very complicated and too difficult for the majority of researcher, especially those lacking a solid background of advanced mathematics. To solve this problem, statisticians suggest using the tailed AUC of a specific distribution (e. g. t-distribution) to replace the probability when the statistic meets this distribution. As is shown in Figure 6.4, the tailed AUC can be estimated in two ways: both sides (AUC highlighted with bright shade) or a single side (AUC covered by the sum of dark shade and right bright shade). In statistics, a hypothesis test based on the tailed AUC containing both sides is called a **two-tailed test** and its associated critical value will be presented as $t_{\frac{\alpha}{2},v}$, while hypothesis test based on single side AUC is called **one-tailed test** and the critical value is $t_{\alpha,v}$.

Although AUC is accepted to be a surrogate of associated p-value in a hypothesis test, its calculation is also quite difficult for researchers without mathematics background. After carefully studying on the principle of a hypothesis test, statisticians find that whether the p-value is no more than α is more important than knowing a specific p-value in a traditional hypothesis test. They also observe that the tailed AUC of a specific distribution is inversely associated with the absolute value of the statistic. So, to help more researchers applying hypothesis test easily, they suggest that we can compare our test statistic with the critical value (e. g. $t_{\frac{\alpha}{2},v}$ or $t_{\alpha,v}$) to know whether the p-value (tailed AUC) is greater than α. In summary, when you want to know whether H_0 can be rejected, you can compare the absolute value of your test statistic, a statistic mainly used in a hypothesis test, with the absolute value of a critical value. If the absolute value of your test statistic is no more than the absolute value of the critical value, e. g. $t \geqslant t_{\frac{\alpha}{2},v}$ (two-sided test) or $t \geqslant t_{\alpha,v}$ (one-sided test), you may think that the p-value $\leqslant \alpha$. So, according to this significant level, you have reason to doubt about the H_0, reject it, and conclude that H_1 will be true. Otherwise, if $t<t_{\frac{\alpha}{2},v}$ or $t<t_{\alpha,v}$, the p-value$>\alpha$. According to the significant level, you have no reason to doubt about H_0 and reject it. Then the conclusion will be that no significant difference among parameters or no significant correlation among variables can be observed in your study.

As is shown in Figure 6.4, the absolute critical value of the test statistic for a two-sided test ($t_{\frac{\alpha}{2},v}$) is much larger than that of a one-sided test ($t_{\alpha,v}$) in a specific distribution. Suppose the test statistic (t-value) of your hypothesis test is between the two critical values ($t_{\frac{\alpha}{2},v}<t<t_{\alpha,v}$), H_0 will be rejected in a one-sided test and will not be rejected in a two-sided test. In other words, type I error will not occur for a two-sided test and is present for a one-sided test in this condition. As stated in the above section (section 6.3.3), we know that type I error should be reduced first when we cannot decrease the two types of error at the same time by means of expanding the sample size. So, we should select a two-sided test instead of a one-sided test in most conditions. This is the reason why two-sided tests are very commonly used in a hypothesis test and one-sided test is only performed in few special conditions, in which researchers are only interested in whether one parameter is greater than or less than that of another.

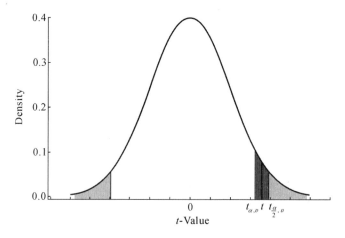

Figure 6.4   Two-Sided and One-Sided Probability

Take t-test as an example. In a two-tailed t-test, the critical values of the test statistic are both $-t_{\frac{\alpha}{2},v}$ and $t_{\frac{\alpha}{2},v}$ and the associated p-value consists of two parts (Figure 6.4, AUC highlighted with bright shade). The H_0 and H_1 are often expressed as follows:

Null hypothesis (H_0): $\mu_1=\mu_2$

Alternative hypothesis (H_1): $\mu_1\neq\mu_2$

When H_0 has been rejected, both $\mu_1>\mu_2$ and $\mu_1<\mu_2$ will be carefully investigated.

In a one-tailed t-test, we only want to know whether one parameter is greater than or less than another, the critical value is only $-t_{\alpha,v}$ or $t_{\alpha,v}$ and its associated p-value only consists of one part (Figure 6.5). The H_0 and H_1 are often expressed as follows:

Null hypothesis (H_0): $\mu_1=\mu_2$

Alternative hypothesis (H_1):　　　　　$\mu_1 > \mu_2$ or $\mu_1 < \mu_2$

In practice, we can perform two types of one-tailed tests: left-tailed test $(\mu_1 < \mu_2)$ and right-tailed test $(\mu_1 > \mu_2)$. In the former, the critical value of the test statistic is $-t_{a,v}$ and the rejected region lies entirely on the left tail of the distribution curve (Figure 6.5(a)). While in a right-tailed test, the critical value of the test statistic is $t_{a,v}$ and the rejected region lies entirely on the right tail of the distribution curve (Figure 6.5(b)).

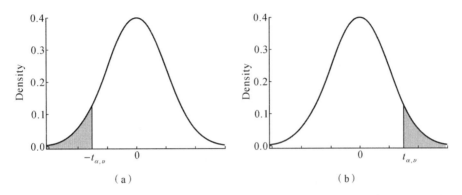

(a)　　　　　　　　　　　　　　　　(b)

Figure 6.5　Principles of the One-Tailed Test

6.3.6　Statistical Significance and Practical Value

When a null hypothesis ("no effect" or "no difference") can be rejected according to a significant level (α), we have evidence to conclude that the effect or difference is **statistically significant**. However, it does not mean that the effect or difference will be very obvious or big in practice. In fact, the conclusion of a hypothesis test is not only depending on the real effect or difference but also highly affected by the sample size. As is shown in Table 6.2, the conclusion of a hypothesis test is greatly affected by both the difference and sample size. In some conditions, although the difference between the two groups is quite small, the H_0 will also be rejected if the sample size is large enough. A **practical value** of a study is mainly determined as to whether the conclusion will be beneficial to the practice. So, the scientific value of a research should be assessed by its statistical significance and practical value at the same time. If it is statistically significant and has little practical value, it means that perhaps your study design is improper and unreasonable or the sample size is too large to overestimate the effect or difference. If the conclusion has obvious practical value and is not statistically significant, it generally indicates that your sample size is insufficient to obtain a proper conclusion or the study design is unreasonable. So, only when the statistical significance and practical value are consistent, will you achieve an appropriate and practical useful conclusion. For example, a researcher wanted to know whether a training program designed to increase the score of College English Test Band 4 (CET-4) is really useful. He collected the CET-4 score of 20,000 undergraduate students who were randomly selected from all students without receiving the program (Group 1), and another 1,000 undergraduate students who have taken the program (Group 2). The scores of both groups all meet normal distribution and $\overline{X}\pm S$ of Groups 1 and 2 are 385. 64±59. 32 and 389. 45± 61. 24, respectively. After a hypothesis test, he concluded that the program can significantly increase the CET-4 scores since the p-value is 0. 048 <0. 05 (Table 6. 3). We say that the difference between the two groups is statistically significant. However, the increased score due to the training program is only 3. 81 and too small to be considered to have practical significance.

Table 6. 2　Influence of the Sample Size on the Final Conclusions

Examples	Intervention	Control	t	P
1	21. 1±2. 2(10)	22. 1±2. 3(10)	0. 99	>0. 05
2	21. 1±2. 2(50)	22. 1±2. 3(50)	2. 22	<0. 05
3	21. 1±2. 2(120)	21. 5±2. 3(120)	1. 38	>0. 05
4	21. 1±2. 2(320)	21. 5±2. 3(320)	2. 25	<0. 05
5	21. 1±2. 2(3,200)	21. 3±2. 3(3,200)	3. 55	<0. 01

Data are presented with mean±standard deviation (sample size)

Table 6. 3　Comparison of the CET-4 Score with Students Receiving Training Program or Not

	Non-training ($n=20,000$)	Training ($n=1,000$)	t	P
CET4 score	385. 64±59. 32	389. 45±61. 24	1. 98	0. 048

Data are presented with mean±standard deviation

6.3.7 Comparison with CI Estimation

(a) A parameter estimation can replace a hypothesis test.

As the major components of a statistical inference, a parameter estimation mainly focuses on inferring the specific value of a parameter, while a hypothesis test is interested in estimating whether there exists statistically significant difference among parameters or statistically significant correlation among several variables. In general, these two statistical inferential approaches are closely correlated though having a different concern. In fact, a parameter estimation can completely replace a hypothesis test. If H_0 (i. e. $\mu_1=\mu_2$) is included in a CI, we have no reason to doubt about H_0 and reject it according to the current significant level (α) since H_0 may be true. Otherwise, if H_0 is not included in the CI, it can be rejected in accordance with the α. Let's compare the hypothesis test with a parameter estimation to better understand their relationship based on Example 6. 1. In a view of a hypothesis test, the test statistic (t) and critical value ($t_{\frac{\alpha}{2},v}$) is 2. 56 and 2. 093, respectively. According to the idea of a hypothesis test, the p-value is less than α and we have reason to reject the H_0. While from the view of a parameter estimation, as $\overline{X}=76$,

$S=7$, and $n = 20$, the 95% CI can be calculated by the formula: $\overline{X} \pm t_{\frac{\alpha}{2},v} S_{\overline{X}} =$

$\left[76 - 2.093 \times \dfrac{7}{\sqrt{20}}, 76 + 2.093 \times \dfrac{7}{\sqrt{20}} \right] = [72.7, 79.3]$. Because $\mu_0 = 72$ is not in the 95%

CI, we have reason to doubt about H_0, reject it and conclude that the difference of the pulse between male residents lived in a mountainous area and the general male adults is statistically significant. This is completely the same as that of a hypothesis test. In fact, a two-tailed hypothesis test based on a significant level α can be replaced by an interval estimation with a confidence level at $1-\alpha$. In other words, we can think that H_0 will also be rejected depending on a two-tailed hypothesis test at a significant level α when it falls outside a CI for μ with a confidence level at $1-\alpha$.

(b) A CI provides more information than a hypothesis test.

In practice, a CI can be applied not only to infer whether H_0 is true or false but also to indicate whether the difference or effect is practically useful or professional significant. As can be seen clearly in Figure 6.6, the examples 1, 2, and 3 (highlighted with grey colors) reveal that the conclusions of associated hypothesis tests will be statistically significant because the H_0 of them are not included in the three CIs. While the H_0 are all included in the CIs of examples 4 and 5 (black color), these two conclusions will be non-statistically significant. Furthermore, among the three examples achieved statistical significance, the conclusion of example 1 is also professional significant since its CI is over the practical value. The conclusion of example 2 is possible professional significant as its CI includes the practical value. While example 3 may be considered as non-professional significant because its CI is under the practical value. As for the two non-statistically significant examples, the CI of example 4 indicates that its sample size is insufficient because it also achieves the practical value. It also illustrates that although the conclusion will be statistically significant by expanding the sample size largely, it is still non-professional significant. Finally, the H_0 of example 5 cannot be rejected because it is included in its CI.

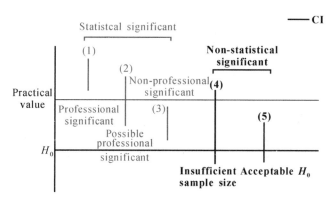

Figure 6.6   Information Provided by a CI

In summary, a researcher should focus on both the statistical significance and professional value of the conclusion in a study, especially the professional significance. An appropriate statistical inference should contain the results of both the hypothesis test and parameter estimation.

(**Meng Qiong，Mao Guangyun**)

Question Bank

Chapter 7 *t*-Test

7.1 Introduction

Student's *t*-test, introduced by W. S. Gossett under the pseudonym of "Student," simply called *t*-test, is used to determine if there is a significant difference between the means of two groups. In *t*-test, the test statistic follows a Student's *t*-distribution under the null hypothesis.

7.2 Categories

There are three different types of *t*-test that can be performed depending on the data: one sample *t*-test, paired-samples *t*-test, and two independent samples *t*-test.

7.2.1 One Sample *t*-Test

One sample *t*-test, also called a single-sample *t*-test, is classically used to test the mean of a single group against a known mean. That is, when a single sample is collected from a population, one-sample *t*-test is used to test whether there is a statistically significant difference between the mean of the population (μ_1) and the mean of another known population (μ_0) or a specified value. In one sample *t*-test, the measurement variable should be continuous and normally distributed. Besides, the sample should be drawn from the population randomly and subjects of samples should be independent.

When the null hypothesis H_0 is true, the *t*-test statistic is:

$$t = \frac{\overline{X} - \mu_0}{S_{\overline{X}}} = \frac{\overline{X} - \mu_0}{\dfrac{S}{\sqrt{n}}}, \quad \upsilon = n - 1 \tag{7.1}$$

where $\overline{X}$ is the sample mean; S is the sample standard deviation; υ is the degree of freedom; and n is the sample size.

Example 7.1 According to large-scale survey data, it is known that the average birth weight of infants is $\mu_0 = 3.30$ kg. A doctor randomly selected 36 dystocia infants and measured their birth weight, and got the sample mean $\overline{X} = 3.43$ kg, the sample standard deviation $S = 0.4$ kg. Is there any difference in birth weight between the dystocia infants and the general infants?

For this example, we can use one-sample *t*-test. The procedures are as follows:

(a) Set up the null hypotheses and alternative hypotheses.

H_0: $\mu_0 = 3.30$ kg, i. e. there is no difference in birth weight between the dystocia infants and the general infants.

H_1: $\mu_0 \neq 3.30$ kg, i. e. there is a difference in birth weight between the dystocia infants and the general infants.

(b) Choose a significant level $\alpha = 0.05$.

(c) Calculate the test statistic.

In this example, we know $n=36$, $\overline{X}=3.45$ kg, $S=0.4$ kg

The test statistic: $t=\dfrac{\overline{X}-\mu_0}{\dfrac{S}{\sqrt{n}}}=\dfrac{3.43-3.30}{\dfrac{0.4}{\sqrt{36}}}=1.95$

$$\upsilon = n-1 = 36-1 = 35$$

(d) Determine the p-value.

From the table of t-distribution critical value (Appendix 2) with $\upsilon=35$, we get the two-sided critical values: $t_{\frac{0.05}{2},35}=2.030$, $t=1.95 < t_{\frac{0.05}{2},35}$, then $P>0.05$.

(e) Make a conclusion.

$P>0.05$, according to the significant level $\alpha=0.05$, we do not reject the null hypothesis H_0, and there is no statistically significant difference between the two populations. So we cannot conclude that there is a difference in birth weight between the dystocia infants and the general infants.

7.2.2　Paired Samples t-Test

A **paired-samples t-test**, also called two related samples t-test, is used to compare two population means based on two paired samples, i. e. when there is only one sample that has been tested twice (repeated measures) or when there are two samples that have been matched or "paired," which includes self-pairing and allogeneic-pairing. (a) **Self-pairing**: two samples are collected from the same individuals at different times, at different sites, or by different methods. For example, individuals collected before and after an intervention in an experimental study, or differences between related sites on the same person (for instance, limbs, eyes, or kidneys), or data from a longitudinal study. (b) **Allogeneic-pairing**: two samples are collected from their matched cases and controls, which are matched with each other according to several important factors, such as age and gender.

In fact, a paired samples t-test, which is similar to one-sample t-test, is used to assess whether the mean difference between paired observations on a particular outcome is significantly different from zero.

The data for each pair of values must be entered on the same row of the spreadsheet. Thus, the number of rows in the data-sheet is the same as the number of individuals when the outcome variable is measured twice for each individual or is the number of individual-pairs when cases and controls are matched. When each individual is measured on two occasions, the effective sample size is the number of individuals or the number of case-control pairs and not the total number of individuals. For this reason, the paired values have to be excluded from the analyses if any one of paired data is loss or inability to recruit matched, which will reduce both power and the generalizability of the paired *t*-test.

Example 7. 2 Serum folate concentrations of 12 women were measured by the ELISA and Radioimmunoassay (RIA) method, respectively, data are shown in Table 7.1. The question is whether there is a difference between the results of the two methods.

Table 7. 1 **Serum Folate Concentrations (nmol/L) of 12 Women Measured by Two Methods**

Number of women (1)	RIA (2)	ELISA (3)	Difference d (4)=(2)−(3)	d^2 (5)
1	16. 5	15. 9	0. 6	0. 36
2	38. 2	36. 5	1. 7	2. 89
3	40. 3	38. 7	1. 6	2. 56
4	45. 1	44. 6	0. 5	0. 25
5	28. 5	27. 6	0. 9	0. 81
6	29. 5	30. 6	−1. 1	1. 21
7	53. 2	52. 1	1. 1	1. 21
8	36. 3	33. 1	3. 2	10. 24
9	14. 5	13. 8	0. 7	0. 49
10	48. 3	45. 1	3. 2	10. 24
11	38. 2	36. 5	1. 7	2. 89
12	32. 5	34. 1	−1. 6	2. 56
Total	—	—	12. 5	35. 71

In this example, the same woman was detected twice using two different methods, and the measurement data obtained were paired quantitative data. The formula of the paired *t*-test is:

$$t = \frac{\overline{d}}{\frac{S_d}{\sqrt{n}}}, \quad v = n - 1 \tag{7.2}$$

In this formula, the differences for each pair must be calculated, n is the number of differences, $\overline{d}$ is the mean of the differences, S_d is the standard deviation of the differences, $\frac{S_d}{\sqrt{n}}$ is the standard error of the mean of the differences, and v is the degree of freedom.

The paired samples *t*-test is really a form of the one-sample *t*-test. Therefore, the procedures of paired samples *t*-test are similar to those of one-sample *t*-test. The typical procedures are as follows.

(a) State the null hypothesis H_0 and the alternative hypothesis H_1.

H_0: $\mu_d = 0$, i. e. there is no statistical difference between the results of two methods.

H_1: $\mu_d \neq 0$, i. e. there is a statistical difference between the results of two methods.

(b) Choose a significant level $\alpha = 0.05$.

(c) Calculate the test statistic.

First, we should calculate the differences of serum folate concentrations between the results of two methods for each woman (see column 4 in Table 7.1).

Then, we know $n = 12$, $\bar{d} = \dfrac{\sum d}{n} = \dfrac{12.5}{12} = 1.04$ (nmol/L), the standard deviation of the differences:

$$S_d = \sqrt{\dfrac{\sum d^2 - \dfrac{\sum d^2}{n}}{n-1}} = \sqrt{\dfrac{35.71 - \dfrac{12.5^2}{12}}{12-1}} = 1.44 \text{ (nmol/L)}$$

The test statistic $t = \dfrac{\bar{d}}{S_d} = \dfrac{\bar{d}}{\dfrac{S}{\sqrt{n}}} = \dfrac{1.0417}{\dfrac{1.44}{\sqrt{12}}} = 2.51$

$$\upsilon = n - 1 = 12 - 1 = 11$$

(d) Determine the p-value.

From the table of t-distribution critical value (Appendix 2) with $\upsilon = 11$, we get the two-sided critical values: $t_{\frac{0.05}{2},11} = 2.201$, $t = 2.51 > t_{\frac{0.05}{2},11}$, then $P < 0.05$.

(e) Make a conclusion.

$P < 0.05$, according to the significant level of $\alpha = 0.05$, we reject the null hypothesis H_0, accept H_1, there is a statistically significant difference between two populations. So we regard that there is a difference in the serum folate concentrations between the two methods.

Example 7.3　In order to study the effects of different temperatures on blood sugar levels in rabbits, one researcher matched 6 pairs of rabbits according to their nests, gender, and weights. Two rabbits in each pair were randomly allocated to Group A with a temperature of 15°C and Group B with a temperature of 30°C, respectively. The blood sugar concentrations (mmol/L) of rabbits were measured and the result is shown in Table 7.2. Is the blood sugar level of rabbits in Group B higher than that of rabbits in Group A?

Table 7.2　Blood Sugar Concentrations (mmol/L) of Rabbits between Two Groups

Nest	Group A	Group B	Difference d	d^2
1	83.21	112.55	29.34	860.8356
2	109.10	139.64	30.54	932.6916
3	101.15	121.10	19.95	398.0025
4	75.20	109.35	34.15	1,166.2225
5	80.23	102.53	22.30	497.2900
6	101.75	137.89	36.14	1,306.0096
Total	—	—	172.42	5,161.0520

The design of this example is allogeneic-pairing; two rabbits in the same nests according to their gender and weights were paired; and then were randomly assigned into Group A and Group B respectively. As the data obtained is paired quantitative data, we use paired samples *t*-test here.

According to the information on this example, we choose one-tailed test.

(a) Set up the null and alternative hypotheses.

H_0: $\mu_d=0$, i. e. there is no statistical difference in the blood sugar levels of rabbits between the two groups.

H_1: $\mu_d>0$, i. e. the blood sugar level of rabbits in Group B is higher than that of rabbits in Group A.

(b) Choose significant level $\alpha=0.05$ (One-sided test).

(c) Calculate the test statistic.

We know that $n=6$, $\bar{d}=\dfrac{\sum d}{n}=\dfrac{172.42}{6}=28.74$ (mmol/L)

The standard deviation of the paired differences:

$$S_d=\sqrt{\dfrac{\sum d^2-\dfrac{\sum d^2}{n}}{n-1}}=\sqrt{\dfrac{5,161.14-\dfrac{28.74^2}{6}}{6-1}}=6.42 \text{ (mmol/L)}$$

The test statistic: $t=\dfrac{\bar{d}}{S_{\bar{d}}}=\dfrac{\bar{d}}{\dfrac{S_d}{\sqrt{n}}}=\dfrac{28.74}{\dfrac{6.42}{\sqrt{6}}}=10.96 \quad \upsilon=6-1=5$

(d) Determine the *p*-value.

From the table of *t*-distribution critical value (Appendix 2) with $\upsilon=5$, we get the one-sided critical values $t_{0.05,5}=2.015$, $t=10.96>t_{0.05,5}$, then $P<0.05$.

(e) Make a conclusion.

According to the significant level $\alpha=0.05$, we reject the null hypothesis H_0, accept H_1. There is a statistically significant difference between the two groups. So we regard that the blood sugar level of rabbits in Group B is higher than that of rabbits in Group A.

7.2.3 Independent Samples *t*-Test with Homogeneity of Variances

The independent samples (unpaired samples, or two samples) *t*-test is used to estimate whether there is a statistically significant difference between the means of two independent samples, which are taken from a single population that has been randomly divided into two subgroups or from two independent populations (e. g. male and female). The two samples are independent, unpaired (i. e. unrelated to each other). For instance, a doctor wanted to evaluate the effect of a medical treatment, and he enrolled 100 subjects into his study. Then these subjects were randomly assigned to the treatment group and to the control group equally. In this case, he had two independent samples and an independent samples *t*-test should be used. The randomization is not essential here—if a researcher contacted 100 people by phone and obtained each person's age and gender, and then he wanted to see whether the mean ages differ by gender or not, this would also be an independent samples t-test, even though the data are observational.

The purpose of the independent samples t-test is to assess whether two sample means are similar enough to have come from the same population or whether their difference is large enough for the two groups to have come from different populations. Rejecting the null hypothesis of the independent samples t-test indicates that the difference in the means of the two samples is large and is not due to either chance or sampling variation.

Let A and B be two populations with means μ_1 and μ_2, respectively. For the independent samples t-test, the null and alternative hypotheses are as follows:

H_0: $\mu_1 = \mu_2$, i. e. the two samples have been drawn from the same population.

H_1: $\mu_1 \neq \mu_2$ (Two-sided test).

Or H_1: $\mu_1 < \mu_2$ or $\mu_1 > \mu_2$ (One-sided test).

When the null hypothesis H_0 is true, the t-test statistic is:

$$t = \frac{\overline{X}_1 - \overline{X}_2}{S_{\overline{X}_1 - \overline{X}_2}} \quad v = n_1 + n_2 - 2 \tag{7.3}$$

Here, $\overline{X}_1$ and $\overline{X}_2$ are the corresponding sample means, and $S_{\overline{X}_1 - \overline{X}_2}$ is the standard error of the difference between two sample means:

$$S_{\overline{X}_1 - \overline{X}_2} = \sqrt{S_c^2 \times \left(\frac{1}{n_1} + \frac{1}{n_2}\right)} \tag{7.4}$$

where S_c^2 is the combined variance of two sample variances S_1^2 and S_2^2, the sample estimates of the population variances σ_1^2 and σ_2^2. If σ_1^2 and σ_2^2 are assumed to be equal, S_c^2 can be obtained using the following equation (the weighted coefficient is the ratio of degree of freedom):

$$S_c^2 = \frac{(n_1 - 1)S_1^2 + (n_2 - 1)S_2^2}{n_1 + n_2 - 1} \tag{7.5}$$

Example 7.4　Table 7.3 shows the waist circumstances between men and women aged over 60 years old. The question is whether the waist circumstances are different between men and women aged over 60 years old?

Table 7.3　Waist Circumstances (cm) between Men and Women Aged over 60 Years Old

Men (X_1) ($n_1 = 11$)	106.5	89.5	112.2	113.0	95.0	84.8	87.5	99.9	108.0	112.8	100.3	—	—
Women (X_2) ($n_2 = 13$)	97.4	90.3	82.4	102.0	95.0	76.2	85.0	72.9	81.6	90.7	86.7	90.6	114.5

For Example 7.4, we use two independent samples t-test, the steps of hypothesis testing are as follows.

(a) Set up the null hypotheses and the alternative hypotheses.

H_0: $\mu_1 = \mu_2$, i. e. there is no statistical difference in the waist circumstances between men and women aged over 60 years old.

H_1: $\mu_1 \neq \mu_2$, i. e. there is a statistical difference in the waist circumstances between men and women aged over 60 years old.

(b) Choose a significant level $\alpha=0.05$.

(c) Calculate the t-test statistic according to Formulae (7.3), (7.4), and (7.5):

In Example 7.4, $n_1=11$, $\overline{X}_1 = \dfrac{\sum X_1}{n_1} = 100.86$, $S_1=10.50$

$$n_2=13, \overline{X}_2 = \frac{\sum X_2}{n_2} = 89.64, S_2=11.07$$

Then $S_c^2 = \dfrac{11\times10.50^2+13\times11.07^2}{11+13-2} = 127.52$

The t-test statistic: $t = \dfrac{100.86-89.64}{\sqrt{127.52\times\left(\dfrac{1}{11}+\dfrac{1}{13}\right)}} = 2.53$

(d) Determine the p-value.

From the table of t-distribution critical value (Appendix 2) with $\upsilon=n_1+n_2-2=11+13$ $-2=22$, we get the two-sided critical values $t_{\frac{0.05}{2},22}=2.074$, $t=2.53>t_{\frac{0.05}{2},22}$, so $P<0.05$.

(e) Make a conclusion.

According to the significant level $\alpha=0.05$, we reject the null hypothesis H_0, and accept H_1. There is a statistically significant difference between the two groups. So we regard that the waist circumstances are different between men and women aged over 60 years old. In other words, we are 95% sure that men have significantly different waist circumstances compared with women.

When the size of each sample is sufficiently large (equal to or greater than 30), u-test can also be used to compare the two independent samples, the test statistic can be calculated as

$$u = \frac{\overline{X}_1-\overline{X}_2}{S_{\overline{X}_1-\overline{X}_2}} = \frac{\overline{X}_1-\overline{X}_2}{\sqrt{\dfrac{S_1^2}{n_1}+\dfrac{S_2^2}{n_2}}} \tag{7.6}$$

where u is the standard normal deviation, in terms of a normal distribution to calculate the p-value and make a conclusion.

Note: As the sample sizes get larger (and the degrees of freedom increase), the t-statistic approaches the u-statistic, i.e. t-test and u-test are essentially the same. But u-tests are preferred to t-tests when standard deviations are known.

Example 7.5   According to large-scale survey data, the statistics of serum cholesterol levels from the male and female groups are as follows. Please try to compare the difference in the serum cholesterol levels between males and females.

Females: $n_1=4,050$, $\overline{X}_1=4.9131$ (mmol/L), $S_1=0.9712$ (mmol/L);

Males: $n_2=4,316$, $\overline{X}_2=5.0288$ (mmol/L), $S_2=1.0143$ (mmol/L).

In Example 7.5, the sample size for each group is greater than 30, so we can perform u-test. The steps of hypothesis testing are as follows.

(a) Set up the null hypotheses and the alternative hypotheses.

H_0: $\mu_1 = \mu_2$, i. e. there is no statistical difference in the average serum cholesterol levels between males and females.

H_1: $\mu_1 \neq \mu_2$, i. e. there is a statistical difference in the average serum cholesterol levels between males and females.

(b) Choose a significant level $\alpha = 0.05$.

(c) Calculate the t-test statistic according to Formula (7.6):

$$S_{\bar{X}_1 \bar{X}_2} = \sqrt{\frac{S_1^2}{n_1} + \frac{S_2^2}{n_2}} = \sqrt{\frac{0.9712^2}{4,050} + \frac{1.0143^{2\,2}}{4,316}} = 0.0217$$

The test statistic: $u = \dfrac{\bar{X}_1 - \bar{X}_2}{S_{\bar{X}_1 - \bar{X}_2}} = \dfrac{4.9131 - 5.0288}{0.0217} = -5.3318$

(d) Determine the p-value.

From the table of standard normal distribution critical value (Appendix 1) or t-distribution critical value (Appendix 2) with $\nu = \infty$, we get the two-sided critical value $u_{\frac{0.05}{2}}$ $= t_{\frac{0.05}{2}, \infty} = 1.96$, $u > u_{\frac{0.05}{2}}$, so $P < 0.05$.

(e) Make a conclusion.

According to the significant level $\alpha = 0.05$, we reject the null hypothesis H_0, and accept H_1. There is a statistically significant difference between the two populations. So we regard that the average serum cholesterol levels between males and females are different.

In actuality, independent samples u-test is rarely used, because the estimate for the standard error for difference used here is biased. Instead, we often use independent samples t-test.

7.2.4 Independent Samples t' Test with Unequal Variances

Independent samples t-test requires that the variances should be equal between two populations. If not, we cannot use t-test, but use approximate t-test (t' test), data transformation or non-parametric test. Here we just introduce the t' test.

As the variances are not equal, the formula of t' test statistic is:

$$t' = \frac{\bar{X}_1 - \bar{X}_2}{\sqrt{\dfrac{S_1^2}{n_1} + \dfrac{S_2^2}{n_2}}} \tag{7.8}$$

The t' test include Satterthwaite's approximate t-test (1946), Welch's approximate t-test (1947), and Cochran & Cox approximate t-test (1950). For the first two t' tests, the test statistic under the null hypothesis is approximated by a t-distribution with approximate degrees of freedom. While for Cochran & Cox approximate t-test, the test statistic is approximated by the approximate t-critical value. Satterthwaite's approximate t-test is a commonly used method in statistical software.

7.2.4.1 Satterthwaite's Approximate t-Test

The adjusted degrees of freedom for the t' test given by Satterthwaite's approximation is:

$$v = \frac{S_{\bar{X}_1}^2 + S_{\bar{X}_2}^2}{\dfrac{S_{\bar{X}_1}^4}{n_1 - 1} + \dfrac{S_{\bar{X}_2}^4}{n_2 - 1}} = \frac{\dfrac{S_1^2}{n_1} + \dfrac{S_2^2}{n_2}}{\dfrac{(\frac{S_1^2}{n_1})^2}{n_1 - 1} + \dfrac{(\frac{S_2^2}{n_2})^2}{n_2 - 1}} \tag{7.9}$$

Then the standard procedure is followed by comparing the t' test statistic with the table of t-distribution critical value (Appendix 2) with the adjusted degrees of freedom in Formula (7.9), the p-value will be obtained.

7.2.4.2   Welch's Approximate *t*-Test

The adjusted degrees of freedom for the t' test given by Welch's approximation is:

$$v = \frac{S_{\bar{X}_1}^2 + S_{\bar{X}_2}^2}{\dfrac{S_{\bar{X}_1}^4}{n_1 - 1} + \dfrac{S_{\bar{X}_2}^4}{n_2 - 1}} - 2 = \frac{\dfrac{S_1^2}{n_1} + \dfrac{S_2^2}{n_2}}{\dfrac{(\frac{S_1^2}{n_1})^2}{n_1 - 1} + \dfrac{(\frac{S_2^2}{n_2})^2}{n_2 - 1}} - 2 \tag{7.10}$$

Similar to the Satterthwaite's approximate t-test, checking the table of t-distribution critical value (Appendix 2) with the adjusted degrees of freedom in Formula (7.10), the p-value will be obtained.

7.2.4.3   Cochran & Cox Approximate *t*-Test

The adjusted t-critical value for the t' test given by Cochran & Cox approximation is:

$$t'_a = \frac{S_{\bar{X}_1}^2 \times t_{a,v_1} - S_{\bar{X}_2}^2 \times t_{a,v_2}}{S_{\bar{X}_1}^2 + S_{\bar{X}_2}^2} = \frac{\dfrac{S_1^2}{n_1} \times t_{a,v_1} - \dfrac{S_2^2}{n_2} \times t_{a,v_2}}{\dfrac{S_1^2}{n_1} + \dfrac{S_2^2}{n_2}} \tag{7.11}$$

where t_{a,v_1}, t_{a,v_2} are the two-sided critical values of t-distribution with $v_1 = n_1 - 1, v_2 = n_2 - 1$, and can be obtained from the table of t-distribution critical value (Appendix 2). Actually, t' is the weighted average of t_{a,v_1} and t_{a,v_2} (use the ratio of variances as the weighted coefficients). If $t' < t'_a$, then $P > a$, do not reject H_0; if $t' \geqslant t'_a$, then $P \leqslant a$, reject H_0 and accept H_1.

In general, the Cochran & Cox approximate t-test tends to be conservative.

Example 7.6   Twelve silicosis stage zero workers (Group A) and ten lung cancer patients (Group B) were randomly selected and their RD values of the right lateral distance of the hilum were measured by X-ray. The results are shown in Table 7.4. The question is whether the average RD value of silicosis stage zero workers is different from that of lung cancer patients.

Table 7.4   RD Values (cm) of Silicosis Stage Zero Workers and Lung Cancer Patients

Group A	3.23	3.50	4.04	4.15	4.28	4.34	4.47	4.64	4.75	4.82	4.95	5.10
Group B	2.78	3.23	4.20	4.87	5.12	6.21	7.18	8.05	8.56	9.60	—	—

In Example 7.6, $n_1 = 12$, $\bar{X}_1 = \dfrac{\sum X_1}{n_1} = 4.36$, $S_1 = 0.57$

$$n_2 = 10, \ \overline{X}_2 = \frac{\sum X_2}{n_2} = 5.98, \ S_2 = 2.32$$

Levene's test of homogeneity of variance shows that the variances between two groups are unequal ($F = 20.455$, $P < 0.001$), and t-test cannot be used. We choose the Satterthwaite's approximate t-test here. The steps are as follows:

(a) Set up the null hypotheses and the alternative hypotheses.

H_0: $\mu_1 = \mu_2$, i. e. there is no statistical difference in the average RD value between silicosis stage zero workers and lung cancer patients.

H_1: $\mu_1 \neq \mu_2$, i. e. there is a statistical difference in the average RD value between silicosis stage zero workers and lung cancer patients.

(b) Choose significant level $\alpha = 0.05$.

(c) Calculate the test statistic according to Formulae (7.8) and (7.9):

The t' test statistic: $t' = \dfrac{\overline{X}_1 - \overline{X}_2}{\sqrt{\dfrac{S_1^2}{n_1} + \dfrac{S_2^2}{n_2}}} = \dfrac{4.36 - 5.98}{\sqrt{\dfrac{0.57^2}{12} + \dfrac{2.32^2}{10}}} = -2.16$

$$\upsilon = \frac{S_{\overline{X}_1}^2 + S_{\overline{X}_2}^2}{\dfrac{S_{\overline{X}_1}^4}{n_1 - 1} + \dfrac{S_{\overline{X}_2}^4}{n_2 - 1}} = \frac{\dfrac{S_1^2}{n_1} + \dfrac{S_2^2}{n_2}}{\dfrac{(\dfrac{S_1^2}{n_1})^2}{n_1 - 1} + \dfrac{(\dfrac{S_2^2}{n_2})^2}{n_2 - 1}} = 9.89 \approx 10$$

(d) Determine the p-value.

From the table of t-distribution critical value (Appendix 2) with $\upsilon = 10$, we get the two-sided critical values $t_{\frac{0.05}{2}, 10} = 2.228$, $t = 2.16 < t_{\frac{0.05}{2}, 10}$, so $P > 0.05$.

(e) Make a conclusion.

According to the significant level $\alpha = 0.05$, we reject the null hypothesis H_0, and accept H_1. There is no statistically significant difference between the two groups. So we cannot conclude that there is a difference in the average RD value between silicosis stage zero workers and lung cancer patients.

7.3　Requirements of t-Test

To conduct a t-test, the following assumptions must be satisfied: independence, normality, and homogeneity of variance.

7.3.1　Independence

The measurement of individuals should be independent, that is the value of one observation does not affect the value of other observations.

7.3.2　Normality

The one-sample t-test assumes that the data are normally distributed. The paired samples *t*-test assumes that the differences between pairs are normally distributed, it is not essential for the original observations to be normally distributed. The independent samples *t*-test assumes that each of the two populations is normally distributed.

In *t*-tests, normality assumption must be satisfied, otherwise, the results of the tests will be unreliable. In this situation, the equivalent non-parametric test or a transformation of the test variable will be needed. However, the *t*-tests are fairly robust to some degree of non-normality if the sample size is large and if there are no influential outliers. The definition of a "large" sample size varies but there is a common consensus that *t*-tests can be used when each group contains at least 30 to 50 individuals.

A normality test is used to determine whether a sample or any group of data has been drawn from a normally distributed population. There are two primary methods for normality testing: graphical methods and mathematical methods. Graphical methods are more intuitive and easy to interpret. Mathematical methods are more precise, hence more objective.

(a) Graphical methods: Stem-and-leaf plots, box plots, histograms, and P-P or Q-Q plots, are useful for visualizing the difference between an empirical distribution and a theoretical normal distribution. For example, if the histogram is bell-shaped, the underlying distribution is symmetric and perhaps approximately normal.

(b) Mathematical methods: There are several mathematical methods. SPSS software provides Shapiro-Wilk test and Kolmogorov-Smirnov test for normality. When the sample size is small ($3 \leqslant n \leqslant 50$), Shapiro-Wilk test is commonly used. However, when the sample size is relatively large ($n > 50$), Kolmogorov-Smirnov test is generally preferred. If $P > 0.1$, we can consider that the data follow a normal distribution; if $P \leqslant 0.1$, then we say that the data do not follow a normal distribution.

7.3.3 Homogeneity of Variance

The independent samples *t*-test assumes that the variances (the square of the standard deviation) of the test variable in the two populations are equal, that is, there is homogeneity of the variances between groups. If the variances are different between the two groups, i. e. there is heterogeneity of variances, the degrees of freedom or the *t*-critical value associated with the independent samples *t*-test should be adjusted.

To determine whether there is homogeneity of variances between two groups, several kinds of hypothesis tests can be used including F-test, Bartlett's test, and Levene's test. Here we use F-test to check if the variances of two populations are equal.

Let A and B be two populations with variances σ_1^2 and σ_1^2, respectively. Let n_1 and n_2 be the sample size, S_1^2 and S_2^2 be the variances of two samples drawn from the populations A and B, respectively. The procedures of F-test for homogeneity of variances are as follows.

(a) Set up the null hypotheses and the alternative hypotheses.

$H_0 : \sigma_1^2 = \sigma_2^2$, the variances of two populations are equal.

$H_1 : \sigma_1^2 \neq \sigma_2^2$, the variances of two populations are different.

(b) Choose a significant level $\alpha = 0.10$.

(c) Calculate the test statistic.

The F-test statistic is defined as:

$$F = \frac{S_1^2}{S_2^2}, \quad \upsilon_1 = n_1 - 1, \quad \upsilon_2 = n_2 - 1 \tag{7.12}$$

where S_1^2 is the bigger variance, S_2^2 is the smaller variance in the two samples, υ_1 and υ_2 are degrees of freedom in two samples, and n_1 and n_2 are the two sample sizes. In general, $S_1^2 > S_2^2$, so $F > 1$ always occurs. When we get F-test statistic, according to the table of F-distribution critical value (Appendix 3-1 or Appendix 3-2) with $n_1 - 1$ and $n_2 - 1$ degrees of freedom at a significant level of α, we can determine the p-value and make a conclusion. If $F \geqslant F_{\frac{\alpha}{2}, n_1 - 1, n_2 - 1}$, $P \leqslant \alpha$, reject H_0; If $F < F_{\frac{\alpha}{2}, n_1 - 1, n_2 - 1}$, $P > \alpha$, do not reject H_0. Noticeably, here we always choose a significant level $\alpha = 0.10$.

Example 7.7 Homogeneity test of variances in Example 7.4.

$H_0 : \sigma_1^2 = \sigma_2^2$, the variances of the two populations are equal;

$H_1 : \sigma_1^2 \neq \sigma_2^2$, the variances of the two populations are different.

$\alpha = 0.10$

Known that $S_1 = 11.07$, $S_2 = 10.49$, $n_1 = 12$, $n_2 = 10$

The test statistic: $F = \dfrac{11.07^2}{10.49^2} = 1.11$

From the F-distribution critical value table (Appendix 3-1) with $\upsilon_1 = 13 - 1 = 12, \upsilon_2 = 11 - 1 = 10$, we get the two-sided critical values $F_{0.20, (12,10)} = 2.28$, $F < F_{0.20, (12,10)}$, $P > 0.20$ (exactly $P = 0.817$, which can be calculated by SPSS software). We do not have enough evidence to reject the null hypothesis H_0 for there is no statistically significant difference between the two variances. Therefore, we regard that the variances of the two populations are equal.

If heterogeneity of variances between the two groups was found, then we should use the t' test (see details in section 7.2.4).

7.4 Variable Transformation

When the data do not follow a normal distribution or the population variances between the two groups are not equal, we cannot use the t-test directly. There are two ways to solve this problem. One is variable transformation and the other is using the non-parametric test (see Chapter 10).

Variable transformation is often necessary to get a more representative variable for the purpose of the analysis. The purpose of variable transformation is to convert the data into a normal distribution or make the data close to the homogeneity of variance. Making the appropriate transformation will often improve the quality of your results.

Usually, variable transformation is to transform the original data by a function. There are many transformations that are used occasionally in biology. Here are three most commonly used variable transformation methods.

7.4.1 Logarithmic Transformation

This transformation consists of taking the log of each observation. The formula is: $Y=\ln X$, where X is the original data. You can use either base-10 logs, base-2 logs or base-e logs, also known as natural logs. We often prefer base-10 logs, because it is possible to look at them and see the size of the original number: $\log(1)=0$, $\log(10)=1$, $\log(100)=2$, etc. The logarithm function tends to squeeze together the larger values in your data set and stretches out the smaller values.

For ease of interpretation, the results of calculations and tests are back-transformed to their original scale. For base-10 logs, the transformed number $x'=\log_{10}(x)$, and back-transformed number is $10^{x'}$. The back-transformed mean is the geometric mean.

If you have zeros or negative numbers in the original data, you cannot take the log; you should add a constant to each number to make them positive and non-zero. In this case, we use this formula: $Y=\ln(X+k)$. After the analysis, you will have to subtract the constant from the results.

Applicability of logarithmic transformation: (a) part of positive skewness data; (b) ratio data; (c) data with little difference between values and mean ratios in each group.

7.4.2 Square Root Transformation

This transformation consists of taking the square root of each observation. The formula is: $Y=\sqrt{X}$. The back transformation is to square the number. If you have negative numbers, you cannot take the square root; you should add a constant to each number to make them all positive: $Y=\sqrt{X+k}$.

The square root transformation is often used when the variable is a count of something, such as bacterial colonies per petri dish, blood cells going through a capillary per minute, mutations per generation.

Applicability of square root transformation: (a) data subject to Poisson distribution; (b) mildly skewed data; (c) the variance and mean of samples are positively correlated; (d) all cases of variable are percentages, and data with values range from 0 to 20% or from 80% to 100%.

7.4.3 Arcsine Square Root Transformation

This transformation consists of taking the arcsine of the square root of a number. The formula is: $Y=\sin^{-1}\sqrt{X}$. The result is given in radians, not degrees, ranging from $-\frac{\pi}{2}$ to $\frac{\pi}{2}$. The back transformation is to square the sine of the number.

This transformation is commonly used for proportions, which range from 0 to 1. Note that this kind of proportion is actually a nominal variable, so it is incorrect to treat it as a measurement variable whether you make an arcsine transform or not. And the original percentages have to be transformed to proportions before the arcsine square root transformation.

(**Zhang Junhui, Liao Qi**)

Question Bank

Chapter 8   Analysis of Variance

8.1   Introduction

Analysis of variance (often referred to as ANOVA) is a collection of methods for comparing multiple means across different groups, which is to test whether the mean of a variable is affected by different types and combinations of factors. Briefly speaking, ANOVA is a hypothesis-testing method used to test the equality of two or more population means by examining the variances of samples that are taken. When the means from two samples are compared using ANOVA, it is actually equivalent to use a t-test to compare the means of independent samples.

ANOVA determines whether the differences between the samples are due to random error (sampling errors) or caused by systematic treatment effects. For example, in the analysis of the effect of four different diets on blood pressure or in the investigation into the effect of three different treatment therapies on the value of glycated haemoglobin in patients with diabetes.

8.2   One-Way ANOVA

One-way ANOVA is the simplest form of ANOVA, which can be regarded as an extension of the independent samples t-test because one source of variation, or factor is investigated. However, ANOVA can be used to compare two more groups or treatments.

The aim of this comparison is to determine the proportion of the variability of the data due to the different treatment levels or random error. In one-way ANOVA, the **total sum of squares** (SS_{total}) for the data are similarly partitioned into a **"between groups" sum of squares** ($SS_{between}$) and a **"within groups" sum of squares** (SS_{within}). The within **groups** sum of squares is also referred to as the random error or residual sum of squares. The **mean squares** (MS), which correspond to variance estimates, are obtained by dividing the **sums of squares** (SS) by their degrees of freedom. The **mean square between** ($MS_{between}$) indicates how much variation there is due to interaction between samples, while the **mean square within** (MS_{within}) is defined as the mean square within samples, which indicates how much variation there is due to differences within individual samples.

The null hypothesis of one-way ANOVA is that the means of multiple populations are equal. Therefore, a significant result means that the means of multiple populations are not the same. The F-ratio equals to the $MS_{between}$ divided by the MS_{within} $(\frac{MS_{between}}{MS_{within}})$, and this ratio follows F-distribution.

When the null hypothesis of equal means is true, the two mean squares estimate the same quantity, and should be of approximately equal magnitude. In other words, their ratio should be close to 1. If the null hypothesis is false, $MS_{between}$ should be larger than MS_{within} and the ratio exceeds an F-value for the test, indicating that there is a significant difference of means between groups. The rejection of the null hypothesis indicates that variation of the data set is due to variation between different treatment levels but not random error. If the null hypothesis is rejected, then we could make the conclusion that the means are different between at least two groups at a defined significant level.

8.2.1 Completely Randomized Design

8.2.1.1 ANOVA for Completely Randomized Design

Example 8.1 In order to investigate the inhibition effect of the different treatments on the weight of the brain tumors, 40 tumor model mice were randomly assigned to be treated with four different drugs. Then, the weights of the tumors were measured. Is there a difference among the weights of four treatments?

In this example, a one-way ANOVA could be conducted. The detailed measured weights of each group are shown in Table 8.1.

Table 8.1 Inhibition Effect of 4 Kinds of Drugs on Tumor Weight (g)

ID	1 Drug A	2 Drug B	3 Drug C	4 Drug D	
1	3.6	3.0	0.6	3.3	
2	4.6	2.5	1.7	1.2	
3	4.2	2.4	2.3	0.4	
4	4.4	1.1	4.5	2.7	
5	3.7	4.0	3.6	3.0	
6	5.7	3.7	1.3	3.2	
7	7.0	2.7	3.2	0.6	
8	4.1	1.9	3.0	1.4	
9	5.2	2.6	2.1	1.2	
10	4.5	1.3	2.5	2.1	
$\sum_j X_{ij}$	47.0	25.2	24.8	19.1	$\sum X = 116.1$
$\sum_j X_{ij}^2$	230.40	71.26	73.34	47.19	$\sum X^2 = 422.19$
n_i	10	10	10	10	$N = 40$
$\overline{X}_i$	4.70	2.52	2.48	1.91	$\overline{X} = 2.9$
S_i	1.08	0.93	1.15	1.09	$S = 1.48$

(a) Set up the null hypotheses and the alternative hypotheses.

H_0: $\mu_A = \mu_B = \mu_C = \mu_D$, i. e. the population means of the four treatments are the same.

H_1: the means are not the same for all groups.

(b) Choose a significant level $\alpha = 0.05$.

(c) Select the testing method and calculate the test statistic.

Total sum of square (SS_{total}): The total sum of square is defined as

$$SS_{total} = \sum_i \sum_j (X_{ij} - \overline{X})^2 = \sum X^2 - C \tag{8.1}$$

$$C = \frac{\left(\sum X\right)^2}{N}$$

$$C = \frac{\left(\sum X\right)^2}{N} = \frac{116.1^2}{40} = 336.98$$

$$SS_{total} = \sum X^2 - C = 422.19 - 336.98 = 85.21$$

Also,

$$SS_{total} = S^2 \times (N-1) = 1.48^2 \times (40-1) = 85.43$$

The SS_{total} can be divided into two parts, which include the sum of square between groups ($SS_{between}$) and sum of square within groups (SS_{within}):

$$SS_{total} = SS_{between} + SS_{within}$$

Sum of square between groups: In Table 8.1, $\overline{X}_i$ represents the mean of the observations in the ith treatment. Here, $\overline{X}_1 = 4.70$, $\overline{X}_2 = 2.52$, $\overline{X}_3 = 2.48$, and $\overline{X}_4 = 1.91$. Therefore, the variation between treatment results can be expressed

$$SS_{between} = \sum_k n_i (\overline{X}_i - \overline{X})^2 \tag{8.2}$$

In our example, the $SS_{between}$ can be calculated

$$SS_{between} = 10 \times (4.7 - 2.9)^2 + 10 \times (2.52 - 2.9)^2 + 10 \times (2.48 - 2.9)^2 + 10 \times (1.91 - 2.9)^2 = 45.409$$

where $SS_{between}$ is sum of square between groups (treatments); and k represents the number of groups. In our example, $k = 4$, because there are 4 treatment classes including drug A, drug B, drug C, and drug D.

Sum of square within groups: In each group, the values of 10 observations are different. This variation is called the variation within groups that is expressed as **the sum of square within groups** (SS_{within}). Because the total sum of square is equal to the sum of squares between groups and the sum of squares within groups, we could also compute the SS_{within}:

$$SS_{within} = SS_{total} - SS_{between} = 85.21 - 45.409 = 39.801$$

The calculation of $MS_{between}$: The above variation decomposition only considers the sum of the variation (sum of squares), and does not consider the influence of the number of groups and the number of individuals within each group on the variation. For example, as the number of individuals within a group increases, the variation within groups will increase. Therefore, it is unsuitable to use $SS_{between}$ and SS_{within} to represent variation between groups and variation within groups respectively. Then the concept of mean square (MS) is derived, which is similar to the variance of a sample. This sum of squares divided by the degrees of freedom ($k-1$) is referred to as the mean square between groups ($MS_{between}$).

$$MS_{between} = \frac{n \times \sum_k (\overline{X}_i - \overline{X})^2}{k-1} \qquad (8.3)$$

When the sample sizes are not all equal, an estimate of variance between groups is provided by

$$MS_{between} = \frac{\sum_k n_i (\overline{X}_i - \overline{X})^2}{k-1} = \frac{\sum_i \frac{(\sum_j X_{ij})^2}{n_i} - C}{k-1} \qquad (8.4)$$

In Example 8.1, we can calculate the mean square between groups:

$$MS_{between} = \frac{SS_{between}}{k-1} = \frac{45.409}{3} = 15.136$$

The calculation of MS_{within}: The variance within groups is the sum of squares within groups divided by the degrees of freedom. Therefore, it is customarily referred to as the mean square within groups (MS_{within}). The mean square within groups (MS_{within}) for our illustrative example is

$$MS_{within} = \frac{SS_{within}}{k-1} = \frac{39.801}{36} = 1.106 \qquad (8.5)$$

The variance ratio (F): Then we need to compare the $MS_{between}$ and MS_{within}. Therefore, we could compute the following variance ratio (F):

$$F = \frac{MS_{between}}{MS_{within}}$$

The variance ratio close to 1 tends to support the hypothesis that the means of the populations are equal. On the other hand, F will be considerably greater than 1, if the $MS_{between}$ is considerably larger than MS_{within}. A value of F which is sufficiently greater than 1 indicates the doubt on the hypothesis of equal population means.

Because of the vagaries of sampling, even when the null hypothesis is true, it is unlikely that $MS_{between}$ and MS_{within} are equal. Therefore, we need to decide how large the observed differences have to be before we can conclude that the difference is due to different treatments other than sampling fluctuation. In other words, how large a value of F is required to conclude that the observed difference between the estimated $MS_{between}$ and MS_{within} is not a result of chance?

The F-test: The ratio of $\frac{MS_{between}}{MS_{within}}$ follows a distribution known as the F-distribution. R. A. Fisher introduced the F-distribution in the early 1920s, which has now become one of the most widely used distributions in modern statistics. The particular F-distribution depends on the degrees of freedom associated with the sample variance in the numerator (numerator degrees of freedom, v_1) and the degrees of freedom associated with the sample variance in the denominator (denominator degrees of freedom, v_2). Here, the sample variance in the numerator is $MS_{between}$ and the sample variance in the denominator is MS_{within}.

The numerator degrees of freedom are equal to the number of groups minus 1, that is $k-1$, and the denominator degrees of freedom value is equal to $N-k$. In Example 8.1:

Numerator degrees of freedom: $k-1=4-1=3$

Denominator degrees of freedom: $N-k=40-4=36$

And, $F=\dfrac{\dfrac{SS_{between}}{k-1}}{\dfrac{SS_{within}}{N-k}}=\dfrac{MS_{between}}{MS_{within}}=\dfrac{15.136}{1.106}=13.685$

Once the appropriate F-distribution has been determined, whether we will reject the null hypothesis of equal population means depends on the significant level chosen. The 2 degrees of freedom and the significant level chosen will determine the critical value of F (Appendix 4), denoted as $F_a(v_1,v_2)$. We usually set a significant level $\alpha=0.05$.

Above all, we could summarize the calculation in Table 8.2, denoted as ANOVA table.

Table 8.2   ANOVA Table for Example 8.1

Source of variation	SS	df	MS	F
Between groups	45.409	3	15.136	13.685
Within groups	39.801	36	1.106	—
Total	85.210	39		

(d) Determine the p-value.

According to F-distribution table in Appendix 4, we could get that $F_{0.05(3,36)}=2.87$. $F=13.691>F_{0.05(3,36)}$, then $P<0.05$.

(e) Make a conclusion.

According to the significant level $\alpha=0.05$, we reject the null hypothesis H_0, and accept H_1. We then could conclude that not all population means are equal, which means the effects of inhibition on the tumor from 4 kinds of drugs are different.

The ANOVA table: The calculations of the ANOVA table can be summarized and displayed in Table 8.3.

Table 8.3   Analysis of Variance Table for the Completely Randomized Design

Source of variation	SS	df	MS	F
Total	$SS_{total}=\sum_i\sum_j(X_{ij}-\bar{X})=(N-1)S^2$	$N-1$	—	—
Between groups	$SS_{between}=\sum_k n_i(\bar{X}_i-\bar{X})^2$	$k-1$	$\dfrac{SS_{between}}{k-1}$	$\dfrac{MS_{between}}{MS_{within}}$
Within groups	$SS_{within}=SS_{total}-SS_{between}$	$N-k$	$\dfrac{SS_{within}}{N-k}$	—

8.2.2　Multiple Comparison

When the analysis of variance leads to a rejection of the null hypothesis, the followed question will naturally arise: Which pairs of means are different? To answer this question, some may suggest carrying out a significance test on every pair of treatment means. For instance, in Example 8.1, if we would like to further compare the mean of one group with the mean of another, we need to do multiple comparisons. In this process, the experimenter must be cautious in testing for significant differences between individual means and need to always think about the validity of the procedure. The critical issue in the procedure is the level of significance. Although the probability α of rejecting a true null hypothesis for the test as a whole is made small, the probability of rejecting at least one true hypothesis when several pairs of means are tested is greater than α.

Several techniques to make multiple comparisons have been suggested over the past years. The first pairwise comparison technique was developed by Fisher in 1935 and is called the least significant difference (LSD) test. This technique can be used only if the ANOVA F-result is significant. The main idea of the LSD is to compute the smallest significant difference (i. e. the LSD) between two means as if these means had been the only means to be compared (i. e. with a t-test) and to declare any significant difference larger than the LSD.

Tukey's multiple comparison analysis method tests each experimental group against the control group. The Tukey method is preferred if there are unequal group sizes among the experimental and control groups. The Tukey method proceeds by first testing the largest pairwise difference. Tukey uses the "q" statistic to determine whether group differences are statistically significant. The "q" statistic is obtained by subtracting the smallest from the largest mean, and dividing that product by the overall group standard error of the mean.

8.2.2.1　Newman-Keuls Test

The Newman-Keuls or Student-Newman-Keuls (SNK) method is similar to Tukey test. However, it is a more powerful test than Tukey because it performs more pairwise comparisons, which is usually referred to as the q-test, makes use of a single value against which all differences are compared. This value is given by

$$q = \frac{|\bar{X}_A - \bar{X}_B|}{\sqrt{\frac{MS_{error}}{2}\left(\frac{1}{n_A}+\frac{1}{n_B}\right)}} \tag{8.6}$$

where MS_{error} is the error mean square from the ANOVA table.

Now we illustrate the use of the q-test in Example 8.1. The first step is to prepare a table of all possible paired means as shown in Table 8.4 (the means should be arranged from the maximum to the minimum).

H_0: any two population means are equal, i. e. $\mu_A = \mu_B$.

H_1: any two population means are not equal, i. e. $\mu_A \neq \mu_B$.

Table 8. 4   All Possible Paired Means

Rank	1	2	3	4
Mean	4. 70	2. 52	2. 48	1. 91
Group	Drug A	Drug B	Drug C	Drug D

Suppose $\alpha = 0.05$.

We could calculate the $MS_{error} = 1.239$.

The hypotheses that can be tested, the value of q, and the statistical decision for each test are shown in Table 8. 5.

Table 8. 5   Multiple Comparison Tests (q-test) of Example 8. 1

A to B	$|\overline{X}_A - \overline{X}_B|$	q	q-critical value $P = 0.05$	q-critical value $P = 0.01$	P
1 to 2	2. 16	6. 35	2. 88	3. 86	<0.01
1 to 3	2. 20	6. 47	3. 47	4. 42	<0.01
1 to 4	2. 79	8. 20	3. 83	4. 76	<0.01
2 to 3	0. 04	0. 12	2. 88	3. 86	>0.05
2 to 4	0. 63	1. 85	3. 47	4. 42	>0.05
3 to 4	0. 59	1. 73	2. 88	3. 86	>0.05

8. 2. 2. 2   Bonferroni Method

The Bonferroni method is a simple method that allows many comparison statements to be made (or CI to be constructed) while still assuring that an overall confidence coefficient is maintained.

The purpose of an adjustment such as the Bonferroni procedure is to reduce the probability of identifying significant results that do not exist, that is, to guard against making type I errors (rejecting null hypotheses when they are true) in the testing process. This potential for error increases with an increase in the number of tests being performed in a given study and is due to the multiplication of probabilities across the multiple tests. To carry out Boferroni procedure, we must select a value for α, which is the confidence level. Typically, we selected $\alpha = 0.05$. In Bonferroni's method, the idea is to divide this familywise error rate (0. 05) among the k-tests (k is the number of tests performed). So each test is done at the $\frac{\alpha}{k}$ level. For example, if you are running 20 simultaneous tests at $\alpha = 0.05$, the correction would be 0. 0025. Therefore, the Bonferroni test, also known as the "Bonferroni correction" or "Bonferroni adjustment" suggests that the "p" value for each test must be equal to alpha divided by the number of tests.

Whether or not to use the Bonferroni correction depends on the circumstances of the study. It should not be used routinely if: (a) a single test of the "universal null hypothesis"

(H_0) that all tests are not significant is required; (b) it is imperative to avoid a type I error; and (c) a large number of tests are carried out without preplanned hypotheses.

Other multiple comparison procedures include the Scheffee method, the Dunnett method, etc.

8.2.3 Requirements

Basically, when we perform the ANOVA, three requirements that are the same for t-test should be satisfied:

(a) The samples are randomly selected and independent of one another (independence);

(b) All populations involved follow a normal distribution (normality);

(c) All populations have the same variance (homogeneity of variance).

8.2.3.1 Independence

The assumption of independence is a critical requirement for the ANOVA test. Independence here means each sample is randomly selected and the value of one observation does not influence or affect the value of other observations. It's essential to getting results from the sample that could reflect what we want to know in a population.

In other words, dependence means a connection between the data. For example, how much the students improved their medicine statistics exams depends upon how many hours they work on this subject. Independence means there isn't a connection. However, the students improved in their medicine statistics exams that are not correlated to what you ate for lunch. The assumption of independence, therefore, means that the data are not connected in any way.

8.2.3.2 Normality

Because ANOVA assumes that the populations involved follow a normal distribution, ANOVA belongs to a category of hypothesis tests which is known as parametric tests. In other words, if the populations involved in ANOVA did not follow a normal distribution, an ANOVA test could not be used to examine the equality of the sample means.

To test the normality of the data involved, we could either use the way of graph such as histogram, or run a test which specifically designed to test for normality. A detailed description of the normality is mentioned in section 7.3.

8.2.3.3 Homogeneity of Variance

The equal variances assumes that different samples have the same variance, even if they came from different populations. This assumption actually can be found in many statistical tests, including ANOVA and Student's t-test.

Conducting a test without checking for equal variances will have a significant impact on the results, and may even invalidate the results completely. How much the results are affected depends on the type of test selected and how sensitive the test is to unequal variances.

We should check whether the assumption of equal variances is true before running the one-way ANOVA. There are many techniques that can be used to test whether the data meets the assumption of equal variances. These include Bartlett's test, Box's M test, Brown-Forsythe test, Hartley's Fmax test and Levene's test.

Bartlett's test for homogeneity of variances is used to test whether the variances are equal for all samples. It is often used when the normality of the data is assured. An alternative test, called Levene's test, is a better choice for data with non-normal distribution.

The null hypothesis for the test is that the variances are equal for all populations. In statistics expressions, that is:

H_0: $\sigma_1^2 = \sigma_2^2 = \cdots = \sigma_k^2$.

H_1: $\sigma_i^2 \neq \sigma_j^2$, for at least one pair (i, j).

The alternative hypothesis can be explained that the variances are not all equal, which means at least two variances are not the same.

The test statistic of Bartlett's test showed as below:

$$X^2 = \frac{(N-k)\ln(S_p^2) - \sum\limits_{i=1}^{k}(n_i - 1)\ln(S_i^2)}{1 + \frac{1}{3(k-1)}\left[\sum\limits_{i=1}^{k}\left(\frac{1}{n_i - 1}\right) - \frac{1}{N-k}\right]} \tag{8.7}$$

where S_i^2 is the variance of the ith group, N is the total sample size, n_i is the sample size of the ith group, k is the number of groups, and S_p^2 is the pooled variance.

The significant level is defined as α.

The variances are judged to be unequal if,

$X^2 > X_{1-\alpha, k-1}^2$

where $X_{1-\alpha, k-1}^2$ is the critical value of the chi-square distribution with $k-1$ degrees of freedom and a significant level of α.

8.3　Randomized Block Design

The randomized block design was developed in 1925 by R. A. Fisher. The statistician firstly divides subjects into different subgroups which are called blocks, that is, individuals within the same block share the same or similar characteristics that may affect the outcome. In this case, the variability within blocks is less than the variability between blocks. Followed by this step, subjects within each block are randomly assigned to different treatment conditions. For example, in many cases of animal experiments, different breeds of animal will respond differently to one treatment, therefore, in this situation, the breed of animal may be used as a blocking factor. And the subjects within each breed are randomly assigned to different treatments.

The technique for analyzing the data from a randomized block design is called "two-way analysis of variance" since an observation is categorized on the basis of two criteria—the block to which it belongs as well as the treatment group to which it belongs. In general, the data from an experiment utilizing the randomized block design may be displayed in a table such as Table 8.6.

Table 8.6 Sample Values for the Randomized Block Design

Blocks	Treatments						$\sum_j X_{ij}$	$\overline{X}_i$
	1	2	3	4	...	k		
1	χ_{11}	χ_{12}	χ_{13}	χ_{14}		χ_{1k}		$\overline{X}_1$
2	χ_{21}	χ_{22}	χ_{23}	χ_{24}		χ_{2k}		$\overline{X}_2$
3	χ_{31}	χ_{32}	χ_{33}	χ_{34}		χ_{3k}		$\overline{X}_3$
$\vdots$	$\vdots$	$\vdots$	$\vdots$	$\vdots$		$\vdots$		$\vdots$
n	χ_{n1}	χ_{n2}	χ_{n3}	χ_{n4}		χ_{nk}		$\overline{X}_n$
$\sum_j X_{ij}$	$T._1$	$T._2$	$T._3$	$T._4$		$T._k$		$\sum X$
$\overline{X}_i$	$\overline{X}_1$	$\overline{X}_2$	$\overline{X}_3$	$\overline{X}_4$		$\overline{X}_k$		$\overline{X}$

Based on this table, and similar with the completely randomized design, SS_{total} could be divided into $SS_{treatment}$, SS_{block}, and SS_{error}.

So, the SS_{total} here could be calculated:

$$SS_{total} = \sum_i \sum_j (X_{ij} - \overline{X})^2 = \sum X^2 - C$$
$$= S^2 \times (N-1) \tag{8.8}$$

and, $C = \dfrac{\left(\sum X\right)^2}{N}$

Sum of square between the blocks (SS_{block}) is

$$SS_{block} = \sum_j k(\overline{X}_i - \overline{X})^2$$
$$= \sum_j \frac{\left(\sum_i X_{ij}\right)^2}{k} - C \tag{8.9}$$

Sum of square between the treatments ($SS_{treatment}$) is

$$SS_{treatment} = \sum_i b(\overline{X}_j - \overline{X})^2$$
$$= \sum_i \frac{\left(\sum_j X_{ij}\right)^2}{b} - C \tag{8.10}$$

Therefore, the sum of square for error (SS_{error}) is

$$SS_{error} = SS_{total} - SS_{block} - SS_{treatment}$$

Example 8.2   A doctor wanted to compare the changes in blood glucose samples in pregnant women during four different times. The blood samples from 8 subjects were placed in room temperature for 0, 45, 90, and 135 minutes and then the blood glucose was tested.

In order to find out the influence of time on the concentration of blood glucose, the data were recorded as Table 8.7 shows.

Table 8.7　Blood Glucose in Different Times (mmol/L)

Block	Time/min 0	45	90	135	Total	Mean
1	5.24	5.27	4.94	4.61	20.06	5.02
2	5.24	5.22	4.88	4.66	20.00	5.00
3	5.88	5.83	5.38	5.00	22.09	5.52
4	5.44	5.38	5.27	5.00	21.09	5.27
5	5.66	5.44	5.38	4.88	21.36	5.34
6	6.22	6.22	5.61	5.22	23.27	5.82
7	5.83	5.72	5.38	4.88	21.81	5.45
8	5.27	5.11	5.00	4.44	19.82	4.96
Total	44.78	44.19	41.84	38.69	169.50	—
Mean	5.60	5.52	5.23	4.84	—	5.30
$\sum_j X_{ij}^2$	251.57	245.07	219.30	187.56	903.49	—

Now, we need to test whether there is a significant difference in blood glucose for these four different times. The procedures are as follow:

(a) Set up the null hypotheses and the alternative hypotheses.

H_0: $\mu_1 = \mu_2 = \mu_3 = \mu_4$, which means the time has no effect on the concentration of glucose in blood sample.

H_1: the mean of the concentration measured four times are not all the same.

(b) Choose a significant level $\alpha = 0.05$.

(c) Select the testing method and calculate test statistic.

First, we calculate the sum of square in total (SS_{total}),

$$C = \frac{(\sum X)^2}{N} = \frac{(169.5)^2}{32} = 897.8203$$

$$SS_{total} = \sum_i \sum_j (X_{ij} - \bar{X})^2 = \sum X^2 - C$$
$$= 903.4908 - 897.8203 = 5.6705$$

We also can use the following formula to calculate SS_{total}.

$$SS_{total} = S^2 \times (N-1)$$
$$= 0.42769^2 \times (32-1)$$
$$= 5.6705$$

Then, we calculate the sum of square between the blocks (SS_{block}),

$$SS_{block} = \sum_j k(\overline{X}_j - \overline{X})^2$$

$$= \sum_j \frac{(\sum_i X_{ij})^2}{k} - C$$

$$= \frac{20.06^2 + 20^2 + 22.09^2 + 21.09^2 + 21.36^2 + 23.27^2 + 21.81^1 + 19.82^2}{4} - 897.8203$$

$$= 900.3527 - 897.8203$$

$$= 2.5324$$

We can also use the following formula to calculate SS_{block}.

$$SS_{block} = \sum_j k(\overline{X}_j - \overline{X})^2$$

$$= 4 \times (5.02 - 5.03)^2 + 4 \times (5.00 - 5.30)^2 + 4 \times (5.52 - 5.30)^2 + \cdots\cdots +$$

$$4 \times (4.96 - 5.30)^2$$

$$= 2.5324$$

Next, we calculate the sum of square between the treatments ($SS_{treatment}$),

$$SS_{treatment} = \sum_i^i b(\overline{X}_j - \overline{X})^2$$

$$= \sum_i \frac{(\sum_j X_{ij})^2}{b} - C$$

$$= \frac{44.78^2 + 44.19^2 + 41.84^2 + 38.69^2}{8} - 897.8203$$

$$= 900.688275 - 897.8203$$

$$= 2.8680$$

Also, we can calculate by the following formula:

$$SS_{treatment} = b \sum_i (\overline{X}_i - \overline{X}_i)^2$$

$$= 8 \times (5.60 - 5.30)^2 + 8 \times (5.52 - 5.30)^2 + 8 \times (4.84 - 5.30)^2$$

$$= 2.8680$$

Therefore, the $SS_{error} = SS_{total} - SS_{block} - SS_{treatment} = 5.6705 - 2.5324 - 2.8680 = 0.2701$

The degrees of freedom is $N-1 = 32-1 = 31$ for total, $b-1 = 8-1 = 7$ for blocks, $k-1 = 4-1 = 3$ for treatments, and $(b-1)(k-1) = (8-1)(4-1) = 21$ for residual (error).

Mean square between blocks (MS_{block}) is

$$MS_{block} = \frac{SS_{block}}{b-1} = \frac{2.5324}{7} = 0.3618$$

Mean square between the treatments ($MS_{treatment}$) is

$$MS_{treatment} = \frac{SS_{treatment}}{k-1} = \frac{2.8680}{3} = 0.956$$

Mean square of error (MS_{error}) is

$$MS_{error} = \frac{SS_{error}}{(b-1)(k-1)} = \frac{0.2701}{21} = 0.0129$$

The value of F for blocks is

$$F_{block} = \frac{MS_{block}}{MS_{error}} = \frac{0.3618}{0.0129} = 28.0465$$

The value of F for treatments is

$$F_{treatment} = \frac{MS_{treatment}}{MS_{error}} = \frac{0.956}{0.0129} = 74.11$$

The results of the calculations for the randomized block design are displayed in Table 8.8.

Table 8.8   ANOVA Table for Randomized Block Design

Source of variation	SS	df	MS	F
Total	$SS_{total} = \sum_i \sum_j (X_{ij} - \bar{X})^2 = (N-1)S^2$	$N-1$		
Blocks	$SS_{block} = \sum_j k(\bar{X}_j - \bar{X})^2$	$b-1$	$\dfrac{SS_{block}}{b-1}$	$\dfrac{MS_{block}}{MS_{error}}$
Treatment	$SS_{treatment} = \sum_i b(\bar{X}_i - \bar{X})^2$	$k-1$	$\dfrac{SS_{treatment}}{k-1}$	$\dfrac{MS_{treatment}}{MS_{error}}$
Error	$SS_{error} = SS_{total} - SS_{block} - SS_{treatment}$	$(k-1)(b-1)$	$\dfrac{SS_{error}}{(k-1)(b-1)}$	

ANOVA table of Example 8.2 is shown in Table 8.9.

Table 8.9   ANOVA Table of Example 8.2

Source of variation	SS	df	MS	F
Total	5.6705	31		
Blocks	2.5324	7	0.3618	28.123
Treatment	2.8680	3	0.9560	74.317
Error	0.2701	21	0.0129	

(d) Determine the p-value.

For the treatment, according to the significant level $\alpha = 0.05$. By looking up the Appendix 4, $F_{0.05(3,21)} = 74.11$, $P < 0.05$.

(e) Make a conclusion.

According to the significant level $\alpha = 0.05$, we reject the null hypothesis H_0, and accept H_1. That is, not all treatment population means are equal, which means that the storing time in room temperature has an influence on the glucose concentration in the blood sample, and it is similar procedure to identify that the glucose concentrations are not equal among different blocks of mice ($P < 0.05$).

8.4   Repeated Measurement Design ANOVA

Repeated measures ANOVA is equivalent to the one-way ANOVA, but for related, not independent groups. We can analyze data by repeated-measures ANOVA in studies to investigate the changes in means over three or more time points. For example, researchers investigated the effect of a 3-month fitness program on weight and therefore wanted to measure the fitness level at 3 separate time points (before, in the middle of, and after the exercise intervention). The important aspect of these designs is that the same people are being measured more than once on the same dependent variable.

In repeated measures ANOVA, the independent variable has categories called **levels** or **related groups**. Where measurements are repeated over time, such as when measuring changes in fitness level due to a fitness program, the independent variable is **time**. Each **level** (or **related group**) is a specific time point. Hence, in this example, there would be three time points and each time point is a level of the independent variable.

Hypothesis for repeated measures ANOVA: The repeated measures ANOVA tests for whether there are any differences between related population means. The null hypothesis H_0 states that fitness level is the same at all time points (before, after 1. 5 months, and after 3 months):

$$H_0 : \mu_1 = \mu_2 = \mu_3 = \cdots = \mu_k$$

where μ is population mean and k is the number of related groups. The alternative hypothesis H_1 states that the related population means are not equal (at least one mean is different to another mean):

H_1: at least two means are significantly different.

The theory of repeated measures ANOVA is that: between-subject ANOVA partitions total variability into between groups variability (SS_{block}) and within groups variability (SS_{within}).

$$SS_{total} = SS_{block} + SS_{within}$$

Here within groups variability (SS_{within}) is defined as the error variability (SS_{error}). Following division by the appropriate degrees of freedom, a mean squares between groups (MS_{block}) and within groups (MS_{within}) are determined and an F-statistic is calculated as the ratio of MS_{block} to MS_{within} (or MS_{error}). Therefore, a repeated measures ANOVA calculates an F-statistic in a similar way.

Example 8. 3　There were 6 different subjects received a test about their fitness level before, in the middle of, and after a fitness intervention continued for 3 months, the detailed data can be found in Table 8. 10.

Table 8. 10　Three Time Repeated Measurements of 6 Participants of Fitness Level

Participants/subjects	Before	In the middle of	After 3 months	Subject means
1	45	50	55	50
2	42	42	45	43
3	36	41	43	40
4	39	35	40	38

				Continued
Participants/subjects	Before	In the middle of	After 3 months	Subject means
5	51	55	59	55
6	44	49	56	49. 5
Mean	42. 8	45. 3	49. 7	45. 9

In this case, there are six subjects who had their fitness level measured on three occasions: before, in the middle of, and after 3 months.

In order to calculate an F-statistic we need to calculate SS_{total} and SS_{error}.

The calculation of SS_{time} is the same as for $SS_{between}$ in an independent ANOVA, and can be expressed as

$$SS_{time}=6[(42.8-45.9)^2+(45.3-45.9)^2+(49.7-45.9)^2]=146.46$$

Notice that because we have a repeated measures design, n_i is the number of subjects in this example. Therefore, we can simply multiply each group by this number.

Calculating SS_{within}: within groups variation is also calculated in the same way as in an independent ANOVA. In our case

$$SS_{within}=715.5$$

Calculating $SS_{subjects}$: we treat each subject as its own block. In other words, we treat each subject as a level of an independent factor called subjects. We can then calculate $SS_{subjects}=658.3$.

Calculating SS_{error}:

As

$$SS_{within}=SS_{subjects}+SS_{error}$$

Then,

$$SS_{error}=SS_{within}-SS_{subjects}=715.5-658.3=57.2$$

Now, determining MS_{time}, MS_{error}, and the F-statistic: to determine the mean squares for time (MS_{time}) we divide SS_{time} by its associated degrees of freedom ($k-1$), where k is the number of time points. In our case

$$MS_{time}=\frac{SS_{time}}{k-1}=\frac{143.44}{2}=71.72$$

We do the same for the mean sum of squares for error (MS_{error}), this time dividing by $(n-1)(k-1)$ degrees of freedom, where n is the number of subjects and k is the number of time points. In our case

$$MS_{error}=\frac{SS_{error}}{(n-1)(k-1)}=5.72$$

Therefore, we can calculate the F-statistic as

$$F=\frac{MS_{time}}{MS_{error}}=12.54$$

We can now look up to ascertain the critical F-statistic for our F-distribution with our degrees of freedom for time (v_{time}) and error (v_{error}) and determine whether our F-statistic indicates a statistically significant result.

We report the F-statistic from a repeated measures ANOVA as

$$F_{(v_{time}, v_{error})} = F\text{-value}, \ p = p\text{-value}$$

which for our example would be

$$F_{(2,10)} = 12.53, \ p = 0.002$$

This means we can reject the null hypothesis and accept the alternative hypothesis. As we will discuss later, there are assumptions and effect sizes we can calculate that can alter how we report the above result. We would report the above findings as there was a statistically significant effect of time on exercise-induced fitness, $F_{(2,10)} = 12.53$, $p = 0.002$.

Tabular Presentation of a Repeated Measures ANOVA: Normally, the result of a repeated measures ANOVA is presented in the written text, as above, and not in a tabular form when writing a report. However, most statistical programs, such as SPSS, will report the result of a repeated measures ANOVA in tabular form. Doing so allows the user to gain a fuller understanding of all the calculations that were made by the program. The table below represents the type of table that you will be presented with and what the different sections mean. The tabular Presentation of a Repeated Measures ANOVA can be found in Table 8.11.

Table 8.11   Tabular Presentation of a Repeated Measures ANOVA

Source of variation	SS	df	MS	F
Conditions	$SS_{conditions}$	$k-1$	$MS_{conditions}$	$\dfrac{MS_{conditions}}{MS_{error}}$
Subjects	$SS_{subjects}$	$n-1$	$MS_{subjects}$	$\dfrac{MS_{subjects}}{MS_{error}}$
Error	SS_{error}	$(k-1)(n-1)$	MS_{error}	
Total	SS_{total}	$N-1$		

The F-statistic found in the first row (time/conditions row) is the F-statistic that will determine whether there was a significant difference between at least two means or not.

8.5   Analysis of Covariance

ANCOVA is a type of ANOVA and regression. By applying the ANCOVA, it can tell additional information by considering one independent variable (factor) at a time, without the influence of the others.

ANCOVA is often used when there are differences between the baseline groups. For example, if the experimenter wants to find out if a new drug has an effect on controlling blood pressure. The study has three treatment groups and one control group. A regular ANOVA can tell you if the treatment works. ANCOVA can control for other factors that might influence the outcome. For example, if we want to investigate whether a new drug works for depression, however, some baseline factors, including family life, job status, or other drug use are confounding variables but not the main focus of the study. In this case, an ANCOVA could be performed to control the effect of the covariate measures from the relationship between the new drug and the dependent variable.

ANCOVA can be used in two ways to control for covariates (typically continuous or variables on a particular scale); and to study combinations of categorical and continuous or variables on a scale as predictors. In this case, the covariate is usually a variable of interest. ANCOVA can explain within-group variance. It takes the unexplained variances from the ANOVA test to explain them with confounding variables (or other covariates).

Requirements for ANCOVA are basically the same as the ANOVA assumptions. It includes that the data involved should be independent variables (minimum of two) and should be categorical variables. The dependent variable and covariate should be continuous variables (measured on an interval scale or ratio scale). Moreover, the observations are independent. The covariate and dependent variable (at each level of independent variable) should be linearly related. The normality and homogeneity of variance could be checked by the methods introduced before.

8.6   Factorial ANOVA

A **factorial ANOVA** compares means across two or more independent variables that split the sample into four or more groups. A factor is another word for an independent variable. Within a factor, there are several levels or groupings. For example, gender is a single factor that has 2 levels (male, female), a study of experimental therapy vs. placebo can be thought of as having a treatment factor with 2 levels. Or a study with two different treatments has the possibility of a two-way design, varying the levels of treatments A and B.

The simplest factorial design is the 2×2 factorial with two factors each being applied in two levels.

For example, we want to investigate the effect of a new drug which developed to control cholesterol. We want to know the effect of quantity of the drug taken and the effect of gender. Therefore, we could say the quantity of the drug is the first factor and gender is the second factor. Suppose that we consider two quantities, with 200 mg and 300 mg of the drug. These two quantities are the two levels of the first factor. Similarly, the two levels of the second factor are male and female. Thus, we have two factors each being applied at two levels. It is exactly a 2×2 factorial design. So, here, we could summarize that we have 4 different treatment groups, one for each combination of levels of factors.

Group 1: 200 mg of the drug applied on male patients.

Group 2: 300 mg of the drug applied on male patients.

Group 3: 200 mg of the drug applied on female patients.

Group 4: 300 mg of the drug applied on female patients.

The results of the factorial ANOVA will be presented in the form of main effects and the interactions among study variables. According to the theory of ANOVA, in a factorial ANOVA design, the SS_{total} could be divided into $SS_A + SS_B + SS_{AB} + SS_{error}$:

$$SS_{total} = SS_A + SS_B + SS_{AB} + SS_{error}$$

And, the corresponding df is:

$$\upsilon_{total} = \upsilon_A + \upsilon_B + \upsilon_{AB} + \upsilon_{error}$$

If the variable A has I levels and variable B has J levels, r represents the repeated observed cases. χ_{ij} represents the mean of the A_i and B_j combination (A_iB_j). The results of the calculations for the factorial ANOVA design was displayed in Table 8.12.

Table 8.12　ANOVA Table for the Factorial ANOVA Design

Source of variation	SS	df	MS	F
Total	$SS_t = \sum\limits_{i=1}^{I}\sum\limits_{j=1}^{J}\sum\limits_{k=1}^{r}(X_{ijk} - \bar{X})^2$	$\upsilon_t = I \times J \times r - 1$		
Factor A	$SS_A = \sum\limits_{i=1}^{I} I \times r(\bar{X}_i - \bar{X})^2$	$\upsilon_A = I - 1$	$MS_A = \dfrac{SS_A}{\upsilon_A}$	$F_A = \dfrac{MS_A}{MS_e}$
Factor B	$SS_B = \sum\limits_{j=1}^{J} I \times r(\bar{X}_j - \bar{X})^2$	$\upsilon_B = J - 1$	$MS_B = \dfrac{SS_B}{\upsilon_B}$	$F_B = \dfrac{MS_{AB}}{MS_e}$
Factor AB	$SS_{AB} = \sum\limits_{i=1}^{I}\sum\limits_{j=1}^{J} r(\bar{X}_{ij} - \bar{X})^2 - SS_A - SS_B$	$\upsilon_{AB} = (I-1) \times (J-1)$	$MS_{AB} = \dfrac{SS_{AB}}{\upsilon_{AB}}$	$F_{AB} = \dfrac{MS_{AB}}{MS_e}$
Error	$SS_e = SS_t - SS_A - SS_B - SS_{AB}$	$\upsilon_e = \upsilon_t - \upsilon_A - \upsilon_B - \upsilon_{AB}$	$MS_e = \dfrac{SS_e}{\upsilon_e}$	

In the example illustrated above, there are three hypotheses to be tested. These are:

H_{01}: main effect "quantity" is not significant.

H_{02}: main effect "gender" is not significant.

H_{03}: interaction effect is not present.

For the main effect gender, the null hypothesis means that there is no significant difference in reduction of cholesterol in males and females. The null hypothesis for the main effect quantity means that there is no significant difference in the reduction of cholesterol whether the patients are given 200 mg or 300 mg of the drug. For the interaction effect, the null hypothesis means that the two main effects of gender and quantity are independent.

(Li Yuping, Lu Guangyu, Liao Qi)

Question Bank

Chapter 9   Chi-Square Test

In Chapters 7 and 8, the methods of hypothesis test for numerical data (t-tests and ANOVA) were presented. In this chapter, we will introduce the methods of hypothesis test for categorical data. χ^2 test, pronounced as *chi-square* test, is a popular hypothesis test that can be used to compare two or more rates (proportions). It can also be used to test for the correlation between categorized variables and goodness-of-fit test for frequency distribution. In addition, Fisher' exact test will be introduced under the case when the data are not satisfied with the conditions of χ^2 test.

9.1   Basic Idea of Chi-Square Test

First, we use the following example to illustrate the base idea and procedure of χ^2 test for completely randomized design 2×2 table.

Example 9.1   Bortezomib plus dexamethasone(BD) and bortezomib, epirubicin plus dexamethasone (PAD) are two chemotherapy regimens for multiple myeloma. The effects of the treatment are shown in Table 9.1. Are the effects of the two chemotherapy regimens different?

Table 9.1   The Effects of Treatment for Multiple Myeloma by BD and PAD Chemotherapy Regimens

Treatment	Effective	Ineffective	Total	Effective rate/%
BD	23 (27.3)	15 (10.7)	38	60.5
PAD	33 (28.7)	7 (11.3)	40	82.5
Total	56	22	78	71.8

The table in the form of Table 9.1 is called 2×2 table or four-fold table as the four cells contain basic values of all the information in the entire table.

23	15
33	7

In Example 9.1, we need to compare two rates. First, we hypothesize that the effective rates of the two chemotherapy regimens are the same and both equal to $\frac{56}{78} \times 100\% = 71.8\%$. According to the effective rate, the theoretical number of effective observations for BD regimen is $38 \times 71.8\% = 27.3$, and that for PAD regimen is $40 \times 71.8\% = 28.7$. Similarly, the ineffective rates of BD and PAD regimens are $\frac{22}{78} \times 100\% = 28.2\%$, and the theoretical

frequency of ineffective cases for BD and PAD regimens are $38 \times 28.2\% = 10.7$ and $40 \times 28.2 = 11.3$ respectively. In practice, the theoretical frequency can be calculated by Formula (9.1).

$$T_{RC} = \frac{n_R n_C}{n} \tag{9.1}$$

in which T_{RC} is the theoretical frequency of the cell in the Rth row and Cth column, n_R is the total number of observations in the Rth row, n_C is the total number of observations in the Cth column, and n is the total number of individuals.

As shown in Table 9.1, the theoretical frequency in the 1st row and 1st column is

$$T_{11} = \frac{38 \times 56}{78} = 27.3$$

Similarly, other theoretical frequencies can be calculated as

$$T_{12} = \frac{38 \times 22}{78} = 10.7 \text{ , } T_{21} = \frac{40 \times 56}{78} = 28.7 \text{ , } T_{22} = \frac{40 \times 22}{78} = 11.3$$

In 2×2 table, the sum of theoretical frequencies in all rows and all columns are equal to the total number of individuals. Therefore, if any of four theoretical frequencies is obtained by Formula (9.1), the others can be calculated by simple subtractions. For example, if it has already calculated that $T_{11} = 27.3$, then $T_{12} = 38 - 27.3 = 10.7$, $T_{21} = 56 - 27.3 = 28.7$, $T_{22} = 40 - 28.7 = 11.3$.

The basic idea of χ^2 test can be explained through the following formula of χ^2 test:

$$\chi^2 = \sum \frac{(A - T)^2}{T} \tag{9.2}$$

A is actual frequency, and T is theoretical frequency, which is calculated on the basis of the null hypothesis H_0. As shown in Formula (9.2), the value of χ^2 reflects the overall difference between the actual frequency and theoretical frequency. If the null hypothesis H_0 is true, the difference between the two sample rates is caused only by the sampling error. Therefore, the value of χ^2 should be close to 0. In the contrary, if the null hypothesis H_0 is wrong, the difference between the two sample rates is caused not only by sampling error, but also the true difference between the two populations. In this case, the value of χ^2 should be large. If the value of χ^2 is too large to be explained only by sampling error, say, greater than the critical value, we may reject H_0 and accept that there is a significant difference between the two rates.

χ^2 distribution is one of the most widely used continuous probability distributions with the only parameter degrees of freedom (v). The degrees of freedom determine the shape of the χ^2 distribution curve. Unlike the normal distribution, the χ^2 distribution is not symmetric. When $v = 1$, the distribution curve looks like an "L." As the degrees of freedom increase, the χ^2 curve approaches a normal distribution. Figure 9.1 shows the curves of the χ^2 distribution with different degrees of freedom (1, 4, 6, 9). When degrees of freedom are given (such as $v=1$), the distribution curve will be fixed. Appendix 5 gives critical values for the χ^2 distribution. The critical value is determined by α and v, denoted as $\chi^2_{\alpha,v}$. For instance, for $v=1$, the 5% critical value is $\chi^2_{0.05,1}=3.84$ (Figure 9.2).

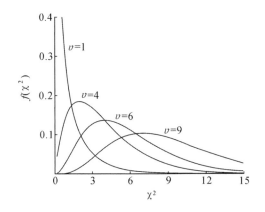

Figure 9.1　The χ^2 Distribution

($v=1$, 4, 6, 9)

Figure 9.2　The χ^2 Distribution ($v=1$)

and Its Critical Value

The critical value should be determined by checking the χ^2 distributions with corresponding degrees of freedom in Appendix 5. The degrees of freedom of χ^2 distribution is

$$N=(R-1)(C-1) \tag{9.3}$$

in which R and C are the number of rows and columns of the table, respectively. As 2×2 table is composed of 2 rows and 2 columns, in Example 9.1, $v=(2-1)(2-1)=1$. If $\chi^2\geqslant\chi^2_{\alpha,v}$, then $P\leqslant\alpha$, we should reject H_0 and accept H_1, the difference is significant statistically. Otherwise, $P>\alpha$, we should not reject H_0 and the difference is not statistically significant.

9.2　Category

χ^2 tests have several common table forms including a completely randomized design 2×2 table, paired design 2×2 table, and $R\times C$ table. To compare effective rates of two different treatments (Examples 9.1 and 9.2), a completely randomized design could be adopted. In the design, each individual is in one of binary statuses: effective or ineffective. Thus, a completely randomized design 2×2 table could be used to count the effective and ineffective individuals in treatment groups. However, if a paired design is constructed to explore whether the results of the two tests are the same (Example 9.3), paired design 2×2 table is generated. If multiple rates (Example 9.4: 3×2 table) or two (or more) proportions (Example 9.5: 2×3 table) are compared, $R\times C$ table is used where the variable in the rows has R categories and the variable in the columns has C categories.

9.2.1　Completely Randomized Design 2×2 Table

9.2.1.1　Routine Formula

Formula (9.2) is the routine formula for a completely randomized design 2×2 table. Use Example 9.1 as an example:

(a) Set up the null hypotheses and the alternative hypotheses.

H_0: $\pi_1 = \pi_2$, the effective rates of two chemotherapy regimens are equal.

H_1: $\pi_1 \neq \pi_2$, the effective rates of two chemotherapy regimens are not equal.

(b) Choose a significant level $\alpha = 0.05$.

(c) Calculate the value of χ^2.

According to Formula (9.1), $T_{11} = \dfrac{38 \times 56}{78} = 27.3$, then $T_{12} = 10.7$, $T_{21} = 28.7$, $T_{22} = 11.3$.

According to Formula (9.2),

$$\chi^2 = \sum \frac{(A-T)^2}{T} = \frac{(23-27.3)^2}{27.3} + \frac{(15-10.7)^2}{10.7} + \frac{(33-28.7)^2}{28.7} + \frac{(7-11.3)^2}{11.3} = 4.685$$

(d) Determine p-value.

The degrees of freedom are $v = (2-1)(2-1) = 1$. By checking the table of χ^2 critical value for $v=1$ (Appendix 5), we can find $\chi^2_{0.05,1} = 3.84$. In this example, $\chi^2 = 4.647 > 3.84$, therefore, $P < 0.05$.

(e) Make a conclusion.

At the significant level $\alpha = 0.05$, we should reject H_0 and accept H_1, for the difference is statistically significant. Then we can think the two chemotherapy regimens have different effective rates for multiple myeloma and PAD regimen is better than BD regimen.

9.2.1.2　Specific Formula

If the frequencies in a 2×2 table are denoted by a, b, c, and d, respectively,

a	b
c	d

then the specific formula calculating χ^2 is:

$$\chi^2 = \frac{(ad-bc)^2 n}{(a+b)(c+d)(a+c)(b+d)} \tag{9.4}$$

Formula (9.4) avoids the complex steps of calculation of theoretical frequency, for example, in Example 9.1:

$$\chi^2 = \frac{(23 \times 7 - 15 \times 33)^2 \times 78}{38 \times 40 \times 56 \times 22} = 4.647$$

The result calculated by Formula (9.4) is the same as that by Formula (9.2).

9.2.1.3　Corrected Formula

χ^2 distribution is a continuous distribution, while the values of categorical variables are discrete. When the sample size is large and the theoretical frequencies in all cells are larger than 5, the approximation is well. But if the sample size is small or at least one theoretical frequency is less than 5, the approximation is bad and the χ^2 calculated by Formula (9.2) will be too large. In this case, we should perform correction for continuity for χ^2. The corrected formulae of routine formule and specific formula for χ^2 test are:

$$\chi^2 = \sum \frac{(\mid A - T \mid - 0.5)^2}{T} \tag{9.5}$$

$$\chi^2 = \frac{\left(\mid ad - bc \mid - \dfrac{n}{2}\right)^2 n}{(a+b)(c+d)(a+c)(b+d)} \tag{9.6}$$

Correction for continuity is used for 2×2 table in usual.

(a) When $n \geqslant 40$ and $T \geqslant 5$ in all cells, there is no need for the correction.

(b) When $n \geqslant 40$ and at least one theoretical frequency satisfies $1 \leqslant T < 5$, use the corrected Formula (9.5) or Formula (9.6) or use Fisher's exact test.

(c) When $n < 40$ or at least one theoretical frequency satisfies $T < 1$, Fisher's exact test should be used.

Example 9.2　Patients treated by PAD chemotherapy regimen from Example 9.1 can be divided into two groups: $\leqslant 4$ chemotherapy regimen cycles and > 4 chemotherapy regimen cycles. Are the effects of the PAD regimen different between two-cycle groups?

Table 9.2　The Effects of Treatment by PAD Regimen for Two-Cycle Groups

Cycles	Effective	Ineffective	Total	Effective rate/%
$\leqslant 4$	14 (16.5)	6 (3.5)	20	70.0
> 4	19 (16.5)	1 (3.5)	20	95.0
Total	33	7	40	82.5

(a) Set up the null hypotheses and the alternative hypothesis.

$H_0: \pi_1 = \pi_2$, i.e. the effective rates of the two cycle groups are equal.

$H_1: \pi_1 \neq \pi_2$, i.e. the effective rates of the two cycle groups are not equal.

(b) Choose significant level $\alpha = 0.05$.

(c) Calculate the value of χ^2.

According to Formula (9.1), $T_{12} = \dfrac{20 \times 7}{40} = 3.5 < 5$, $T_{22} = \dfrac{20 \times 7}{40} = 3.5 < 5$, $n = 40$, therefore, we should use Formula (9.6):

$$\chi^2 = \frac{\left(\mid 14 \times 1 - 6 \times 19 \mid - \dfrac{40}{2}\right)^2 \times 40}{(14+6)(19+1)(14+19)(6+1)} = 2.771$$

(d) Determine p-value.

The degrees of freedom are, $\upsilon = (2-1)(2-1) = 1$

By checking the table of χ^2 critical value for $\upsilon = 1$ (Appendix 5), we can find $\chi^2_{0.05,1} = 3.84$. In the example, $\chi^2 = 2.771 < 3.84$, therefore, $P > 0.05$.

(e) Make a conclusion.

At the significant level $\alpha = 0.05$, we should not reject H_0, the difference is not statistically significant. Thus we cannot conclude that the effective rates of two-cycle groups are not equal.

If we use the uncorrected formula of χ^2 test, the value of statistic χ^2 is 4.329, we may make a contrary conclusion wrongly.

9.2.2 Paired Design 2×2 Table

Paired design 2×2 table is the table form of paired-samples design for binary data. In the table, the tested hypothesis is usually whether the results of the two tests are the same.

Example 9.3 A hundred systemic lupus erythematosus (SLE) serum samples were examined by chemiluminescent immunoassay (CLIA) and line immnuoassay (LIA) to test the autoantibodies to ribonucleoprotein (RNP). The examination records are listed in Table 9.3. Please evaluate whether two assays have equal positive rates.

Table 9.3 The Autoantibodies to RNP Results Examined by CLIA and LIA

No.	CLIA	LIA
1	+	−
2	+	+
3	−	−
4	−	+
...	...	...
100	+	+

The original records can be re-arranged to the form of Table 9.4.

Table 9.4 The Comparison of the Testing Results by Two Assays

CLIA	LIA +	LIA −	Total
+	28(a)	2(b)	30
−	4(c)	66(d)	70
Total	32	68	100

Table 9.4 shows four types of testing results combined by two tests: CLIA (+) & LIA (+), CLIA (−) & LIA (−), CLIA (+) & LIA (−), CLIA (−) & LIA (+). The number of cases for these four types are a, d, b, and c, respectively. The previous two types are concordant results (both positive a and both negative d) while the latter two types are discordant results (one positive and the other negative). The positive testing rates of CLIA and LIA are $\frac{a+b}{a+b+c+d}$ and $\frac{a+c}{a+b+c+d}$, respectively. To compare the two positive

testing rates, we only need to compare b and c. If the testing results of two tests are equal, B and C in the population should be equal (B and C are the corresponding values of b and c in the population). Since there is a sampling error between population and sample, b may not be equal to c. Thus, χ^2 test for paired-samples data or so-called McNemar's test (Formula (9.7) or Formula (9.8)) should be performed to test the hypothesis whether the difference between b and c is caused by the sampling error.

$$\chi^2 = \frac{(b-c)^2}{b+c} \tag{9.7}$$

$$\upsilon = 1$$

The condition of Formula (9.7) is $b+c \geqslant 40$.

If $b+c < 40$, the continuity correction Formula (9.8) should be used.

$$\chi^2 = \frac{(\mid b-c \mid -1)^2}{b+c} \tag{9.8}$$

$$\upsilon = 1$$

The steps of McNemar's test are as below.

(a) Set up the null hypotheses and the alternative hypothesis.

H_0: the positive testing rates of two tests are equal.

H_1: the positive testing rates of two tests are not equal.

(b) Choose a significant level $\alpha = 0.05$.

(c) Calculate the value of χ^2.

In example $b=2$, $c=4$, $b+c=6 < 40$, Formula (9.8) is followed.

$$\chi^2 = \frac{(\mid b-c \mid -1)^2}{b+c} = \frac{(\mid 2-4 \mid -1)^2}{2+4} = 0.167$$

(d) Determine the p-value.

$$\chi^2 = 0.167 < 3.84, \ P > 0.05.$$

(e) Make a conclusion.

At the significant level $\alpha = 0.05$, we should not reject H_0, the difference is not statistically significant. We cannot conclude that the positive testing rates of the two assays are not equal.

9.2.3   R × C Table

R × C table or contingency table refers to the table with more than two rows or columns. χ^2 test for contingency table is used to compare multiple (two or more) rates or proportions.

The theory of χ^2 test for $R \times C$ table is the same as that of 2×2 table and the formula of χ^2 test for contingency table can follow Formula (9.2). To simplify the calculation process, Formula (9.9) can also be used and the results of these two formulae are equal.

$$\chi^2 = n\left(\sum \frac{A^2}{n_R n_C} - 1 \right) \tag{9.9}$$

$$\upsilon = (R-1)(C-1)$$

In the formula, n is the sample size or total number; A indicates the actual frequency of the cell in the Rth row and Cth column; n_R refers to the overall frequencies of the Rth row; and n_C is the overall frequencies of the Cth column.

9.2.3.1 χ^2 Test for the Comparison of Multiple Rates

Example 9.4   Ninety-five acute pancreatitis patients were divided into three groups: mild acute pancreatitis (MAP), moderately severe acute pancreatitis (MSAP), and severe acute pancreatitis (SAP). Table 9.5 lists the incidence rates of pleural effusion for these three acute pancreatitis groups. Please evaluate whether the incidence rates of the three groups are equal.

Table 9.5   Comparison of Incidence Rates of Pleural Effusion among Acute Pancreatitis Groups

Groups	Pleural effusion		Total	Incidence rate/%
	Yes	No		
MAP	6	45	51	11.8
MSAP	6	18	24	25.0
SAP	10	10	20	50.0
Total	22	73	95	23.2

The steps for χ^2 test:

(a) Set up the null hypothesis and alternative hypothesis.

H_0: $\pi_1 = \pi_2 = \pi_3$, the incidence rates of pleural effusion for the three groups are equal.

H_1: at least two of π_1, π_2, π_3 are not equal.

(b) Choose a significant level $\alpha = 0.05$.

(c) Calculate the value of χ^2.

Use Formula (9.9):

$$\chi^2 = n\left(\sum \frac{A^2}{n_R n_C} - 1\right)$$

$$= 95 \times \left(\frac{6^2}{51 \times 22} + \frac{45^2}{51 \times 73} + \frac{6^2}{24 \times 22} + \frac{18^2}{24 \times 73} + \frac{10^2}{20 \times 22} + \frac{10^2}{20 \times 73} - 1\right) = 11.864$$

(d) Determine the p-value.

$\upsilon = (3-1)(2-1) = 2$

From the table of χ^2 critical value with $\upsilon = 2$ (Appendix 5), $\chi^2_{0.05,2} = 5.99$, $\chi^2 = 11.864 > 5.99$, $P < 0.05$.

(e) Make a conclusion.

At the significant level $\alpha = 0.05$, H_0 should be rejected. At least two of the three groups have different incidence rates.

9.2.3.2 χ^2 Test for the Comparison of Two or More Proportions

Example 9.5   A hundred and sixty five esophageal squamous cell carcinoma (ESCC) patients were divided into two groups (early group and late group) according to the biochemical indices. Table 9. 6 lists the proportions of the positions of carcinomas in the esophagus for two ESCC groups. Please evaluate whether the proportions of the two groups are equal.

Table 9. 6   The Positions of Carcinomas in the Esophagus of ESCC Patients

Groups	Upper	Middle	Lower	Total
Early	20	34	7	61
Late	30	63	11	104
Total	50	97	18	165

The steps for χ^2 test:

(a) Set up the null hypothesis and alternative hypothesis.

H_0: the proportions of the positions of carcinomas are equal between the early group and the latter group.

H_1: the proportions of the positions of carcinomas are not equal between the early group and the latter group.

(b) Choose a significant level $\alpha = 0.05$.

(c) Calculate the value of χ^2.

Use Formula (9. 9):

$$\chi^2 = n\left(\sum \frac{A^2}{n_R n_C} - 1\right)$$

$$= 165 \times \left(\frac{20^2}{61 \times 50} + \frac{34^2}{61 \times 97} + \frac{7^2}{61 \times 18} + \frac{30^2}{104 \times 50} + \frac{63^2}{104 \times 97} + \frac{11^2}{104 \times 18} - 1\right)$$

$$= 0.379$$

(d) Determine the p-value.

$$\upsilon = (2-1)(3-1) = 2$$

$\chi^2_{0.05,2} = 5.99$, $\chi^2 = 0.379 < 5.99$, $P > 0.05$.

(e) Make a conclusion.

At the significant level $\alpha = 0.05$, H_0 should not be rejected. We cannot conclude that the proportions of the positions of carcinomas are not equal between the early group and the latter group.

9.2.3.3   Notes for χ^2 Test for $R \times C$ Table

χ^2 test for $R \times C$ table should avoid the following cases: more than 20 percent of cells have a theoretical frequency of less than 5, or one (or more) theoretical frequency less than 1. If such cases are met, one may use the following solutions:

(a) Improve the sample size to increase theoretical frequencies.

(b) Merge the row (or column) that has a small theoretical frequency with the nearby row (or column).

(c) Delete the row (or column) that has a small theoretical frequency.

(d) Fisher's exact test.

For the χ^2 test involved more than 2 rates or proportions, the rejection of H_0 only indicates that at least two of rates or proportions are different in the population. Multiple testing procedures can be performed to test whether each pair of groups have different rates or proportions. One of the most popular multiple testing methods for χ^2 test is Bonferroni correction. As an example, for a $k \times 2$ table, we can split it into $\dfrac{k(k-1)}{2}$ 2×2 tables. Therefore, the Type I error will increase if we perform a χ^2 test for each 2×2 table. Significant level of the tests should be corrected as $\alpha' = \dfrac{\alpha}{\dfrac{k(k-1)}{2}} = \dfrac{2\alpha}{k(k-1)}$.

9.3 Fisher's Exact Test

9.3.1 Fisher's Exact Test for 2 × 2 Table

When $n < 40$ or at least one *theoretical frequency* satisfying $T < 1$, the chi-square test introduced above is likely to be biased, therefore we use the Fisher's exact test. The test is attributed to R. A. Fisher, who describes it in his design of experiments text (Fisher, 1935). The exact p-values from this test can be determined easily (by enumerating all the more extreme tables and their probabilities under the null hypothesis).

Firstly, we use the following example to illustrate the steps of Fisher's exact test for four-fold table data.

Example 9.6 This is a randomized, double-blind, placebo-controlled study in patients. In total, 17 patients received new drug and 14 placebo. After a course of treatment, the effects of treatment are assessed (Table 9.7). Question: Are the effects of treatment by the two treatments different?

Table 9.7 Comparison of Effective Rates by Two Treatments

Group	Effective	Ineffective	Total	Effective rate/%
New drug	2	15	17	11.76
Placebo	4	10	14	28.57
Total	6	25	31	19.35

(a) Make a null hypothesis and an alternative hypothesis.

H_0: $\pi_1 = \pi_2$, i.e. the effective rates of two different treatments are equal.

H_1: $\pi_1 \neq \pi_2$, i.e. the effective rates of two different treatments are not equal.

(b) Select a significant level $\alpha = 0.05$.

(c) Calculate the probability P.

Before we proceed with the Fisher's exact test, we first introduce some notations. We represent the cells by the letters a, b, c, and d, call the totals across rows and columns marginal totals, and represent the grand total by n. So the table now looks like this:

Table 9.8　Basic 2×2 Contingency Table for Fisher's Exact Test

	Column 1	Column 2	Total
Row 1	a	b	$a+b$
Row 2	c	d	$c+d$
Total	$a+c$	$b+d$	$a+b+c+d\ (=n)$

Let m be the cell value for column 1, row 1 in a 2×2 contingency table with the constraints that the row 1 total is $a+b$ and the column one total is $a+c$, with $a+b$ and $a+c$ less than or equal to the grand total n. The hypergeometric distribution used for calculating test statistic for Fisher's exact test is given in Formula (9.10). Then for $x=0, 1, \cdots$, min $((a+b),(a+c))$, $i=1, 2, 3,\cdots$,

$$P_i = P(m=x) = \frac{(a+b)!(a+c)!(b+d)!(b+c)!}{a!b!c!d!n!} \tag{9.10}$$

The calculation steps for Fisher's exact test are listed as follows:

(a) Under the condition of fixed row and column totals, we list all 2×2 tables (Table 9.9) with row 1, column 1 cell values equal to or smaller than 6 (min(17,6));

(b) Use Formula (9.10) to calculate the values of P for both these tables under the null hypothesis;

e.g. The probability of Table 9.7 (listed as ID$=3$ in Table 9.9) can be obtained by Formula (9.10);

$$P_3 = P(m=2) = \frac{6!14!17!25!}{2!4!15!10!31!} = 0.1849$$

(c) Find all p-values, which are equal to or smaller than 0.1849;

(d) Add them together.

This gives a two-tailed test, with P approximately

$P_1+P_2+P_3+P_6+P_7=0.0041+0.0462+0.1849+0.1177+0.0168=0.3697$

For an one-tailed test, both of the definition of p-value and an alternative hypothesis (H_1) are different. This includes two kinds of situations:

• When $H_1: \pi_1<\pi_2$, the p-value of a one-tailed test is,

$P_1+P_2+P_3=0.0041+0.0462+0.1849=0.2352$

• When $H_1: \pi_1>\pi_2$, the p-value is,

$P_3+P_6+P_7=0.1849+0.1177+0.0168=0.3194$

The purpose of this study is to test whether the effects of two treatments are different, so the p-value of a two-tailed test is selected for conclusion.

Table 9.9   2×2 Contingency Tables for Fisher's Exact Test

ID		Effective	Ineffective	P
1	New drug	0	17	0.0041
	Placebo	6	8	
2	New drug	1	16	0.0462
	Placebo	5	9	
3	New drug	2	15	0.1849
	Placebo	4	10	
4	New drug	3	14	0.3362
	Placebo	3	11	
5	New drug	4	13	0.2942
	Placebo	2	12	
6	New drug	5	12	0.1177
	Placebo	1	13	
7	New drug	6	11	0.0168
	Placebo	0	14	

(e) Make an inferring conclusion.

At the significant level $\alpha = 0.05$, we should not reject H_0, the difference is not significant statistically. That is to say the two treatments have no different effective rates.

9.3.2   Fisher's Exact Test for $R \times C$ Table

For hand calculations, the test is only feasible in the case of a 2×2 contingency table. However the principle of the test can be extended to the general case of an $R \times C$ contingency table, as proposed by Freeman & Halton, and some statistical packages provide a calculation (sometimes using a Monte Carlo method to obtain an approximation) for the more general case.

9.4   Goodness-of-Fit Test

The goodness-of-fit of a statistical model describes whether an observed frequency distribution differs from a theoretical distribution, such as Normal distribution, Binomial distribution, Poisson distribution, and so on. Pearson's chi-square test, as a common goodness-of-fit test method, can be used to test whether outcome frequencies follow a specified distribution.

Firstly, we use the following example to illustrate the basic idea and the steps of goodness-of-fit test.

Example 9.7   There is a random sample of 119 boys from somewhere, and their heights are listed below:

119.3	121.2	116.6	126.4	120.0	115.5	119.9	116.5	121.6	116.9	122.1
123.4	119.2	117.3	114.4	119.9	118.7	123.2	119.8	122.3	122.6	127.6
110.4	115.9	129.4	115.2	115.9	113.0	126.3	125.3	114.6	122.4	125.7
124.0	130.4	118.9	122.1	118.6	117.2	116.7	121.3	115.6	120.5	125.2
122.2	112.8	117.3	125.3	116.7	132.2	119.3	116.4	118.2	121.7	118.6
115.2	118.0	109.7	120.5	110.3	117.2	113.7	120.0	117.0	121.3	112.9
110.2	116.1	118.5	120.0	120.7	121.4	119.6	114.2	121.7	123.6	120.6
112.7	119.8	123.4	122.3	113.2	120.1	124.3	120.5	127.8	123.7	125.9
108.9	119.7	114.3	127.8	120.3	114.5	130.6	120.8	120.5	114.6	119.1
114.5	121.9									

Question: Do the heights of the 119 boys follow the normal distribution?

(a) Calculate the sample statistics.

First, the mean and standard deviation of this data set are estimated.

$$\bar{x} = 119.54 \quad s = 4.77$$

(b) Make a null hypothesis and an alternative hypothesis.

H_0: the population distribution is normal distribution $N(119.54, 4.77^2)$.

H_1: the population distribution is not normal distribution $N(119.54, 4.77^2)$.

(c) Select a significant level $\alpha = 0.05$.

(d) Calculate the statistic χ^2.

If the null hypothesis is true, the test statistic will be drawn from a chi-square distribution with $k-q-1$ degrees of freedom, where k is the number of non-empty cells and q is the number of parameters estimated from the data to compute the expected number T. The calculation steps of χ^2 for goodness-of-fit test are listed as follows:

• We divide the range of possible values for a random variable into connected disjoint intervals.

• For each interval, we count the number of observations from the observed data that fall in that interval.

• We compute an expected number (T) for the normal distribution $N(119.54, 4.77^2)$. Here T_i is obtained by:

$$P_i = pr(l_i \leqslant X < u_i) = pr(Z < \frac{u_i - u}{\sigma}) - pr(Z < \frac{l_i - u}{\sigma}) \quad i = 1, 2, \cdots, k$$

(9.11)

$$T_i = N \times P_i \quad i = 1, 2, \cdots, k$$

(9.12)

where $pr(Z)$ is the cumulative probability of the standard normal distribution, u_i is the upper limit for class i, l_i is the lower limit for class i, and N is the total sample size.

• As with the other chi-square tests described in this chapter, we compute the quantities $\frac{(A-T)^2}{T}$ for each interval i and sum them up over all the intervals $i = 1, 2, \cdots,$

9. The resulting computations for this case are given in Table 9. 10. According to Formula (9. 2), the value of the chi-square statistic is:

$$\chi^2 = \sum \frac{(A-T)^2}{T} = 3.17$$

Since $k = 9$ and $q = 2$, the degrees of freedom are $k-q-1=6$.

Table 9. 10　Chi-Square Test for Normal Distribution

Interval	Observed (A)	Expected (T)	$\frac{(A-T)^2}{T}$
107~	2	1. 87	0. 0090
110~	6	6. 31	0. 0152
113~	16	14. 53	0. 1487
116~	19	22. 82	0. 6395
119~	30	24. 45	1. 2598
122~	14	17. 86	0. 8342
125~	10	8. 90	0. 1360
128~	3	3. 02	0. 0001
131~	1	0. 70	0. 1286
Total	101	—	3. 17

(e) Make a conclusion.

From the chi-square table we see that the p-value is higher than 0. 05. So we cannot reject the null hypothesis of a normal distribution. The data seem to fit the normal distribution reasonably well.

(Dong Changzheng, Liu Liya, Wu Siying)

Question Bank

Chapter 10 Non-parametric Tests

In the former chapters, we have learned that when we want to compare whether there are significant difference(s) for some special variables in two or more populations, we usually select t-test, F-test (also may be called ANOVA), or χ^2 test (chi-square test). These most commonly used methods usually assume that we have already known the distribution type of the variables and they also must meet normal distribution (Figure 10.1) and independent in the population or populations from which we get our data. Unfortunately, the distribution types of the populations usually are unknown or may not be exactly normal distribution (Figure 10.2). So the results of these usual methods for inference about the population would not be quite robust to moderate lack of normality. Therefore, they are not the most suitable methods for inference and cannot be the first selection in that situation. What can we do if the data distribution is a non-normal distribution, especially when the sample size is quite small? Finally, statisticians push out non-parametric tests to overcome these problems.

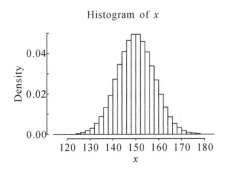

Figure 10.1   Normal Distribution

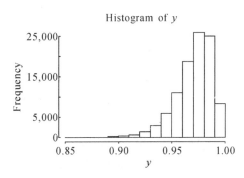

Figure 10.2   Non-normal Distribution

Non-parametric test is a branch of methods which concerned with non-parametric statistical models and non-parametric inference. In statistics, they are often referred to as distribution free methods as they do not rely on assumptions that the data are drawn from a given probability distribution. It means that the term of non-parametric statistics refers to statistics that do not assume the population has any characteristic structure or parameters. For example, non-parametric statistics are suitable for examining the order of runners completing a race, while parametric statistics would be more appropriate for looking at the actual race times (which may possess parameters such as a mean and standard deviation). In other words, the order (or "rank") of the values is used rather than the actual values themselves in non-parametric test.

Compared with most commonly used parametric tests including *t*-test, *F*-test, etc. , the major characteristics of non-parametric tests are as follows:

(a) Need not to consider the distribution type of data;

(b) Need not to conduct the statistical inference of population parameters;

(c) Need not to test whether the distribution types of populations are equal;

(d) Hypothesis test conducted with the rank of data, not with the data itself.

(e) Efficiency of a non-parametric test is often lower than a parametric test if the data are analyzed by them at the same time.

Non-parametric tests are mainly used for:

(a) Population with distribution not known;

(b) Data that do not meet the requirement of a normal distribution or/and homogeneity of variance;

(c) Ordinal data;

(d) Data with uncertain values at one or both ends (<0.1, >10, etc.).

In general, non-parametric tests consist of Wilcoxon signed-rank test, Wilcoxon Mann-Whitney *U*-test, Kruskal-Wallis *H*-test, Friedman test, Spearman rank correlation, non-parametric regression, etc. This chapter mainly focuses on the former three tests.

10. 1　Wilcoxon Signed-Rank Test

The **Wilcoxon signed-rank test** is a non-parametric test that is used for comparing two related samples, matched samples, or repeated measurements on a single sample to assess whether their population mean ranks differ (i. e. it is a paired design). It can be used as an alternative to the paired Student's *t*-test for matched pairs, or the *t*-test for dependent samples when the population cannot be assumed to be normally distributed.

It has been widely accepted that an appropriate example is the best way to learn a new method of inference. So let's take an example to learn the principles and procedures of the Wilcoxon signed-rank test.

Example 10. 1 An ophthalmologist wanted to assess the efficacy of a new operation on the visual acuity improvement. He randomly selected 12 of her inpatients and measured the visual acuity before and after the operation, respectively. Table 10. 1 shows the data of 12 subjects' visual acuity in the study.

Table 10. 1　Visual Acuity of 12 Subjects before and after Operation

Patients	1	2	3	4	5	6	7	8	9	10	11	12
Pre-operation	4. 3	4. 1	4. 5	4. 1	4. 5	4. 7	4. 0	4. 1	5. 2	4. 1	4. 1	4. 8
Post-operation	4. 1	4. 6	4. 5	4. 2	4. 5	4. 5	4. 4	4. 3	4. 7	4. 2	4. 1	4. 7

The first step of data analysis in this example is to decide which method for inference is

Chapter 10   Non-parametric Tests   • 133 •

more suitable to assess the efficacy of the operation. Because this is a matched pairs design and visual acuity is a continuous variable, we base our inference on the differences of visual acuity between pre- and post-operation for each subject. If the difference satisfies a normal distribution as Figure 10. 1, the most commonly used method for inference should be paired t-test. But in this example, the distribution of the 12 differences is not normal (Figure 10. 3). So we should not compare the efficacy with paired t-test but rank sum test. Firstly, we should organize the data as Table 10. 2.

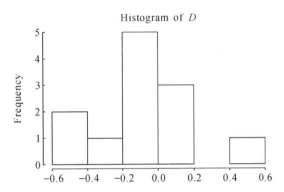

Figure 10. 3   Distribution of the Difference between Pre- and Post-operation for 12 Patients

Table 10. 2   Visual Acuity of 12 Participants between Pre- and Post-operation

Patient (1)	Pre-operation (2)	Post-operation (3)	Difference (4)=(2)−(3)	Rank (5)
1	4. 3	4. 1	0. 2	4
2	4. 1	4. 6	−0. 5	−8. 5
3	4. 5	4. 5	0	/
4	4. 1	4. 2	−0. 1	−2
5	4. 5	4. 5	0	/
6	4. 7	4. 5	0. 2	5
7	4. 0	4. 4	−0. 4	−7
8	4. 0	4. 3	−0. 3	−6
9	5. 2	4. 7	0. 5	8. 5
10	4. 1	4. 2	−0. 1	−2
11	4. 1	4. 1	0	/
12	4. 8	4. 7	0. 1	2

$T_+=19.5,\ T_-=25.5$

10.1.1　Typical Procedures of Wilcoxon Signed-Rank Test

(a) Set up the hypothesis.

H_0: $M_d = 0$, i. e. there is no difference between pre- and post-operation.

H_1: $M_d \neq 0$, i. e. there is a significant difference between pre-and post- operation.

(b) Choose a significant level $\alpha = 0.05$.

(c) Calculate the differences of the visual acuity between pre- and post-operation for each subject (see column 4).

(d) Rank the difference (see column 5):

• If the difference equals to 0, there is no need to rank it (patients 3, 5, and 11);

• Ascending rank each difference strictly according to the absolute value, not the difference itself;

• If the absolute value of several differences are equal, give the same average rank to each of them (patients 2 and 9; patients 4, 10, and 12) when the symbols are of difference, otherwise, ordinary rank or average rank will be fine;

• If the difference is less than 0, add a negative sign before the rank (patients 2, 4, 7, 8, and 10). If the difference is larger than 0, you may or may not add a positive sign before the rank as you want.

(e) Calculate the rank sum for positive difference and negative difference, respectively.

(f) Decide the test statistic:

• When it is a two-sided test, we can select the smaller absolute value of the two rank sums as the statistic. When it is a right-tailed or left-tailed test, we can select a positive or negative rank sum as the statistic (T_+ or T_-).

• In this example, it is a two-sided test, so we should select the smaller absolute rank sum ($T_+ = 19.5$) as the statistic.

(g) Review the T-critical value table for Wilcoxon signed-rank test and make a decision.

• In the T-critical value table for Wilcoxon signed-rank test, the upper and lower critical values are listed for two-sided test with the level of $\alpha = 0.05$. If either T-value $\leqslant$ the lower critical value or T-value $\geqslant$ the upper critical value at the level of 0.05, the result is statistically significant. Otherwise, the result is not statistically significant.

• In this example, it is a two-sided test and the critical T-value interval is (5, 40). Because 19.5 is between 5 and 40, which means the statistic is in the interval, we should say $P > 0.05$ and have no reason to reject the H_0. So, the final decision of this example will be that we cannot find the necessity of the operation for these patients based on the sample.

10.1.2　The Principle of the Wilcoxon Signed-Rank Test

In this example, if there is no significant difference between pre- and post-operation (H_0 is true), the location of the distribution of the visual acuity for pre- and post-operation will be equal. So, the differences of visual acuity must meet a symmetry distribution (Median of the difference is equal to 0).

When we rank the differences according to the absolute value and give a negative sign (if the difference <0) or positive sign (if the difference >0), the absolute value of the theoretical positive rank sum may be equal to that of negative rank sum.

In almost all studies, we usually assumed that our samples are taken from the populations randomly. Even if $\sum d \neq 0$, it might be only caused by randomized error and not to be too large. However, if $\sum d$ is large enough to exceed the limitation, the probability of this happening is very low, in other words, we have no reason to believe that were fully explained by randomized error anymore and have to reject the null hypothesis (H_0) and receive the conclusion that the operation is necessary for these 12 patients.

10. 2　Wilcoxon-Mann-Whitney Test

In statistics, the **Wilcoxon-Mann-Whitney test** (also called the Mann-Whitney-Wilcoxon (MWW), Wilcoxon rank-sum test, or Wilcoxon-Mann-Whitney U-test) is another kind of non-parametric test. The null hypothesis is that the locations of the two populations are the same as an alternative hypothesis. It has greater efficiency than the t-test on non-normal distributions. MWW is suitable for cases where the distributions of two independent samples do not distribute as a normal distribution.

10.2.1　Two Independent Measurement Data

Example 10. 2　A researcher wanted to know whether the protein level in the food will affect the weight. He randomly selected 19 rats from the university animal center and randomly assigned them into two groups. One group was given high-protein food and the other was fed with low-protein food. The weight of each rat at baseline and 3 months later was measured respectively. The additive weight of rats is shown in Table 10. 3.

Table 10. 3　Additive Weight of Rats after Supplemented with Low- or High-Protein Food

Rats	1	2	3	4	5	6	7	8	9	10	11	12
Low-protein food	6	118	93	85	107	119	94	—	—	—	—	—
High-protein food	134	146	104	120	124	161	107	8	113	129	97	123

The objective of this example is to infer whether there is a significant difference for the additive weights of the rats after supplementation with low- and high-protein food. Because this is a completely randomized design and the additive weights of two groups are continuous variables. If the additive weight meets normal distribution and has equal variances, two independent samples t-test may be the best choice to infer the difference of additive weights between two groups. Otherwise, we should use Wilcoxon-Mann-Whitney test. So at first, we should conduct the normality test (Figure 10. 4) and homogeneity test for variance.

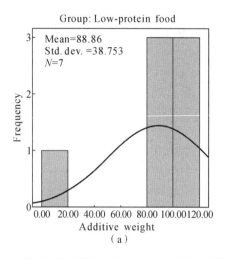 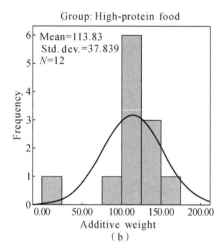

Figure 10. 4 The Distributions of the Additive Weights of Rats after Supplemented with Low-Protein Food (a) or High-Protein Food (b)

From Figure 10. 4, we can clearly find that the data of this example does not meet normal distribution. So, we should use Wilcoxon-Mann-Whitney test to infer whether there is a significant difference in the additive weights after supplemented with low- and high-protein food. We should also organize the data as Table 10. 4.

Table 10. 4 Additive Weights of Rats after Supplemented with Low- and High-Protein Food

High-protein food		Low-protein food	
Additive weight/g	Ranks	Additive weight/g	Ranks
134	17	6	1
146	18	118	11
104	7	93	4
120	13	85	3
124	15	107	8. 5 [ε]
161	19	119	12
107	8. 5 [ε]	94	5
8	2	—	—
113	10	—	—
129	16	—	—
97	6	—	—
123	14	—	—
$N_1 = 12$	$R_1 = 145. 5$	$N_2 = 7$	$R_2 = 44. 5$

[ε]*Average rank*

10. 2. 1. 1   The Typical Procedures of Wilcoxon-Mann-Whitney Test

(a) Set up the hypothesis.

H_0: $M_1 = M_2$, i. e. the overall distribution of additive weight between the two groups were the same.

H_1: $M_1 \neq M_2$, i. e. the overall distribution of additive weight between the two groups were different.

(b) Determine a significant level $\alpha = 0.05$.

(c) Rank the differences.

• Combine the data from the two groups, and ascendingly rank all the additive weights together according to the value itself.

• If a set of observations has the same value, then assign the average rank for each observation in the set.

• Calculate the rank sum of each group (R_1 or R_2), respectively.

(4) Decide the test statistic.

• If the sample sizes of the two samples are equal, you can select any rank sum (R_1 or R_2) as the statistic.

• If the sample sizes of the two samples are different, we should select the rank sum with a smaller sample size as the statistic. In this example, you may select 44. 5 as the statistic because the sample size of this group ($N_2 = 7$) is smaller than that of another group ($N_1 = 12$).

(5) Review the T-critical value table (Wilcoxon-Mann-Whitney test) and make the decision.

• In Wilcoxon-Mann-Whitney test, the lower and upper T-critical values at the level of significant level forms an interval. If the statistic (R-value) is not in the interval, we should say that $P < 0.05$ and have reason to reject the null hypothesis and think that the operation is necessary for these patients. If the statistic (R-value) is in the interval, we should say that $P > 0.05$ and cannot reject the null hypothesis that the operation is not necessary for these patients.

• In this example, it is a two-sided test and the critical value interval is (46, 94). Because 44. 5 is not within the interval, which means $P < 0.05$ and we have reason to reject the null hypothesis. The final decision is that protein level in the food will affect the weights of rats significantly.

10. 2. 1. 2   The Principle of Wilcoxon-Mann-Whitney Test

In this example, if there is no significant difference in the additive weight between low- and high-protein food (H_0 is true), the location of the distribution of the additive weight for low-and high-protein food supplementation will be equal. So, the differences in the additive weight must meet asymmetry distribution ($M_1 = M_2$).

We combined all the data and ranked them according to the values themselves. If the null hypothesis H_0 is true, the rank sum of Group 1 must be equal to that of Group 2.

Just like the previous example, we also assumed that our samples are taken from the populations randomly. Even if the two samples come from the same population under H_0, the two medians may still have a small difference because of sampling error. However, the difference between the two medians ($\sum d$) should not be too big. If $\sum d$ is large enough to exceed the limitation, we have no reason to think it is fully caused by randomized error anymore, have to reject the null hypothesis (H_0), and conclude that the protein contents affect the rats' weight significantly.

10.2.2   Two Independent Ordinal Data

In clinical research, we will not always want to compare the difference of measurements between the two groups. In some conditions, we need to assess whether there is a significant difference in the efficacy, which may be defined as excellent, valid, and invalid. Because the outcomes such as excellent, valid, and invalid are highly related and been called ordinal data, independent samples t-test or chi-square test will not be suitable for inferring the difference of efficacy between two groups. Under this circumstance, we can also perform Wilcoxon-Mann-Whitney test to compare the efficacy.

Example 10.3   A physician wanted to know whether treatment A is different from a reference treatment for essential hypertension (EH) patients. He randomly selected 200 EH patients and assigned them into two groups in a random manner. Then all these 200 subjects were given treatment A (TRT group) or the reference treatment (Control group) for 6 months. Table 10.5 is the outcome of the two groups.

Table 10.5   Comparison of the Efficacy of Two Treatments in EH Patients

Group	Excellent	Valid	Invalid
TRT	50	30	20
Control	30	40	30

This is a completely randomized designed study and the outcomes are ordinal data. So, we can conduct Wilcoxon-Mann-Whitney test to assess the difference in the efficacy between the two groups.

(a) Organize the data as Table 10.6.

Table 10.6   Efficacy of Two Treatments in EH Patients

Efficacy (1)	TRT (2)	Control (3)	Total (4)	Range (5)	Mean rank (6)
Invalid	20	30	50	1~50	25.5
Valid	30	40	70	51~120	86.5
Excellent	50	30	80	121~200	160.5
T_i	11,100	9,000	—	—	—

(b) Set up the hypothesis.

$H_0: M_1 = M_2$

$H_1: M_1 \neq M_2$

(c) Determine a significant level $\alpha = 0.05$.

(d) Rank the efficacy and calculate the rank sum and mean rank sum of each level of efficacy:

- Calculate the total number of subjects for each level of efficacy (column 4)
- Give the range of the ranks for each level of efficacy (column 5)
- Calculate the average rank for each level of efficacy (column 6)
- Calculate the rank sum of each level of efficacy (T_i) based on the sum of the number

$\times$ mean rank, respectively.

For example, for TRT group: $T_1 = 20 \times 25.5 + 30 \times 85.5 + 50 \times 160.5 = 11,100$.

(e) Decide the test statistic.

Calculate U-score with the following equation:

$$U = \frac{T - \dfrac{n_i(N+1)}{2}}{\sqrt{\dfrac{n_1 n_2(N+1)}{12}\left[1 - \dfrac{\sum(t_j^3 - t_j)}{N^3 - N}\right]}} \tag{10.1}$$

where $N = n_1 + n_2$; n_1 and n_2 indicate the sample size of each group, respectively. T means the rank sum of the group with a smaller sample size.

(f) Make decision.

- Use U-score as the statistic and compare it with the critical value ($\alpha = 0.05$).
- If U-score is less than the critical value, we say that $P > 0.05$, and have no reason to reject it according to the significant level $\alpha = 0.05$. It means that we cannot conclude that the efficacy between TRT and control groups is different.
- Otherwise, if U-score is more than the critical value, we should say that $P \leqslant 0.05$ and the null hypothesis is false, and have reason to reject it according to the significant level $\alpha = 0.05$. It means that the difference of efficacy between two groups reaches the statistical significant level.

In this example, it is a two-sided test, the statistic $U = 2.739$ and the critical value $t_{0.05,\infty} = 1.96$. Therefore, we may say that $P < 0.05$, H_0 is false and there is a statistically significant difference in the efficacy between the two treatments. Because the rank sum of group TRT is larger than that of the control, the final conclusion of this example is that the efficacy of TRT for EH patients is statistically significantly higher than the reference treatment.

10.3　Comparison of Multiple Independent Samples

In statistics, the Kruskal-Wallis H-test (also called Kruskal-Wallis one-way analysis of variance by ranks) is a non-parametric method for testing whether several samples originate from the same population. It is used for comparing more than two samples that are independent, or not related. The parametric equivalent of the Kruskal-Wallis test is the one-way analysis of variance (ANOVA). When the Kruskal-Wallis test leads to significant results, then at least one of the samples is different from the other samples significantly. The test does not identify where the differences occur or how many differences have really occurred. It is an extension of the Mann-Whitney U-test to 3 or more groups. Since it is a non-parametric method, the Kruskal-Wallis H-test does not assume a normal distribution, unlike the analogous ANOVA. However, the test does assume a Kruskal-Wallis is also used when the examined groups are of an unequal number of participants (Wikipedia definition).

Kruskal-Wallis H-test usually is used to infer whether the distributions of 3 or more populations (measurement data or ordinal data) reached a statistically significant level based on the samples randomly selected from the above-mentioned populations.

10.3.1   Multiple Comparisons of Measurement Data

Example 10.4   A physician wanted to know whether nutrient X is good for the growth of children. She randomly selected 120 primary school students from the childhood population in a city. All these 120 children were also randomly assigned into 4 groups and given placebo or different doses of the nutrient. Before the intervention, every kid's height would be measured twice, strictly following the standard operating procedure (SOP). A year later, the height of each student was measured again. The average changes of height for each student between pre- and post-intervention were used to assess the efficacy of nutrient X on children's growth and development (Table 10.7).

Table 10.7   Changes of Height (cm) among Different Groups

ID	Placebo	Low dose	Medium dose	High dose
1	8.43	8.79	9.05	9.40
2	8.39	8.99	8.95	9.43
3	8.37	8.89	8.81	9.22
4	8.30	8.90	8.93	9.36
5	8.34	8.86	8.83	9.30
6	8.26	8.65	8.84	9.32
⋮	⋮	⋮	⋮	⋮
22	8.33	8.79	8.51	9.03
23	8.21	8.66	9.01	9.31
24	8.21	8.90	8.97	9.41
25	8.34	8.84	8.86	9.31
26	8.26	8.89	8.92	9.44

				Continued
ID	Placebo	Low dose	Medium dose	High dose
27	8. 33	8. 79	8. 89	9. 41
28	8. 05	8. 77	9. 00	9. 41
29	8. 25	8. 89	8. 83	9. 41
30	8. 41	8. 74	9. 00	9. 26

The objective of this example is to infer whether there is a significant difference in the change of height for the supplementation with nutrient X or not. It is a completely randomized designed data of 4 groups and the primary variable is a continuous variable. In general, to infer the differences between 4 groups reach the statistically significant level or not, one-way analysis of variance (ANOVA) or Kruskal-Wallis H-test should be considered. If the changes of height meet normal distribution and equal variances, ANOVA would be a better selection. Otherwise, we should use Kruskal-Wallis H-test rather than ANOVA to perform the comparisons. So, normality assessment should be applied first (Figure 10. 5).

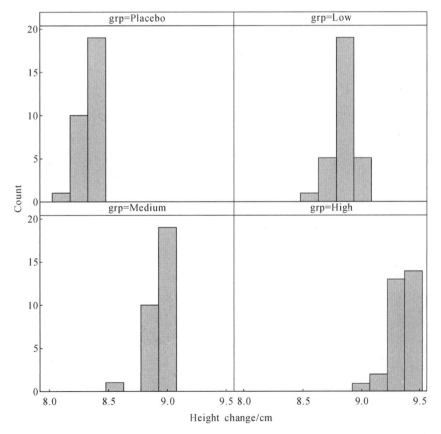

Figure 10. 5   The Distributions of the Height Changes after Supplemented with or without Different Contents of Nutrient X

As we can see from Figure 10.5, the distributions of 4 groups' height changes are significantly skewed. So Kruskal-Wallis H-test should be the best option for the inference on the difference of height changes among groups. To conduct H-test, we may organize the data and rank them first (Table 10.8) and follow the following typical procedures.

Table 10.8   Changes of Height and Ranks among Different Groups

ID	Placebo		Low dose		Medium dose		High	
	Raw data	Ranks	Raw data	Ranks	Raw data	Ranks	Raw data	Ranks
1	8.43	28.5	8.79	39	9.05	90.5	9.40	111
2	8.39	22.5	8.99	77	8.95	73	9.43	119
3	8.37	19.5	8.89	59.5	8.81	41.5	9.22	93
4	8.30	10.5	8.90	63.5	8.93	68	9.36	104
5	8.34	16	8.86	51.5	8.83	44	9.30	96
6	8.26	7.5	8.65	33	8.84	48	9.32	99
7	8.41	26	8.87	54	9.05	90.5	9.13	92
8	8.45	30	8.84	48	9.02	86	9.41	114.5
9	8.39	22.5	8.81	41.5	8.97	74.5	9.33	100
10	8.41	26	8.93	68	8.94	71	9.35	101.5
11	8.35	18	8.53	32	9.02	86	9.37	106
12	8.34	16	8.89	59.5	8.89	59.5	9.35	101.5
13	8.30	10.5	8.94	71	9.01	83	9.39	109
14	8.29	9	8.92	65.5	9.04	89	9.36	104
15	8.19	2	8.84	48	8.99	77	9.36	104
16	8.21	4	8.84	48	8.99	77	9.39	109
17	8.37	19.5	8.94	71	9.02	86	9.38	107
18	8.39	22.5	8.87	54	9.00	80	9.41	114.5
19	8.33	13	8.70	35	9.01	83	9.24	94
20	8.39	22.5	8.93	68	8.83	44	9.39	109
21	8.43	28.5	8.88	56	8.87	54	9.42	118
22	8.33	13	8.79	39	8.51	31	9.03	88
23	8.21	4	8.66	34	9.01	83	9.31	97.5
24	8.21	4	8.90	63.5	8.97	74.5	9.41	114.5
25	8.34	16	8.84	48	8.86	51.5	9.31	97.5
26	8.26	7.5	8.89	59.5	8.92	65.5	9.44	120
27	8.33	13	8.79	39	8.89	59.5	9.41	114.5
28	8.05	1	8.77	37	9.00	80	9.41	114.5
29	8.25	6	8.89	59.5	8.83	44	9.41	114.5
30	8.41	26	8.74	36	9.00	80	9.26	95

10.3.1.1   The Typical Procedures of Kruskal-Wallis H-Test

(a) Set up the hypothesis.

H_0: $M_1 = M_2 = M_3 = M_4$, i. e. there is no difference among 4 groups.

H_1: Medians of four groups are not equal or not completely equal.

(b) Determine a significant level $\alpha = 0.05$.

(c) Rank the changes of the height.

• Rank all data from all groups together, i. e. rank the data from 1 to N ignoring group membership.

• If the values among the 4 groups are equal, assign the average rank to these tied observations. If the values in the same sample are equal, rank them accordingly.

• Calculate the rank sum of each group respectively.

(d) Determine the statistic.

• Calculate H-score with the following equation:

$$H = \frac{12}{N(N+1)} \left(\sum \frac{R_i^2}{n_i} \right) - 3(N+1) \tag{10.2}$$

where N is equal to the total sample size of 4 groups, in this example $N = 120$. The n_i ($i=1$, 2, 3, 4) indicates the sample size of each group respectively. R_i^2 means the rank sum of each group respectively.

• If there exists the same rank among different groups, H-score calculated by the above formula will be smaller than expected. Under this circumstance, H-score should be corrected with the following equation to get the H_C-score:

$$H_C - \frac{H}{C_n}, \quad C = 1 - \frac{\sum (t_j^3 - t_j)}{N^3 - N} \tag{10.3}$$

where t_j refer to the number of the number of observations (i. e. the frequency) with the same value in the jth cluster of tied observations. This correction usually makes little difference in the value of H unless there are many ties.

(e) Make decision.

• Because H or H_C-scores meet χ^2 distribution ($\upsilon = g-1$, g indicates the number of groups), we can use H or H_C score as the statistic and compare it with the critical value ($\alpha = 0.05$).

• If H or H_C-score less than the critical value, we say that $P > 0.05$, and we have no reason to the reject it according to significant level $\alpha = 0.05$. It means that we cannot conclude that the height change among the 4 groups is different.

• Otherwise, if H or H_C score is greater than the critical value, we say that $P \leqslant 0.05$, the null hypothesis is false, and we have reason to reject it according to the significant level $\alpha = 0.05$. It means that the difference in height changes among 4 groups is significant.

• In this example, it is a two-sided test, the statistic $H_C = 103.920$, and the critical value is 7.81 ($\upsilon = g-1 = 4-1 = 3$). Because $H_C > 7.81$, we say that $P < 0.05$, H_0 is false, and there is a statistically significant difference in the height changes among the 4 groups.

We may conclude that nutrient X is effective in the children's growth and development.

10.3.1.2 Nemenyi Test

Like Example 10.4, when the H_0 is rejected, it only means that the 4 locations of the population are different. We do not know whether they are pairwise different. Like ANOVA, if the H_0 is rejected, post-hoc test should also be considered to identify the differences among groups one by one. For Kruskal-Wallis H-test, Nemenyi test will be a good choice for post-hoc test.

In statistics, the Nemenyi test (also called Nemenyi-Damico-Wolfe-Dunn test) is a post-hoc test, which intends to investigate the differences one by one among several groups when the null hypothesis has been rejected in a multiple comparison (such as the Kruskal-Wallis H-test). The test, named after Peter Nemenyi, makes pairwise tests of performance.

10.3.1.3 The Principle of the Nemenyi Test

Suppose g is the number of all groups in a special example. We will conduct C_2^2 chi-square tests to compare the differences among all the groups based on partitions of the chi-square method.

(a) Use the following formula to calculate the chi-square value:

$$\chi_{i,j}^2 = \frac{(R_i - R_j)^2}{\dfrac{N(N+1)}{2}\left(\dfrac{1}{n_i} + \dfrac{1}{n_j}\right)C} \tag{10.4}$$

$$v = g - 1, \ C = 1 - \frac{\sum(t_j^3 - t_j)}{N^3 - N}$$

where $\overline{R_i}$ and $\overline{R_j}$ indicate the mean rank sum of Group i and Group j, respectively. n_i and n_j indicate the sample size of Group i and Group j, respectively. N means the total sample size of all the groups. t_j means the number of tied values that are tied at a specific value. This correction usually makes little difference in the value of H unless there are many ties.

(b) Compare $\chi_{i,j}^2$ with the critical value $\chi_{0.05,v}^2$. If $\chi_{i,j}^2 < \chi_{0.05,v}^2$, we may say the difference between Group i and Group j does not reach the statistically significant level. Otherwise, if the $\chi_{i,j}^2 \geqslant \chi_{0.05,v}^2$, we think that there is a significant difference between Group i and Group j.

(c) Repeat the above steps until all the comparisons were finished.

Because Nemenyi test is quite complicated, we cannot use some famous statistical software such as SAS, SPSS, and STATA to perform the Nemenyi test directly. Recently, some statisticians believe that we can also follow the following steps to conduct the pairwise tests instead of the Nemenyi test when the null hypothesis is rejected in Kruskal-Wallis H-test:

- Rank all the raw data together from 1 to N based on the values;
- Perform one-way ANOVA test based on the ranks of the raw data;
- Perform the post-hoc test to conduct the pairwise tests based on the ranks.

10.3.2 Multiple Comparisons of Ordinal Data

Besides the comparison of the difference for measurement data among 3 or more groups, sometimes we also want to know whether there are statistically significant differences for ordinal data among several groups. What should we do? Is one-way ANOVA OK anymore?

As we all know, the requirements of one-way ANOVA consist of: (a) normality; (b) equal variance; and (c) independence. For ordinal data, because they are not independent (also called related data), one-way ANOVA is not suitable for the comparison of the differences among several groups even if the distribution of the test variables meets normal distribution. For ordinal data, Kruskal-Wallis H-test is also a good choice to infer the differences among groups.

Example 10. 5　A physician wanted to know whether the efficacy of a special treatment significantly differs among doses. She randomly selected 240 participants from her outpatients and inpatients. Then she randomly assigned these patients into 4 groups and gave them different doses of the treatments for 6 months. Table 10. 9 shows the outcomes of the research.

Table 10. 9　Efficacy of the Treatment at Different Doses

Doses	Excellent	Valid	Invalid
A	10	20	30
B	20	30	10
C	30	20	10
D	40	10	10

This is a completely randomized design and the outcome (efficacy of the treatments) is ordinal data. So, we can use Kruskal-Willas H-test to infer the differences in the efficacy among 4 groups according to the following steps.

(a) Organize the data as in Table 10. 10.

Table 10. 10　Efficacy of the Treatment among Four Different Doses

Efficacy (1)	Dose A (2)	Dose B (3)	Dose C (4)	Dose D (5)	Total (6)	Range (7)	Average rank (8)
Invalid	30	10	10	10	60	1~60	30. 5
Valid	20	30	20	10	80	61~140	100. 5
Excellent	10	20	30	40	100	141~240	190. 5
R_i	4,830	7,130	8,030	8,930	—	—	—
n_i	60	60	60	60	—	—	—
$\overline{R}_i$	80. 5	118. 8	133. 8	148. 8	—	—	—

(b) Set up the hypothesis.

H_0: $M_1 = M_2 = M_3 = M_4$, i. e. there is no difference among 4 groups.

H_1: Medians of 4 groups are not equal or not completely equal.

(c) Determine a significant level $\alpha = 0.05$.

(d) Rank the efficacy and calculate the rank sum and mean rank sum of each dose.

• Calculate the total number of subjects for each level of efficacy (column 6);

• Give the range of the ranks for each level of efficacy (column 7);

• Calculate the average rank for each level of efficacy (column 8);

• Calculate the rank sum of each dose based on the sum of the number × mean rank (row R_i), respectively.

For example, for dose A: $R_A = 30 \times 30.5 + 20 \times 100.5 + 10 \times 190.5 = 4,830$

• Calculate the mean rank sum of each dose of the treatment, respectively.

(e) Decide the test statistic.

• Calculate the H-score with the following equation:

$$H = \frac{12}{N(N+1)} \left(\sum \frac{R_i^2}{n_i} \right) - 3(N+1) \tag{10.5}$$

where N is equal to the total sample size of 4 groups, in this example $N = 120$. The n_i ($i = 1, 2, 3, 4$) indicates the sample size of each group respectively. R_i^2 means the rank sum of each group respectively.

• Because there exist many same ranks among different doses, H-score calculated by the above formula should be corrected with the following equation to get the H_C-score:

$$H_C = \frac{H}{C}, C = 1 - \frac{\sum (t_j^3 - t_j)}{N^3 - N} \tag{10.6}$$

where t_j refers to the number of the number of observations (i. e. the frequency) with the same value in the jth cluster of tied observations. This correction usually makes little difference in the value of H unless there are many ties.

(f) Make decision.

• Use H_C-score as the statistic and compare it with the critical value ($\alpha = 0.05$).

• If H_C-score is within the interval of critical value (ICV), we say that $P > 0.05$, and have no reason to reject it according to the significant level $\alpha = 0.05$. It means that we cannot conclude that the height change among the 4 groups is different.

• Otherwise, if H_C-score is not within ICV, we say that $P \leqslant 0.05$ and the null hypothesis is false, and we have reason to reject it according to the significant level $\alpha = 0.05$. It means that the difference of height changes among the 4 groups reaches a statistically significant level.

In this example, it is a two-sided test, the statistic $H_C = 36.751$, and the critical value $\chi^2_{0.05,3} = 7.81$ ($\upsilon = g - 1 = 4 - 1 = 3$). Because $H_C > \chi^2_{0.05,3}$, we say that $P < 0.05$, H_0 is false, and there is a statistically significant difference in the efficacy of the treatment among their different doses.

In a multiple comparison of several groups, when the H_0 is rejected we may conduct a post-hoc test to do the pairwise tests among these groups. In non-parametric test, Nemenyi test is a good choice for multiple comparisons of measurement data. But for ordinal data, Nemenyi test cannot be used anymore. We could choose Ridit score analysis because the data are collected from several related samples and are not independent.

10.4　Summary

Non-parametric tests are a branch of methods associated with non-parametric statistical models and non-parametric statistical tests. These methods are often referred to as distribution free methods as they do not rely on assumptions that the data are drawn from a given probability distribution. Unlike parametric tests, they are not to conduct the statistical inference of population parameters such as mean, standard deviation, variance, or rates. They are only used to test whether the locations of population distributions are the same and the hypothesis test conducted with the rank of data, not with the data itself.

In general, the most commonly used methods for inference about the means of quantitative response variables assume that the variables in question have normal distributions in the population or populations from which we draw our data. In practice, of course, no distribution is exactly normal. Because of the reliance on fewer assumptions, non-parametric tests are more robust and easier to use than parametric methods. Due both to this simplicity and to their greater robustness, non-parametric methods are seen by some statisticians as leaving less room for improper using and misunderstanding. In a word, as non-parametric tests make fewer assumptions, their applicability is much wider than the parametric methods, especially under the circumstances as: (a) population distribution is unknown; (b) data do not meet normal distribution and homogeneity of variance; (c) data are hard to precisely measured, such as ordinal data; (d) data are with uncertain values at one or both ends (<0.1, >10, etc.). However, the test efficiency of a non-parametric test is usually lower than that of parametric test. So, it is only suggested to be applied when a routine parametric test cannot be used for the inference.

(Mao Guangyun, Wang Tao, Shi Hongying)

Question Bank

Chapter 11　Linear Correlation and Regression

11.1　Simple Linear Correlation

11.1.1　Introduction

In many studies, the purpose of the research is to assess the relationship between two variables (x, y). For example, height and weight, temperature and pulse rate, drug dose and reaction time, etc. Therefore, we frequently need to observe whether there is any statistical relationship between two variables (x, y).

Correlation analysis is a statistical method that is utilized to observe and study the non-definitive relationship between two variables. There appears to be a rough relationship between two variables (x, y). As x increases, y increases or decreases accordingly. Since the relationship is not precisely one to one, we want to summarize how much of the variability the relationship explains, or a summary quantity which tells us how closely the two variables are related.

Let us consider how x and y vary together. Two variables (x, y) are positively correlated if as x increases, y tends to increase, whereas as x decreases, y tends to decrease. Two variables (x, y) are negatively correlated if as x increases, y tends to decrease, whereas as x decreases, y tends to increase. The correlation can also be divided into linear correlation and non-linear correlation. In this section we mainly discuss the linear correlation.

11.1.2　Scatter Plot

If we let each pair of numbers (x, y) be represented by a dot in a diagram with the x's on the horizontal axis and the y's on the vertical axis, we now have a figure called scatter diagram, as seen in Figure 11.1. A scatterplot shows the relationship between two quantitative variables (x, y) measured on the same individuals. Each individual in the data appears as the point in the plot fixed by the values of both variables for that individual. When we graph the observed value of y (body mass index, BMI) versus x (waist circumference), the points do not fall perfectly on any line. Figure 11.1 gives a scatterplot that displays the relationship between the response variable, BMI, and the explanatory variable, waist circumference. The plot confirms our idea that a higher BMI should be associated with a higher waist circumference. Figure 11.1 plots the (x, y) data with a fitted straight line. The line helps us to see and to evaluate the linear form of the relationship. The relationship in Figure 11.1 also has a clear direction: this is a positive association between the two variables. The strength of a relationship in a scatterplot is determined by how closely the points follow a clear form. In brief, the scatter diagram is a useful diagnostic tool for checking the validity of features of simple linear correlation.

If the dots fall around a curve, not a straight line, the linearity assumption may be violated (Figure 11.2). In addition, the model stipulates that for each level of x, the normal distribution of y has a constant variance not depending on the value of x. That would lead to a scatter diagram with dots spreading out around the line evenly across levels of x.

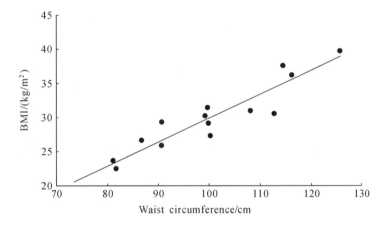

Figure 11.1 Scatter Plot of BMI Versus Waist Circumference with a Fitted Straight Line

11.1.3 Correlation Coefficient

A scatterplot displays the form, direction, and strength of the relationship between two quantitative variables. Linear (straight-line) relations are particularly important because a straight line is a simple pattern that is quite common. We say a linear relationship is strong if the points lie close to a straight line, and weak if they are widely scattered about a line. Our eyes are not good judges of how strong a relationship is. We need to follow our strategy for data analysis by using a numerical measure to supplement the graph. **Correlation coefficient** is the measure we use.

The **Pearson** product-moment correlation coefficient, which briefly designates the correlation coefficient, is a useful indicator to express the linear correlation degree and direction between the two variables. The sample correlation coefficient is represented by the symbol "r," and "ρ" (which is pronounced rho) represents the population correlation coefficient. The correlation coefficient is a useful tool for quantifying the relationship between variables (x, y).

The BMI versus waist circumference of n adults were measured, for the ith individual, the BMI was x_i and the waist circumference was y_i. The sample correlation coefficient (r) is defined by

$$r = \frac{\sum(x_i - \bar{x})(y_i - \bar{y})}{\sqrt{\sum(x_i - \bar{x})^2 \sum(y_i - \bar{y})^2}} = \frac{l_{xy}}{\sqrt{l_{xy}l_{yy}}} \qquad (11.1)$$

The corrected sum of squares for x is denoted by l_{xx} and defined by

$$l_{xx} = \sum(x_i - \bar{x})^2 = \sum x_i^2 - \frac{\left(\sum x_i\right)^2}{n} \qquad (11.2)$$

The corrected sum of squares for y is denoted by l_{yy} and defined by

$$l_{yy} = \sum(y_i - \bar{Y})^2 = \sum y_i^2 - \frac{\left(\sum y_i\right)^2}{n} \qquad (11.3)$$

The corrected sum of cross products which is denoted by l_{xy} is defined by

$$l_{xy} = \sum(x_i - \bar{x})(y_i - \bar{Y}) = \sum x_i y_i - \frac{\left(\sum x_i\right)\left(\sum y_i\right)}{n} \qquad (11.4)$$

where l_{xy} refers to the sum of the deviation from average between x and y.

The correlation coefficient, is a pure number and is independent from the units of measurement. It tends to lie between -1.0 and 1.0, which indicates the degree and direction of the correlation.

If $r > 0$, it indicates a positive correlation between x and y, i. e. when x increases, y tends to increase, and vice versa (Figure 11. 2a). When $r = 1$, it indicates a perfect positive correlation, i. e. there is a direct function between the two variables and each variable can be perfectly calculated by the other variable (Figure 1. 1b). If $r < 0$, it indicates a negative correlation, i. e. when x increases, y tends to decrease (Figure 11. 2c). When $r = -1$, a perfect negative correlation exists between two variables (Figure 11. 2d). If $r = 0$, it indicates there is no or little linear correlation relationship between x and y (Figure 11. 2e, f, g, h).

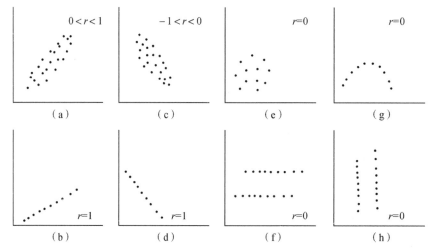

Figure 11. 2   Diagram of Correlation Coefficient

Meanwhile, the correlation coefficient provides a quantitative measurement of the dependence between two variables. This can be applied when the basic relationship between the two variables is linear, namely, when the tendency for one variable to increase is accompanied by an increase or decrease of the other variable accordingly. The absolute value of r thus gives the degree of relationship. The closer $|r|$ is to 1, the closer two variables are related; if $|r| = 1$, one variable can be calculated exactly by the other variable.

Example 11.1   Consider 15 adults for each of whom has a measurement of BMI versus waist circumference, we have found that the scatter plot has a linear tendency which means a linear relationship between BMI versus waist circumference (Figure 11.1). Please create the correlation analysis (Table 11.1).

Table 11.1   BMI (y, kg/m^2) and Waist Circumference (x, cm) of 15 Adults

No.	x (1)	y (2)	x^2 (3)	y^2 (4)	xy (5)
1	99.9	29.1	9,980.01	846.81	2,907.09
2	81.6	22.56	6,658.56	508.9536	1,840.896
3	90.7	29.39	8,226.49	863.7721	2,665.673
4	108	30.94	11,664	957.2836	3,341.52
5	112.8	30.62	12,723.84	937.5844	3,453.936
6	100.3	27.33	10,060.09	746.9289	2,741.199
7	86.7	26.68	7,516.89	711.8224	2,313.156
8	81	23.68	6,561	560.7424	1,918.08
9	125.7	39.76	15,800.49	1,580.8576	4,997.832
10	90.6	25.93	8,208.36	672.3649	2,349.258
11	114.5	37.6	13,110.25	1,413.76	4,305.2
12	73.4	19.44	5,387.56	377.9136	1,426.896
13	116.1	36.16	13,479.21	1,307.5456	4,198.176
14	99.3	30.23	9,860.49	913.8529	3,001.839
15	99.8	31.42	9,960.04	987.2164	3,135.716
Total	1,480.4	440.84	149,197.28	13,387.408	44,596.467

(a) Draw the scatter plot.

According to the actual measure values (x, y), we can draw 15 dots in the Cartesian coordinate (Figure 11.3). The scatter plot appears to be a rough, but linear tendency between the two variables. As waist circumference (x) increases, BMI (y) also increases, this is considered a positive and linear tendency.

When we inspect these plots, it appears that children with larger waist circumference tended to have a larger BMI.

(b) Calculate the sample correlation coefficient r.

Firstly, 5 values need to be calculated from the raw data:

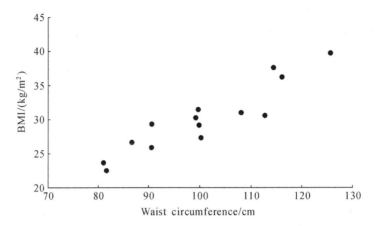

Figure 11.3   Scatterplot of BMI Versus Waist Circumference

$$\sum x_i = 1480.4, \quad \sum x_i^2 = 149,197.28, \quad \sum y_i = 440.84, \quad \sum y_i^2 = 13,387.4084,$$

$$\sum x_i y_i = 44,596.467$$

Secondly, by Formulae (11.2), (11.3), and (11.4), the average value, quadratic sum of the deviation from average, and sum of the deviation from the average of x and y need to be calculated.

$$l_{xx} = 3,091.6693, \quad l_{yy} = 431.4147, \quad l_{xy} = 1,088.4979$$

$$\bar{x} = 98.6933, \quad \bar{y} = 29.3893$$

Finally, according to Formula (11.1), we can obtain the correlation coefficient:

$$r = \frac{1,088.4979}{\sqrt{3,091.6693 \times 431.4147}} = 0.9425$$

11.1.4   Coefficient of Correlation Inferences

The sample correlation coefficient r, like other statistics, has the sampling error of ρ. Even if r is randomly sampled from a population of $\rho = 0$, the sample correlation coefficient is not always equal to 0, which means we cannot make a conclusion that there is or is not a correlation between x and y only using the r-value. We should make a hypothesis test to find out whether r comes from the population of $\rho = 0$ or not. The hypothesis test would be naturally based on the sample correlation coefficient r. H_0 would be rejected if $|r|$ is significant from 0. We would utilize a t-test.

$$t_r = \frac{|r|}{s_r} = \frac{|r|}{\sqrt{\dfrac{1-r^2}{n-2}}} \tag{11.5}$$

In this formula, $\sqrt{\dfrac{1-r^2}{n-2}}$ refers to the standard error of r, which is defined by s_r. We can infer from the distribution of t, freedom degree $v = n - 2$.

To test the hypothesis for Example 11.1, use the following procedure:

(a) Set up the hypothesis.

H_0: $\rho=0$, i. e. there is no correlation between BMI and waist circumference.

H_1: $\rho\neq0$, i. e. there is a correlation between BMI and waist circumference.

(b) Choose a significant level $\alpha=0.05$.

(c) By Formula (11.5), we can calculate the testing statistic t:

$$t = \frac{|r|}{\sqrt{\frac{1-r^2}{n-2}}} = \frac{0.9425}{\sqrt{\frac{1-0.9425^2}{15-2}}} = 10.1672$$

$$\upsilon=n-2=15-2=13$$

From Appendix 2, $t_{0.05,13} = 2.160$, $t_{0.01,13} = 3.012$, we can say that $P<0.001$ and therefore, we have a reason to reject H_0. It is considered that there is a positive correlation between BMI and waist circumference of adults, and the correlation degree is 0.9435.

When $\leqslant50$, we can also verify the Appendix 6 (r-boundary value table) according to υ. If $|r|\geqslant r_{(\alpha,\upsilon)}$, then $P\leqslant\alpha$; if $|r|<r_{(\alpha,\upsilon)}$, then $P>\alpha$. According to the r-boundary value table, we can obtain the two-sided $r_{(0.05,13)}=0.514$, $|r|>r_{(0.05,13)}$, $P<0.05$. This means that there is a correlation between BMI and waist circumference.

11.1.5   Interval Evaluation of the Population Correlation Coefficient ρ

Sampling from the population of $\rho=0$, the sampling distribution of r is symmetric. And when the sample size is large, it is similar to the normal distribution. However, sampling from the population of $\rho\neq0$, the sampling distribution of r is skewed. An easy method for obtaining the confidence limits for ρ can be derived based on the approximate normality of Fisher's z-transformation of r. Suppose we have a sample correlation coefficient r based on a sample of n pairs of observations. To obtain a two-sided $100\%\times(1-\alpha)$ CI for the population correlation coefficient (ρ):

Firstly, compute Fisher's z-transformation

$$r = z = \frac{1}{2}\ln\left(\frac{1+r}{1-r}\right) \tag{11.6}$$

Secondly, a two-sided $100\%\times(1-\alpha)$ CI is given for $z_\rho = (z_1,z_2)$ where

$$z_1 = z - \frac{z_{1-\frac{\alpha}{2}}}{\sqrt{n-3}}, \ z_2 = \frac{z + z_{1-\frac{\alpha}{2}}}{\sqrt{n-3}} \tag{11.7}$$

and $z_{1-\frac{\alpha}{2}}=100\%\times(1-\frac{\alpha}{2})$ percentile of an $N(0, 1)$ distribution.

Thirdly, a two-sided $100\%\times(1-\alpha)$ CI for ρ is then given by (ρ_1,ρ_2) where

$$\rho_1 = \frac{e^{2z_1}-1}{e^{2z_1}+1}, \ \rho_2 = \frac{e^{2z_2}-1}{e^{2z_2}+1} \tag{11.8}$$

Example 11.2   Now we can take the data of Example 11.1, and try to calculate the 95% and 99% CI of the population correlation coefficient ρ.

Due to $r=0.9579$, from Formula (11.6) we can obtain:

$$z = \frac{1}{2}\ln\left(\frac{1+0.9425}{1-0.9425}\right)= 1.7580 \qquad \frac{1}{\sqrt{n-3}} = \frac{1}{\sqrt{15-3}} = 0.2887$$

So, the 95% CI of value $z_\rho = (z_1, z_2)$: $1.9198 \pm 1.96 \times 0.3780 = (1.1789, 2.6607)$.

From Formula (11.8), we can construct a 95% CI of value ρ: $0.8312 - 0.9810$. The CI does not include zero. So the difference between the correlation coefficient and 0 has a statistical significance, which is consistent with the conclusion of the hypothesis test.

11.1.6 Spearman Rank Correlation

Sometimes we may want to look at the relationship between two variables, but one or both variables are either ordinal or have a distribution that is far from normal. Significance tests based on the Pearson correlation coefficient will then no longer be valid, and non-parametric analogs to these tests are needed. There are many methods to make an analysis for the non-parametric correlation, the most common one is the Spearman rank correlation.

11.1.6.1 Spearman Rank Correlation

The basic idea of Spearman rank correlation is:

(a) Make the rank transformation for the two values of x_i and y_i respectively, which can be represented by p_i and q_i.

(b) Calculate the correlation coefficient r of p_i and q_i, according to Formula (11.1). The sample rank correlation coefficient can be represented by r_s, and the population rank correlation coefficient can be represented by ρ_s.

Example 11.3   Please analyze whether there is relationship between burn area and length of stay of burn patients.

Table 11.2   Burn Area and Length of Stay of 12 Burn Patients

Case no.	Burn area x_i (1)	Length of stay y_i/d (2)	p_i (3)	q_i (4)	p_i^2 (5)	q_i^2 (6)	$p_i q_i$ (7)
1	Large	92	9	12	81	144	108
2	Large	83	9	11	81	121	99
3	Large	79	9	10	81	100	90
4	Severe	68	11.5	9	132.25	81	103.5
5	Severe	55	11.5	8	132.25	64	92
6	Small	11	3	5	9	25	15
7	Small	30	3	6	9	36	18
8	Small	35	3	7	9	49	21
9	Middle	9	6.5	3	42.25	9	19.5
10	Middle	10	6.5	4	42.25	16	26
11	Small	2	3	1	9	1	3
12	Small	3	3	2	9	4	6
Total			78	78	637	650	601

The analysis procedure is as follows:

(a) Sort the x and y values in ascending order, and calculate the rank of x and y. Please see the columns 3 and 4 of Table 11. 2. If x and y have the same value, take the average rank respectively.

(b) Through Formula (11. 9), we can calculate the rank correlation coefficient r_s.

$$r_s = \frac{\sum (p_i - \bar{p})(q_i - \bar{q})}{\sqrt{\sum (p_i - \bar{p})^2 \sum (q_i - \bar{q})^2}} = \frac{l_{pq}}{\sqrt{l_{pq} l_{qq}}} \tag{11.9}$$

After replacing the relative data of Table 11. 2 into the above formula, we can obtain:

$$r_s = \frac{601 - 78 \times 78/12}{\sqrt{(637 - \frac{78^2}{12})(650 - \frac{78^2}{12})}} = 0.6894$$

The calculation Formula (11. 9) of Spearman rank correlation coefficient is similar to the calculation Formula (11. 1) of linear correlation coefficient, we just need to replace x, y in Formula (11. 1) with Rank p, q.

11. 1. 6. 2   Hypothesis Testing of Rank Correlation

To determine whether the population rank correlation coefficient ρ_s is 0, there are two methods that can be used according to the size of sample n. When n is small, we use the checking table method. When n is large, we use the hypothesis test method.

(1) Checking table method

When $n \leqslant 50$, we verify with Appendix 7 (r_s boundary value table) according to n. If $|r_s| \geqslant r_{s(a,n)}$, then $P \leqslant \alpha$, in other words, there is a rank correlation between the two variables; if $|r_s| < r_{s(a,n)}$, then $P > \alpha$, i. e. there is not a rank correlation between the two variables.

We test the rank correlation coefficient of data in Example 7. 3, $n = 12$. According to the r_s value table, we can obtain the two-sided $r_{s(0.05,12)} = 0.587$, $|r_s| > r_{s(0.05,12)}$, $P < 0.05$. This means that there is a rank correlation between burn area and length of stay.

(2) Hypothesis test method

The statistic value t can also be calculated according to Formula (11. 5):

$$t = \frac{|r|}{\sqrt{\frac{1 - r^2}{n - 2}}} = \frac{0.6894}{\sqrt{\frac{1 - 0.6894^2}{12 - 2}}} = 3.009$$

Using Appendix 2, $P < 0.05$, which means there is a positive rank correlation between burn area and length of stay of burn patients.

11.2   Simple Linear Regression

11.2.1   Introduction

Correlation analysis involves measuring the degree and direction of the relationship between two random variables. Sometimes, we want to explore the linear relationship between two variables. We want to estimate the regression line of two variables, test the significance of the relationship and predict one variable as a function of another variable.

11.2.2   Structure of Simple Linear Regression Model

Linear regression is the simplest relationship between two variables, which is also called simple regression. It differs from linear correlation; two variables x and y have different positions in linear regression. The variable y being predicted is called the dependent variable or response variable, the variable x used to predict the y is called the independent variable, or the explanatory variable.

In some instances, we can only observe the independent variable x and use the regression model to predict the expected mean value μ_y of the dependent variable y. The regression model describes the mean of the normally distributed dependent variable y as a function of the predictor or independent variable x:

$$\mu_y = \beta_0 + \beta_1 x_i \tag{11.9}$$

The model above is referred to as the simple linear regression model. It is simple because it contains only one independent variable. The parameters β_0 and β_1 are called the regression coefficient. The parameter β_0 is the intercept of the regression line to represent the point at which the regression line crosses the Y axis (when $x = 0$); the parameter β_1 is the slope of the regression line, and $\beta_1 > 0$ represents the increase (or decrease, if β_1 is negative) in the mean of y associated with a 1-unit increase in the value of x. If $\beta_1 = 0$, regression line parallels to the X axis which means there is no linear regression between x and y.

In linear regression, μ_y and x are on the regression line, but since the individual observed values y_i are not always equal to their mean μ_y, the relationship between the individual value of y and its overall mean μ_y is as follows: $y_i = \bar{\mu}_y + e_i$, in which e_i is a random error term distributed as normal with mean zero and variance σ^2.

11.2.3   Parameter Estimation

The question remains as how to obtain a regression line, or how to estimate β_0 and β_1 equivalently. To find good estimates of the unknown parameters β_0 and β_1 , statisticians use a method called least squares, which means the sum of squared distances between each measured value y and $\hat{y}$ from the regression line $\sum (y - \hat{y})^2$ will be minimized. According to the method of least squares, good estimates of β_0 and β_1 are values b_0 and b_1, respectively. At this criterion, least-squares estimation of b_1 value is given by:

$$b_1 = \frac{\sum(x_i - \bar{x})(y_i - \bar{y})}{\sum(x_i - \bar{x})^2} = \frac{l_{XY}}{l_{XX}} \tag{11.10}$$

As the regression line crosses the dot $(\bar{x}, \bar{y})$, the estimation of a-value is given by:

$$b_0 = \bar{y} - b_1\bar{x} \tag{11.11}$$

Example 11.2　Derive the estimated regression line for the data in Example 11.1.

(a) Draw the scatter plot.

Similar to correlation analysis, regression analysis also needs to draw the scatter plot to determine whether there is a linear tendency between the two variables. Figure 11.1 shows the linear tendency between waist circumference and BMI.

(b) Calculate b_0 and b_1 values of the linear regression function.

For Example 11.2, we have the following quantities:

$\bar{x} = 98.69$, $\bar{x} = 29.39$, $l_{xx} = 3{,}091.6693$, $l_{yy} = 431.4147$, $l_{xy} = 1{,}088.4979$

The slope b_1 is:

$$b_1 = \frac{1{,}088.4979}{3{,}091.6693} = 0.3521$$

And the intercept b_0 is:

$$b_0 = 29.39 - 0.3521 \times 98.69 = -5.3581$$

Thus the regression line is given by:

$$\hat{y} = -5.3581 + 0.3521x$$

(c) Draw the regression line.

Two points $(x_1, \hat{y}_1)$, $(x_2, \hat{y}_2)$ which are relatively far from each other can be calculated using the regression function, and a straight line will be drawn through the two points. $\hat{y} = -5.3581 + 0.3521x$, if $x_1 = 90$, $\hat{y}_1 = 26.3309$; if $x_2 = 110$, $\hat{y}_2 = 33.3729$. This fitted regression line is shown in Figure 11.4.

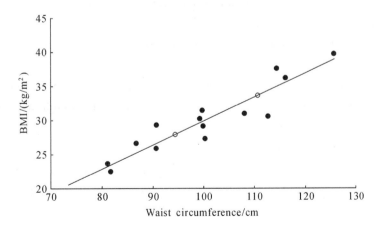

Figure 11.4　Regression Line of Waist Circumference and BMI of 15 Adults

11.2.4 Hypothesis Test

11.2.4.1 t-Test of $\beta_1 = 0$

The hypothesis test here is based on the sample regression coefficient β_1. If we are randomly sampling from the population of a $\beta_1 = 0$, the sample regression coefficients are not always equal to 0. So, we cannot make a conclusion. There is the regression relationship between x and y, only by the b_1 value. We should make a hypothesis test to determine whether b_1 is from the population of $\beta_1 = 0$ or not. An alternative method for testing the hypothesis $H_0 : \beta_1 = 0$ vs. $H_1 : \beta_1 \neq 0$ is presented. This method is based on the t-test, which is widely used and also provides an interval estimation for β_1.

The t-test uses the following procedure:

(a) Set up the hypothesis.

$H_0 : \beta_1 = 0$

$H_1 : \beta_1 \neq 0$

(b) Choose a significant level $\alpha = 0.05$.

(c) Calculate the test statistic by Formulae (11.13) to (11.15):

$$t_{b_1} = \frac{|b - 0|}{S_{b_1}}, \quad \upsilon = n - 2 \tag{11.13}$$

where S_{b_1} is the standard error of sample regression coefficients;

$$S_{b_1} = \frac{S_{y \cdot x}}{\sqrt{l_{xx}}} \tag{11.14}$$

where $S_{y \cdot x}$ is the standard deviation of the regression or the standard error of estimation of the regression;

$$S_{y \cdot x} = \sqrt{\frac{\sum (y_i - \hat{y}_i)^2}{n - 2}} \tag{11.15}$$

where $S_{y \cdot x}$ is often used to evaluate the fitting precision of the regression function.

Using Appendix 2, we can obtain the p-value and make an inference conclusion according to the significant level α.

To test the hypothesis for Example 11.2, we use the following procedure:

(a) Set up the hypothesis.

$H_0 : \beta_1 = 0$, i.e. there is no regression between waist circumference and BMI.

$H_1 : \beta_1 \neq 0$, i.e. there is a regression between waist circumference and BMI.

(b) Choose a significant level $\alpha = 0.05$.

(c) Calculate the test statistic.

$n = 15$; $l_{xx} = 3,091.6693$; $b_1 = 0.3521$; $\sum (y_i - \hat{y}_i)^2 = 48.1823$.

Using Formulae (11.13), (11.14), and (11.15), we can calculate the testing statistic value t:

$$S_{y \cdot x} = \sqrt{\frac{48.1823}{15 - 2}} = 1.9252; \quad S_{b_1} = \frac{1.9252}{\sqrt{3,091.6693}} = 0.0346$$

$$t_{b_1} = \frac{0.3521}{0.0346} = 10.1763; \, v = 15 - 2 = 13$$

From Appendix 2 ($t_{0.05,8} = 2.306$, $t_{0.01,8} = 3.355$), we can say that $P < 0.001$. Searching for the level of $\alpha = 0.05$, the H_0 hypothesis is therefore rejected and H_1 hypothesis is accepted. It can be considered that there is a linear regression between the waist circumference and BMI of 15 adults. Reviewing Example 11.1, you can verify that the t-test statistics for the correlation coefficient and regression coefficient are equal, $t_{b_1} = t_r = 10.1716$.

11.2.4.2　ANOVA of the Regression Coefficient

A hypothetical regression line and a representative sample point have been drawn. First, note that the point $(\bar{x}, \bar{y})$ falls on the regression line. If a typical sample point $P(x, y)$ is selected and a line is drawn through this point parallel to the Y axis, then the representation in Figure 11.5 is obtained.

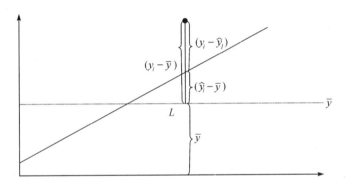

Figure 11.5　Variation Decomposition of $y_i - \bar{y}$

The total deviation of y_i about $\bar{y}$ defined by $y_i - \bar{y}$ has been partitioned additively into two components. One is the regression component, $\hat{y}_i - \bar{y}$; and the other is the residual component, $y_i - \hat{y}_i$.

$$y_i - \bar{y} = (\hat{y}_i - \bar{y}) + (y_i - \hat{y}_i) \tag{11.16}$$

To square the total deviations of the mean, sum them all up, and decompose this sum of squares into regression and residual components.

$$\sum(y_i - \bar{y})^2 = \sum(\hat{y}_i - \bar{y})^2 + \sum(y_i - \hat{y}_i)^2 \tag{11.17}$$

(a) The total sum of squares, or SS_{total}, is the sum of square of the deviations of all the individual sample points from the sample mean: $\sum(y_i - \bar{y})^2$.

(b) The regression sum of squares, or SS_{reg}, is the sum of squares of the regression components: $\sum(\hat{y}_i - \bar{y})^2$.

It denotes the component of the total sum of squares of y which can be explained by the linear effect of x.

(c) The residual sum of squares, or SS_{res}, is the sum of squares of the residual components: $\sum(y_i - \hat{y}_i)^2$.

It denotes the component of the total sum of squares of y which cannot be explained by the linear effect of x.

$$SS_{total} = SS_{reg} + SS_{res} \tag{11.18}$$

(d) Associated with each sum of squares is a degree of freedom (df or v) which can also be partitioned as follows:

$$v_{total} = v_{reg} + v_{res}; \quad v_{total} = n-1, \quad v_{reg} = 1, \quad v_{res} = n-2 \tag{11.19}$$

The decomposition of the total variation of the dependent variable, which is the same as the decomposition principle of variance analysis, can be used for analysis if there is a statistical significance for the influence of x to y, or whether there is a regression relation between x and y. The following terms are introduced to describe the hypothesis test.

The regression mean square, or MS_{reg} is the SS_{reg} divided by the number of predictor variables in the model (not including the constant). Thus, $MS_{reg} = \dfrac{SS_{reg}}{v_{reg}}$. We have been discussing $v_{reg} = 1$ in Formula (11.19) and thus $MS_{reg} = SS_{reg}$.

The residual mean square, or MS_{res} is the ratio of the SS_{res} divided by $n-2$, $MS_{res} = \dfrac{SS_{res}}{n-2}$.

Calculate the test statistic:

$$F = \frac{MS_{reg}}{MS_{res}} \tag{11.20}$$

Example 11.3 F-test for Example 11.2, use the following procedures:

(a) Set up the hypothesis and significant level.

H_0: $\beta=0$, i.e. there is no regression between waist circumference and BMI;

H_1: $\beta\neq0$, i.e. there is a regression between waist circumference and BMI.

(b) Set a significant level $\alpha=0.05$.

(c) Calculate the statistic value:

$l_{xx} = 3,091.6693$, $l_{yy} = 431.4147$, $l_{xy} = 1,088.4979$, $SS_{total} = l_{yy} = 431.4147$

By Formulae (11.18) and (11.3), $SS_{res} = 431.4147 - \dfrac{1,088.4979^2}{3,091.6693} = 48.1823$

$SS_{reg} = SS_{total} - SS_{res} = 431.4147 - 48.1823 = 383.2324$

These results are summarized in the ANOVA table (Table 11.3).

Table 11.3　ANOVA Table of Example 11.1

Variation	SS	v	MS	F
Regression	383.2324	1	383.2324	103.40
Residual	48.1823	13	3.7063	—
Total variation	431.4147	14	—	—

$F = 89.01$, $v_1 = 1$, $v_2 = 8$, from Appendix 4, $F_{(0.05,1,8)} = 5.32$, $F_{(0.01,1,8)} = 11.26$, therefore $P<0.01$. H_0 is rejected and the alternative hypothesis, namely that the slope of the regression line is significantly different from 0, is accepted, implying a significant linear relationship between waist circumference and BMI. Example 11.2 verifies that $\sqrt{F} = t_{b_1} = 10.1716$. Therefore, the hypothesis tests whether the overall regression coefficient β_1 is not 0 for the same data, and the analysis of variance and t-test are consistent in linear regression.

11.2.5 CIs for Individual Observations

Suppose we wish to make a prediction from a regression line for an individual observation with an independent variable x that was not used in constructing the regression line. The standard deviation of the distribution of observed y values for the subset of individuals with independent variable x is given by:

$$S_y = S_{y \cdot x} \sqrt{1 + \frac{1}{n} + \frac{(x_i - \bar{x})^2}{\sum (x_i - \bar{x})^2}} \tag{11.22}$$

Furthermore, $100\% \times (1-\alpha)$ of the observed values will fall within the interval

$$\hat{y}_1 \pm t_{a, n-2} S_{y_i} \tag{11.23}$$

This interval is sometimes called a 100% $(1-\alpha)$ prediction interval for y.

For Example 11.2, S_{y_i} is given by

$$S_{y_i} = 1.9252 \sqrt{1 + \frac{1}{15} + \frac{(110 - 98.69)^2}{3,091.6693}} = 2.0265$$

The regression function for waist circumference and BMI is given by $\hat{y} = -5.3581 + 0.3521x$. Thus the estimated BMI for a waist circumference of 110 cm is 33.3729 kg/m². $t_{0.05,13} = 2.160$. The 95% CI is given by

$$33.3729 \pm 2.160 \times 2.0265 = 28.9957 \sim 37.7501 \ (\text{kg/m}^2)$$

Therefore, 95% of adults with a waist circumference of 110 cm will have a BMI between 28.9957 and 37.7501 kg/m².

11.2.6 CIs for Population Predicted Mean

For a fixed value of x_i, $\mu_{\hat{y}_l}$ is the population predicted mean of $\hat{y}_l$ at the point x_i. If we want to assess the mean value of BMI for a large number of adults of a particular waist circumference rather than for one particular participant, how can we estimate the mean value of BMI, $\mu_{\hat{y}_l}$, and the standard error of the estimation? The best estimate of $\mu_{\hat{y}_l}$ for a given x_i is $\hat{y}_l = b_0 + b_1 x_1$. Its standard error, denoted by $S_{\hat{y}_l}$, is given by:

$$S_{\hat{y}_l} = S_{y \cdot x} \sqrt{\frac{1}{n} + \frac{(x_i - \bar{x})^2}{\sum (x_i - \bar{x})^2}} \tag{11.24}$$

Furthermore, a two-sided $100\% (1-\alpha)$ CI for $\mu_{\hat{y}_l}$ is

$$\hat{y}_l \pm t_{a, n-2} S_{\hat{y}_l} \tag{11.25}$$

The best estimate of the mean value of BMI is the same as the estimate given above, which is 33.3729 kg/m². However, the standard error is computed differently.

$$S_{\hat{y}_i} = 1.9252 \sqrt{\frac{1}{15} + \frac{(110 - 98.69)^2}{3,091.6693}} = 0.6328$$

Therefore, a 95% CI for $\mu_{\hat{y}_i}$ over a large number of adults with a waist circumference of 110 cm is given by

$$33.3729 \pm 2.160 \times 0.6328 = 32.0060 \sim 34.7398 \ (kg/m^2)$$

Notice that this interval (32.0060, 34.7398) is much narrower than the predicted interval (28.9957, 37.7501) for y_i, which is a range encompassing approximately 95% of individual BMI. This disparity reflects the intuitive idea that it is much more precise when estimating the mean value of y for a large number of adults with the same waist circumference x than when estimating y for one particular waist circumference x. From Figure 11.6, for every x value, we can calculate $\hat{y}$, and two 95% CIs. Therefore, we can obtain the 95% CI bands for population means and 95% CI bands for a future observation, which are called the "five-line bands."

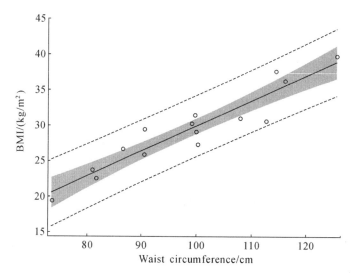

Figure 11.6　95% CI Bands for Population Means (Shaded Area) and 95% CI Bands for a Future Observation (Dashed)

A 95% CI band for the population mean is represented by the shaded area inside in Figure 11.6, which refers to the population mean of y for a given x value will be within the given band. The other 95% CI band for future observations is represented by dashed lines in Figure 11.6. This band means that we are 95% certain that the next observation at the fixed point x will be within the given band. Note that the curvature is not nearly as marked.

11.3　Comparison between Correlation and Regression

In this chapter, we introduced the methods of statistical inference that are appropriate for investigating the relationship between two variables, which are denoted as regression and correlation.

If we are interested in the association between the two continuous variables meeting normal distribution, then the linear regression or correlation analysis can be used. If we simply want to look at the association between two normally distributed variables, then a Pearson correlation analysis is more appropriate. If both variables are continuous but are not normally distributed, or are ordinal variables, then rank correlation analysis should be used instead.

If only two variables, both of which are continuous, are being studied, and we wish to predict one variable (the dependent variable) as a function of the other variable (the independent variable), then a simple linear-regression analysis is used.

In many instances, we are interested in more than two variables and we want to predict the value of one variable (the dependent variable) as a function of several independent variables. If the dependent variable is normally distributed, then multiple-regression methods can be used. Multiple-regression analysis can be a very powerful tool because the independent variables can be either continuous or categorical, or a combination of both.

(Sun Hongpeng, Wu Siying, Minyao Ng Derry)

Question Bank

Chapter 12　Multiple Linear Regression

12. 1　Introduction

In statistics, linear regression is a statistical technique used for modeling the relationship between a response (dependent variable) and one or more explanatory variables (independent variables). When there is only one explanatory variable, it is called simple linear regression. Since things are influenced by many other things, the change of a dependent variable may be influenced by many other independent variables. For example, the change in a patient's blood pressure can be simultaneously attributed to many factors, such as age, emotional stress, obesity, genetic mutation, exercise, and so on.

Therefore, to provide a more comprehensive analysis, it is desirable to consider a large number of factors and sort out which ones are most important for the prediction of a response variable. In this section, we discuss a multivariate method for this type of risk determination. For more than one explanatory variable, the process is called multiple linear regression. The goal of constructing the multiple linear regression model is to assess the linear relationship between one continuous dependent variable and a set of independent variables.

12. 2　Structure

In multiple linear regression, there are p explanatory variables, and the relationship between the dependent variable (Y) and the explanatory variables (X, Table 12. 1) is represented by

$$Y = \beta_0 + \beta_1 X_1 + \beta_2 X_2 + \cdots + \beta_p X_p + \varepsilon \qquad (12. 1)$$

following multiple linear regression model.

Table 12. 1　Data Form of Multiple Linear Regression

ID	X_1	X_1	$\cdots$	X_p	Y
1	X_{11}	X_{12}	$\cdots$	X_{1p}	Y_1
2	X_{21}	X_{22}	$\cdots$	X_{2p}	Y_2
$\vdots$	$\vdots$	$\vdots$	$\vdots$	$\vdots$	$\vdots$
n	X_{n1}	X_{n2}	$\cdots$	X_{np}	Y_n

In the above model, the dependent variable Y can be denoted, the linear function of independent variables approximate $(X_1, X_2, \cdots, X_p)$. β_0 is the constant, $\beta_1, \beta_2, \cdots, \beta_p$ are partial regression coefficients, denote that when other dependent variables hold the line, X_i increase or decrease one unit that means average variation of Y. The residual ε, is random error that excludes m entries independent variables influence to Y.

Similar to simple linear regression, we use the method of least squares estimation (LSE) to obtain estimators of the regression coefficients β_i. Let

$$b_0, b_1, b_2, \cdots, b_p$$

denote the estimators of the parameters:

$$\beta_0, \beta_1, \beta_2, \cdots, \beta_p$$

For the ith observation, the predicted response is

$$\hat{y} = b_0 + b_1 X_1 + b_2 X_2 + \cdots + b_p X_p \tag{12.2}$$

The application of multiple linear regression models needs to meet the conditions:

(a) Linear: there is a linear relationship between Y and $X_1, X_2, \cdots, X_p$.

(b) Independence: the measured value $Y_i (i=1, 2, \cdots, n)$ of each case is independent.

(c) Normality: $\varepsilon_i \sim N(0, \sigma^2)$, $i=1, 2, \cdots, n$.

(d) Equal variance: $\mathrm{Var}(i) = \sigma^2$, $i=1, 2, \cdots, n$. That is to say that residual ε is independent and normally distributed with mean 0 and variance σ^2, it equates to that for any independent variables $X_1, X_2, \cdots, X_p$ the dependent variable Y has the same variance, and obeys normal distribution.

We often use the abbreviation of LINE for the above four assumptions.

12.2.1   Intercept

The parameter β_0 is the intercept of the regression line. If the scope of the model includes $X=0$, β_0 gives the mean of Y when $X=0$. When the scope of the model does not cover $X=0$, β_0 does not have any particular meaning as a separate term in the regression model.

12.2.2   Partial Regression Coefficient

$\beta_1, \beta_2, \cdots, \beta_p$ are partial regression coefficients. The average increase (or decrease, if β_i is negative) in the mean of Y associated with a 1-unit increase in the value of X_i, $X_i = X+1$ versus $X_i = X$. For an m-unit increase in the value of X_i, say $X_i = X+m$ versus $X_i = X$, the corresponding increase (or decrease) in the mean of Y is $m\beta_i$ assuming that other independent variables are fixed. In other words, β_i represents the additional contribution of X_i in the explanation of variation among Y values.

Partial regression coefficients differ from simple linear regression coefficients. The latter represents the average increase in Y per unit increase in X, without considering any other independent variables. If there are strong relationships among the independent variables in a multiple regression model, then the partial regression coefficients may differ considerably from the simple linear regression coefficients obtained from considering each independent variable separately.

12.2.3　Standardization Partial Regression Coefficient

We are often interested in ranking the independent variables according to their predictive relationship with the dependent variable Y. It is difficult to rank the variables based on the magnitude of the partial regression coefficients because the independent variables are often in different units.

The standardization regression coefficient (b') is given by $b \times \dfrac{S_x}{S_y}$. It represents the estimated average increase in Y (expressed in standard deviation units of Y) per standard deviation increase in X, after adjusting for all other variables in the model.

Thus, the standardized regression coefficient is a useful measure for comparing the predictive value of several independent variables because it tells us the predicted increase in standard deviation units of Y per standard deviation increase in X. By expressing the changes in standard deviation units of X, we can control for differences in the units of measurement for different independent variables.

Example 12.1　Suppose systolic blood pressure (SBP), age, BMI, and serum albumin (ALB) are measured for 8,366 subjects and the data is as shown in Table 12.2.

Table 12.2　Sample Data for SBP, Age, BMI, and ALB for 8,366 Cases

ID	Age (X_1) /years	BMI (X_2) /(kg/m²)	ALB (X_3) /(g/L)	SBP (y) /mmHg
5	49	29.10	45	122
6	19	22.56	51	114
7	59	29.39	45	123
...	...	...	...	...
41,466	58	33.65	44	151
41,468	66	26.44	44	148
41,472	34	26.23	50	127

Here we use the SPSS to obtain the least squares estimates which are given in Table 12.3.

Table 12.3   Regression Analysis Results of Example 12.1

Variable	Partial regression coefficient	Coefficients SE	Standardization regression coefficient	t	P
Intercept	67.621	2.332	—	29.002	<0.001
Age	0.488	0.008	0.528	57.630	<0.001
BMI	0.482	0.030	0.151	16.289	<0.001
ALB	0.441	0.046	0.090	9.662	<0.001

SE is the abbreviation of standard error.

The linear regression model is given by

$$\hat{y} = 67.621 + 0.488X_1 + 0.482X_2 + 0.441X_3$$

(a) The partial regression coefficient for age: $b_1 = 0.488$ mmHg/year represents the estimated average increase in SBP per year increase in age for people with the same BMI and ALB.

The regression coefficient for BMI: $b_2 = 0.482$ mmHg/(kg/m^2) represents the estimated average increase in SBP per kg/m^2 increase in BMI for people of the same age and ALB.

The regression coefficient for ALB: $b_3 = 0.441$ mmHg/(g/L) represents the estimated average increase in SBP per g/L increase in ALB for people of same age and BMI.

(b) According to the standardization regression coefficient column, $b'_1 = 0.528$, $b'_2 = 0.151$, $b'_3 = 0.090$.

Thus the average increase in SBP is 0.528 standard deviation units of blood pressure per standard deviation increase in age, holding BMI and ALB constant, and 0.151 standard deviation units of blood pressure per standard deviation increase in BMI, holding age and ALB constant, and 0.090 standard deviation units of blood pressure per standard deviation increase in ALB, holding age and BMI constant. Thus, age appears to be the most important variable after controlling for three variables simultaneously in the multiple linear regression model.

12.3   Parameter Estimation

To find good estimates of the $k+1$ unknown parameters β_0 and β_i in the model, statisticians use the same method of least squares estimation described earlier. The method of least squares is a standard approach in regression analysis. Although there are other ways of estimating the parameters in the regression model, the least squares criterion has several desirable statistical properties, most notably, that the estimates are maximum likelihood (ML) if the residuals are normally distributed. We will use the least squares criterion to estimate the equations so that we minimize the sum of squares of the differences between the actual and predicted values for each observation in the sample. The most important application is in data fitting. The best fit in the least-squares sense minimizes the sum of squared residuals (a residual is the difference between an observed value and the fitted value provided by a model).

$$Q = \sum_{i=1}^{n}(y_i - \hat{y}_i)^2 = \sum_{i=1}^{n}[y_i - (b_0 + b_1 x_{i1} + b_2 x_{i2} + \cdots + b_p x_{ip})]^2 \qquad (12.3)$$

According to the differentiation, the partial derivatives of the $(k+1)$ parameters b_0 and b_i are obtained and equalized to 0, and the normal equations which can obtain p equations are solved:

$$\begin{cases} l_{11}b_1 + l_{12}b_2 + \cdots + l_{1p}b_p = l_{1Y} \\ l_{21}b_1 + l_{22}b_2 + \cdots + l_{2p}b_p = l_{2Y} \\ \vdots \\ l_{p1}b_1 + l_{p2}b_2 + \cdots + l_{pp}b_p = l_{pY} \end{cases} \qquad (12.4)$$

$$b_0 = \bar{Y} - (b_1 \bar{X}_1 + b_2 \bar{X}_2 + \cdots + b_p \bar{X}_p) \qquad (12.5)$$

$$l_{jk} = \sum_{i}(X_{ij} - \bar{X}_j)(X_{ik} - \bar{X}_k) \quad j,k = 1,2,\cdots,p \qquad (12.6)$$

$$l_{jY} = \sum_{i}(Y_i - \bar{Y})(X_{ij} - \bar{X}_j) \quad j = 1,2,\cdots,p \qquad (12.7)$$

We estimate the regression model to get the estimations of partial regression coefficients.

For Example 12.1, if we estimate the regression model we get:

$$\hat{y} = 67.621 + 0.488X_1 + 0.482X_2 + 0.441X_3 \qquad (12.8)$$

The age regression coefficient is 0.488 mmHg/year indicating that when other factors are fixed, the average SBP increased by 0.488 mmHg for a one-year increase in age. The regression coefficient of ALB showed that after fixing other factors, the average SBP increased by 0.441 mmHg as ALB increased by one g/L.

In this section, we have have learned how to fit regression lines using the method of least squares based on the linear regression model. Note that the method of least squares is appropriate whenever the average residual for each given value of x is 0, that is when $\varepsilon(e|X = X) = 0$. The normality of the residuals is not strictly required. However, the normality assumption is necessary to perform hypothesis tests concerning regression parameters, as discussed in the next section.

12.4 Hypothesis Test

A multiple regression model is fitted and estimates for the various parameters of interest are obtained. Then we want to answer questions about the contributions of various factors to the prediction of the continuous response variable.

There are two types of test questions:

(a) Overall regression test. Taken collectively, does the entire set of explanatory or independent variables contribute significantly to the prediction of the response?

(b) Test for the value of a single factor. Does one particular variable of interest promote significantly to the prediction of response?

12.4.1 Overall Regression Tests

12.4.1.1 Analysis of Variance

The first question stated above is considered concerning an overall test for a model containing i factors together. The null hypothesis for this test may be stated as: "All i independent variables considered together do not explain the variation in the responses."

$$H_0: \beta_1 = \beta_2 = \cdots = \beta_p = 0$$

The alternative hypothesis H_1 is that at least one coefficient relating the X variable to the Y variable is not equal to zero. In other words, there is some kind of relationship between X and Y.

$$H_1: \text{at least one } \beta \neq 0$$

The total sum of squares (SS), or total SS is the sum of the squares of the deviations of the individual sample points from the sample mean of Y:

$$\sum_{p=1}^{n} (y_p - \bar{y})^2 \tag{12.9}$$

Decomposition of the total sum of squares into regression and residual components:

$$\sum_{p=1}^{n} (y_p - \bar{y})^2 = \sum_{p=1}^{n} (\hat{y}_p - \bar{y})^2 + \sum_{p=1}^{n} (y_p - \hat{y}_p)^2 \tag{12.10}$$

The regression mean square, or MS_{reg} is the SS_{reg} divided by the number of predictor variables (p) in the model. Thus $MS_{reg} = \dfrac{SS_{reg}}{p}$. We will refer to p as the degrees of freedom for the regression sum of squares, or df_{reg}.

The residual mean square, or MS_{res}, is the ratio of the SS_{res} divided by $n-p-1$, or $MS_{res} = \dfrac{SS_{res}}{n-p-1}$. We refer to $n-p-1$ as the degrees of freedom for the residual sum of squares, or df_{res}.

$$MS_{reg} = \frac{SS_{reg}}{p} \tag{12.11}$$

$$MS_{res} = \frac{SS_{res}}{n-p-1} \tag{12.12}$$

Compute the F-statistics:

$$F = \frac{MS_{reg}}{MS_{res}} \tag{12.13}$$

which follows an $F_{p, n-p-1}$ distribution under H_0.

Table 12.4　Frame of Multiple Linear Regression Analysis of Variance

Source of variation	SS	df	MS	F	P
Regression	SS_{reg}	p	$\dfrac{SS_{reg}}{p}$	$\dfrac{MS_{reg}}{MS_{res}}$	—
Residual	SS_{res}	$n-p-1$	$\dfrac{SS_{res}}{n-p-1}$	—	—
Total variation	SS_Y	$n-1$	—	—	—

Under H_0, $F=\dfrac{MS_{reg}}{MS_{res}}$ follows an F-distribution with p and $n-p-1$ degree of freedom, respectively. H_0 should be rejected for large values of F value. Thus, for a level α test, H_0 will be rejected if $F>F_{p,n-p-1,1-\alpha}$, and otherwise there is no reason to reject H_0.

For Example 12.1, a test for the significance of the regression model is derived for the SBP with age, BMI, and ALB data.

Table 12.5　Frame of Multiple Linear Regression Analysis of Variance

Source of variation	SS	df	MS	F	P
Regression	817,502.169	3	272,500.723	1,264.206	<0.001
Residual	1,802,436.825	8,362	215.551	—	—
Total variation	2,619,938.994	8,365	—	—	—

From the F bound value we get $P<0.05$, at $\alpha=0.05$ level; and we can reject H_0, accept H_1, and consider that the regression model has statistical significance, implying significant linear relationships.

12.4.1.2　R^2

R^2, a statistic, is the proportion of the variation of the response variable Y that is explained by a set of explanatory variables $(X_1, X_2, \cdots, X_p)$ in a multiple linear regression.

$$R^2=\frac{SS_{reg}}{SS_{total}}=1-\frac{SS_{res}}{SS_{total}} \tag{12.14}$$

The closer R^2 is to 1, the better the model is responsible for data.

If $R^2=1$, then all variation in Y can be explained by variation in X, and all data points fall on the regression line. If $R^2=0$, then X gives no information about Y, and the variance of Y is the same with or without knowing X. In this case:

$$R^2=\frac{817,502.169}{2,619,938.994}=0.312$$

That indicates 31.2% of the variance in SBP is predictable from age, BMI, and ALB.

12.4.1.3　Multiple Correlation Coefficient

It can be used to measure the degree of the relationship between the dependent variable Y and a set of independent variables, which is the degree of the relationship between observation Y and $\hat{Y}$.

$$R = \sqrt{R^2} \tag{12.15}$$

For Example 12.1, $R = \sqrt{0.312} = 0.559$. If $p=1$, $R = |r|$, where r is a simple correlation coefficient.

12.4.2　Tests for a Single Variable

12.4.2.1　t-Test

Assuming that we want to test whether the addition of one particular independent variable of interest adds significantly to the prediction of the response over and above that achieved by other factors already present in the model. The null hypothesis for this test may be stated as: "Factor X_i does not have any value added to the prediction of the response given that other factors are already included in the model."

$$H_0 : \beta_i = 0$$

To test such a null hypothesis, one can use:

$$t_i = \frac{\hat{\beta}_i}{SE(\hat{\beta}_i)} \quad (i = 1, 2, \cdots, p) \tag{12.16}$$

in a t-test with $n - p - 1$ degrees of freedom, where $\hat{\beta}_i$ is the corresponding estimated regression coefficient and $SE(\hat{\beta}_i)$ is the estimate of the standard error of $\hat{\beta}_i$.

For Example 12.1, the test results of three independent variables can be calculated by SPSS as shown in Table 12.3.

From Table 12.3, we get $P_1 < 0.05$, $P_2 < 0.05$, and $P_3 < 0.05$, at $\alpha = 0.05$ level; we can reject H_0 and consider that age, BMI, and ALB have statistical significance, respectively, implying significant linear relationships.

12.4.2.2　Sum of the Squared for Partial Regression

In the model, sum of the squared for partial regression of one of independent variables X_j means that when there are other $p-1$ independent variables, the contribution of this independent variable to the dependent variable Y. That is, after X_j is excluded from the equation, the sum of the squared regression decreases. That is, on the basis of $p-1$ independent variables, when X_j increases, the sum of squared regression increases, as shown in Formula (12.17):

$$F_j = \frac{\dfrac{SS_{reg}(X_j)}{1}}{\dfrac{SS_{res}}{n-p-1}} \tag{12.17}$$

$$\upsilon_1 = 1, \upsilon_2 = n - p - 1$$

where $SS_{reg}(X_j)$ is the sum of the squared for partial regression, and the bigger, the more important its corresponding independent variable.

In general condition, the effect of $m-1$ independent variables to the sum of the squared for partial regression of Y should be obtained from the new equation, rather than exclude from the equation of m independent variables simply.

For Example 12.1, the sum of the squared for partial regression of each independent variable can be accounted according to different regression models drawing up from different independent variables. Table 12.6 gives some part result of the case.

Table 12.6 Partial Regression Results of Multiple Linear Regression Model

Independent variables	Sum of the squared	
	SS_{reg}	SS_{res}
X_1, X_2, X_3	817,502.169	1,802,436.825
X_2, X_3	101,600.464	2,518,338.531
X_1, X_3	760,312.641	1,859,626.353
X_1, X_2	797,378.304	1,822,560.691

Calculate the partial regression squared sum of the respective variables based on the results above.

$$SS_{reg}(X_1) = SS_{reg}(X_1, X_2, X_3) - SS_{reg}(X_2, X_3)$$
$$= 817,502.169 - 101,600.464$$
$$= 715,901.705$$
$$SS_{reg}(X_2) = SS_{reg}(X_1, X_2, X_3) - SS_{reg}(X_1, X_3)$$
$$= 817,502.169 - 760,312.641$$
$$= 57,189.528$$
$$SS_{reg}(X_3) = SS_{reg}(X_1, X_2, X_3) - SS_{reg}(X_1, X_2)$$
$$= 817,502.169 - 797,378.304$$
$$= 20,123.865$$

The F-test results of the partial regression squared sum:

$$F_1 = \frac{\dfrac{SS_{reg}X_1}{1}}{\dfrac{SS_{res}}{8,366-3-1}}$$
$$= \frac{715,901.705}{215.551}$$
$$= 3,321.26$$

$$F_2 = \frac{\dfrac{SS_{reg}X_2}{1}}{\dfrac{SS_{res}}{8,366-3-1}}$$
$$= \frac{57,189.528}{215.551}$$
$$= 265.32$$

$$F_3 = \frac{\dfrac{SS_{reg}X_3}{1}}{\dfrac{SS_{res}}{8,366-3-1}}$$

$$=\frac{20,123.865}{215.551}$$

$$=93.36$$

From the F bound value, we get $P_1<0.05$, $P_2<0.05$, and $P_3<0.05$, at $\alpha=0.05$ level; we can reject H_0, accept H_1, and consider that age, BMI, and ALB all have statistical significance, implying significant linear relationships. It is seen from the squared sum of the two variables that the regression contribution of age is relatively large.

12.4.2.2   Standardization Regression Coefficient

A standardization variable is when you subtract the mean of the corresponding variable from the original data, then divide by the standard deviation of the variable.

$$X'_j = \frac{X_j - \overline{X}_j}{S_j} \qquad (12.18)$$

As discussed previously, the standardization regression coefficient (b'_j) is given by $b_j\frac{S_x}{S_y}$. So if it does not have a unit, then it can be used to compare with the effective intension of each independent variable X_j to Y. Generally, if there is a statistical significance, the larger the absolute value of the standardization regression coefficient is, the more important the effect of the correspondent independent variable to Y.

For this example, calculate the standardization regression coefficients of the respective variables:

$$b'_1 = 0.528, b'_2 = 0.151, b'_3 = 0.090$$

As the result shows, the size of the factors affecting SBP can be ranked as follows: age (X_1), BMI (X_2), and ALB (X_3). Thus, age appears to be the most important variable after controlling for the other two variables simultaneously in the multiple regression model.

12.5   Independent Variables Selection

In many applications, our major interest is to identify the most important risk factors. In other words, we wish to identify a small subset of factors that relate to the outcome (e.g. the disease under investigation) significantly from many available factors.

How does one select the "best" model for describing a relationship or for predicting a dependent variable when multiple independent variables are available but some of them may not be needed or useful? There is no simple answer. A statistician chooses from several different techniques when selecting a model, depending on the particular situation. This section will briefly illustrate the use of two standard methods: all possible regressions and stepwise selection.

12.5.1   All Possible Regressions

(a) Revise coefficient of determination choosing method.

R_c^2 can be expressed as

$$R_c^2 = 1 - (1 - R^2) \frac{n-1}{n-p-1} = 1 - \frac{MS_{res}}{MS_{reg}} \tag{12.19}$$

where n is sample size. R^2 is the coefficient of determination of the regression model, which includes $p(p \leqslant m)$ independent variables. The change rule of is: when R^2 are equal, the greater number of nonsignificant independent variables are, the smaller R_c^2 is. By mean of "the best" regression model, R_c^2 is the largest.

(b) Choose C_p:

$$C_p = \frac{(SS_{res})_p}{(MS_{res})_m} - [n - 2(p+1)] \tag{12.20}$$

where $(SS_{res})_p$ is the sum of squared errors of regression from $p(p \leqslant m)$ of independent variables, $(MS_{res})_m$ is the residual mean square that comes from the regression model of total m of independent variables.

When the model with p of independent variables is the best theoretically, the expected value of C_p is $p+1$, so the regression model in which C_p is the closest to $p+1$ should be chosen as the optimum model. The C_p should not be applied to choose independent variables if there is no variable that has the main effect on Y within all the independent variables.

12.5.2   Stepwise Selection

12.5.2.1   Forward Selection

The forward selection technique is based on the intuitive idea that one starts with the single best predictor variable and then proceeds by adding the "next best" predictor followed by the next best, and so on, one will eventually arrive at the best prediction model. This method is often used when it is not feasible or practical to compute all possible regressions.

Here are the steps to follow:

(a) Fit a simple linear regression model to each factor, one at a time.

(b) Select the most important factor according to a certain predetermined criterion.

(c) Test for the significance of the factor selected in step b and determine, according to a certain predetermined criterion, whether or not to add this factor to the model.

(d) Repeat steps b and c for those variables not yet included in the model. At any subsequent step, if none meets the criterion in step c, no more variables are included in the model and the process is terminated.

12.5.2.2   Backward Elimination

The backward elimination procedure is similar to the forward selection procedure. It is based on the idea that one should start with the model with all the predictor variables and then eliminate those variables that do not add significantly to the prediction. The user must first specify the significant level to retain. This value is usually small; the values 0.15 and 0.10 are used frequently. The procedure starts with a model using all available independent variables and then discards variables one at a time until all the remaining variables are significant at this level.

Here are the steps to follow:

(a) Fit the multiple regression model containing all available independent variables.

(b) Select the least important factor according to a certain predetermined criterion, which is done by considering one factor at a time and treat it as though it was the last variable to enter.

(c) Test for the significance of the factor selected in step b and determine, according to a certain predetermined criterion, whether or not to delete this factor from the model.

(d) Repeat steps b and c for those variables still in the model. At any subsequent step, if none meets the criterion in step c, no more variables are removed from the model and the process is terminated.

12.5.2.3 Stepwise Regression

Stepwise regression is on the basis of the two approaches hereinbefore. Essentially speaking, it is a way of forward selection that permits a reexamination, at every step, of the variables incorporated in the model in previous steps. A variable entered at an early stage may become superfluous at a later stage because of its relationship with other variables now in the model; the information it provides becomes redundant. That variable may be removed if it meets the elimination criterion, and the model is refitted with the remaining variables, and the forward process goes on. The entire process, one step forward followed by one step backward, continues until no more variables can be added or removed.

For Example 12.1, the results of the forward selection, the backward elimination, and the stepwise regression are the same which are shown in Table 12.3.

From the results, all variables enter the model, where the older the age is and the higher the BMI and the ALB are, the higher the blood pressure is.

12.6　Goodness-of-Fit for the Model

12.6.1　Coefficient of Determination

One measure of goodness-of-fit is the coefficient of determination (R^2), which is always between 0 and 100%. R-squared does not indicate whether a regression model is adequate. You can have a low R-squared value for a good model, or a high R-squared value for a model that does not fit the data. R^2 can never decrease when another independent variable is added to a regression, and will usually increase. Because R^2 usually increases with the number of independent variables, it is not a good way to compare models. This problem can be avoided by doing an F-test of the statistical significance of the increase in the R^2, or by using the adjusted R^2 instead.

12.6.2   Adjusted R-Squared

If a model has too many predictors and higher-order polynomials, it begins to model the random noise in the data. This condition is known as overfitting the model and it produces misleadingly high R-squared values and a reduced ability to make predictions. The adjusted R-squared is a modified version of R-squared that has been adjusted for the number of predictors in the model. The adjusted R-squared increases only if the new term improves the model more than would be expected by chance. It decreases when a predictor improves the model by less than expected by chance. The adjusted R-squared can be negative, but it is usually not. It is always lower than the R-squared.

12.6.3 F-Test

The criterion for goodness-of-fit used is the ratio of the regression sum of squares to the residual sum of squares. A large ratio indicates a good fit, whereas a small ratio indicates a poor fit.

Goodness-of-fit test and F-test are two kinds of test from different principles, but they are correlated: goodness-of-fit test is based on the model to test the degree of fit to samples, while F-test is based on samples to test significance of total linear relationship. F-test and goodness-of-fit test are correlated both based on the analyzing of decomposition to deviation of response. We can see: when $R^2 = 0$, $F = 0$; when $R^2 = 1$, $F \rightarrow \infty$; when R^2 is greater, F-value is greater.

$$F = \frac{\dfrac{R^2}{k-1}}{\dfrac{1-R^2}{n-k}} = \frac{n-k}{k-1} \frac{R^2}{1-R^2} \tag{12.21}$$

12.6.4   Residual Analysis

Residual analysis is a useful tool for checking whether the data meet the conditions of a model. Because a linear regression model is not always appropriate for the data, we should assess the appropriateness of the model by defining residuals and examining residual plots.

The residuals from a fitted model are defined as the differences between the response data and the fit to the response data at each predictor value.

Residual = Observed value − Predicted value, that is:

$$e_i = Y_i - \hat{Y}_i, \sum e = 0 \tag{12.22}$$

Under regular circumstances, the residuals e_i are normally distributed. The mean of this normal distribution is zero, and the variance equals to σ^2. The residuals plot is composed of standardized residuals as the vertical line and independent variable as the horizontal line.

$$e_i' = \frac{e_i}{\sqrt{MS_{res}}} \tag{12.23}$$

12.7　Application and Its Considerations

12.7.1　Application

12.7.1.1　Analysis of the Related Factors

For example, there are many factors that can affect hypertension, such as age, diet, habit, smoking, tension, family history, and so on. So, among those, it is necessary to find which factors are related and which can be discarded.

During clinical practice, it is sometimes difficult to ensure the agreement of all parameters of all groups, because of lots of complicated conditions. For example, the regression model can be used for comparing two different therapies, with the disagreement on age, the state of illness, and so on. An easy method to control confounding factors is to include these into a regression model and analyze them with other major variables.

12.7.1.2　Estimation and Prediction

For example, linear regression can be used to estimate the lung capacity by their weight and height; predicting infants' weights by their gestational age, diameter of head, diameter at breast height (DBH), and abdomen girth (AG).

12.7.1.3　Statistical Control, Back Run Estimation

For instance, when we use radio frequency therapy to treat brain tumors, the impaired diameter of pallium has linear relationship with the temperature of radio frequency and the exposure time. The regression model is established and it can help determine the optimal control of the temperature of radio frequency and the exposure time, by giving the impaired diameter of pallium in advance.

12.7.2　Considerations

12.7.2.1　Dummy Variables in Regression

Many important variables are not continuous but are measured as discrete categories and thus cannot be used as independent variables without adjustments. Examples of such variables include race, marital status, region, smoking, drug use, union membership, social class, and so on.

Dummy variable codes "1" to indicate the presence of an attribute and "0" its absence. The method of generating dummy variables for discrete variables: (a) Create and name one dummy variable for each of the K categories of the original discrete variable. (b) For each dummy variable, code a respondent "1" if he/she has that attribute, and "0" if lacking that attribute. (c) Every respondent will have a "1" for only one dummy, and "0" for the $K-1$ other dummy variables.

Given K dummy variables, if you know respondent's codes for $K-1$ dummies, then you also know that person's code for the Kth dummy! This linear dependency is similar to the degrees of freedom problem in ANOVA. Thus, to use a set of K dummy variables as predictors in a multiple regression model, you must omit one of them. Only $K-1$ dummies can be used in a regression model. For example, if the BMI is divided into three indicators: low weight, normal, and overweight, then only two dummies are needed. The results of the assignment of the dummies are as follows:

$$X_1 = \begin{cases} 1, \text{low-weight} \\ 0, \text{others} \end{cases} \qquad X_2 = \begin{cases} 1, \text{over-weight} \\ 0, \text{others} \end{cases}$$

Table 12.7　Dummy Variable Scheme

BMI	Dummy variable	
	X_1	X_2
Low weight	1	0
Overweight	0	1
Normal	0	0

If $X_1 = X_2 = 0$, that is, in the "other" item, it means "normal." We could use this dummy variable scheme, where "normal" is the reference category.

12.7.2.2 Multicollinearity

Multicollinearity is a high degree of correlation between supposedly independent variables in a multiple regression model. For example, diabetic nephropathy and age, weight, the levels of blood glucose, and so on. Those explanatory variables are strongly related which makes the LSE out of use in linear regression model.

By carrying out a correlation analysis before we fit the regression models, we can see which, if any, of the explanatory variables are very highly correlated, and try to avoid this problem (or at least this will indicate why estimates of regression coefficients may give values very different from those we might expect). For pairs of explanatory variables which have very high correlations—variance inflation factor (VIF) > 10 or tolerance < 0.1, we could consider dropping one of the explanatory variables from the model.

Multicollinearity can lead to skewed or misleading results:

(a) Standard error of the test statistic becomes large; therefore, t-value becomes small.

(b) Regression model becomes unstable. The estimation of regression coefficients could change significantly when the observed datum is increased or decreased.

(a) Inaccuracy of t-test can cause some important variables to be discarded when they should be involved in the model.

(d) There are inconsistent positive and negative estimations compared with the objective reality.

The methods of elimination of multicollinearity include discarding the explanatory variable which makes collinearity, rebuild the regression equation, and use stepwise regression.

Table 12. 8   Multicollinearity Statistics

Variable	Condition index	VIF	Tolerance
Age	5. 718	1. 021	0. 979
BMI	11. 398	1. 051	0. 952
ALB	36. 949	1. 050	0. 952

Using SPSS to obtain the condition index, VIF, and tolerance of Example 12. 1. The results are given in Table 12. 8: the VIF is less than 10, so it can be considered that there is no multicollinearity in the data of this example.

12. 7. 2. 3   The Interaction between Variables

In order to test whether there is a multiplicative interaction between the two independent variables, we usually add the product of them into the equation.

In analyzing the data in Table 12. 2, we have chosen three variables: age (X_1), BMI (X_2), and ALB (X_3). And now we add $X_1 \times X_2$ into the model. If the product $(X_1 \times X_2)$ is statistically significant, it means that there is an interaction between the age and the BMI. Therefore, we should define the new variable $Z(Z = X_1 \times X_2)$, and estimate the test statistic according to the new model $(Y_{hat} = b_0 + b_1 X_1 + b_2 X_2 + b_3 X_3 + b_z Z)$. If the hypothetic test is rejected $H_0: \beta_Z = 0$, it could be concluded that there exists an interactive effect outside the main effect of X_1 and X_2. In this case, the conclusion is that the use of Z is statistically significant $(P = 0. 047)$. $Y_{hat} = 63. 684 + 0. 574 X_1 + 0. 620 X_2 + 0. 447 X_3 - 0. 003 Z$, which means that the effect of BMI in populations relies on the age.

12. 7. 2. 4   Stepwise Regression

Do not trust the result of stepwise blindly. The so called "best" regression equation is not by all means the best. The variable excluded from the model does not mean that it has no statistical significance. Which regression model to use is decided by experience.

(Wu Siying, Yi Honggang, Maria Haleem)

Question Bank

Chapter 13　Multiple Logistic Regression

13. 1　Introduction

The purpose of many medical research projects is to assess the relationships among a set of variables and regression techniques often used as statistical analysis tools in the study of such relationships. In most cases, one variable is usually the response or dependent variable. That is, a variable to be predicted from or explained by other variables. The other variables are called predictors, explanatory variables, or independent variables.

In multiple linear regression, the dependent variable of interest is a continuous variable which we assume, perhaps after an appropriate transformation, to be normally distributed. However, in a variety of other applications, the dependent variable of interest is not on a continuous scale; it may have only two possible outcomes, and therefore can be represented by an indicator variable taking on values 0 and 1. This kind of variable, such as ill and healthy, dead and alive, recover and not recover, do not follow a normal distribution. In this situation, logistic regression is a choice.

13. 2　Binary Logistic Regression Model

Logistic regression is a mathematical modeling approach that can be used to describe the relationship of several predictor variables X_1, X_2, $\cdots$, X_m to a dichotomous dependent variable Y, where Y is typically coded as 1 or 0 for its possible categories. The logistic model describes the expected value of $Y(E(Y))$ in terms of the following "logistic" formula:

$$E(Y) = \frac{1}{1 + \exp[-(\beta_0 + \beta_1 X_1 + \beta_2 X_2 + \cdots + \beta_m X_m)]} \tag{13.1}$$

For $(0,1)$ random variables, such as Y, it follows from basic statistical principles about expected values that $E(Y)$ is equivalent to the probability $P(Y=1)$; so the formula for the logistic model can be written in a form that describes the probability of occurrence of one of two possible outcomes of Y(denoted as $P=P(y=1)$), as follows:

$$P = P(Y = 1) = \frac{1}{1 + \exp[-(\beta_0 + \beta_1 X_1 + \beta_2 X_2 + \cdots + \beta_m X_m)]} \tag{13.2a}$$

or

$$P = P(Y = 1) = \frac{\exp[(\beta_0 + \beta_1 X_1 + \beta_2 X_2 + \cdots + \beta_m X_m)]}{1 + \exp[(\beta_0 + \beta_1 X_1 + \beta_2 X_2 + \cdots + \beta_m X_m)]} \tag{13.2b}$$

or

$$\ln(\frac{P}{1-P}) = \beta_0 + \beta_1 X_1 + \beta_2 X_2 + \cdots + \beta_m X_m \tag{13.2c}$$

or

$$\text{logit}(P) = \beta_0 + \beta_1 X_1 + \beta_2 X_2 + \cdots + \beta_m X_m \tag{13.2d}$$

where $\frac{P}{1-P}$ is so-called odds, and $\ln \frac{P}{1-P}$ is the logarithm of odds, called "logit of P."
Formula (13.2c) is called the logit form of the model.

Then set up a linear regression for Z, that is,

$$Z = \beta_0 + \beta_1 X_1 + \beta_2 X_2 + \cdots + \beta_m X_m \tag{13.3}$$

The relationship between Z and P is shown as Figure 13.1, the Z varies from $-\infty$ to $+\infty$, the values of P range from 0 to 1.

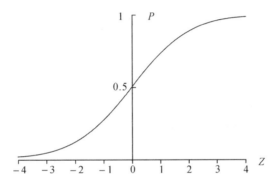

Figure 13.1　The Relationship between Z and P

13.3　Estimating the Odds Ratio Using Logistic Regression

To obtain an expression for the odds ratio from a logistic model, we must compare the odds for two groups of individuals. For example, if Y denotes lung cancer status (1=yes, 0=no) and there is only one (i.e. $m=1$) predictor X_1—say, smoking statues (1=smoker, 0=non-smoker)—then the logistic model can be written equivalently in logit form as

$$\ln(\frac{P}{1-P}) = \ln(\text{odds}) = \beta_0 + \beta_1 (\text{smoking status})$$

Thus for this example, the ln (odds) for smokers and non-smokers can be written as

$$\ln(\text{smokers}) = \beta_0 + \beta_1 \times 1 = \beta_0 + \beta_1$$

and

$$\ln(\text{non-smokers}) = \beta_0 + \beta_1 \times 0 = \beta_0$$

respectively. It follows that the odds ratio comparing smokers to non-smokers is given by

$$OR_{\text{S vs. NS}} = \frac{\text{odds(smokers)}}{\text{odds(non-smokers)}} = \frac{e^{\beta_0 + \beta_1}}{e^{\beta_0}} = e^{\beta_1} \tag{13.4}$$

In other words, for the simple example involving one (0−1) predictor, the odds ratio compares the two categories and the predictor is obtained by exponentiating the coefficient of the predictor in the logistic model.

Generally, when computing an odds ratio, we can define the two groups (or individuals) that are to be compared in terms of two different specifications of the set of predictors X_1, X_2, $\cdots$, X_m. We do this by letting $X_A = (X_{A1}, X_{A2}, \cdots, X_{Am})$ and $X_B = (X_{B1}, X_{B2}, \cdots, X_{Bm})$ denote the collection of X's for groups (or individuals) A and B, respectively. To obtain a general formula for the odds ratio, we must divide the odds for group (or individual) A by the odds for the group (or individual) B and then substitute the logit form of the logistic model given by Formula (13.2c), to obtain an expression involving the logistic model parameters. From the algebra, the following result is obtained:

$$OR_{X_A \text{ vs. } X_B} = \frac{\text{Odds for } X_A}{\text{Odds for } X_B} = \frac{e^{(\beta_0 + \sum_{j=1}^{m} \beta_j X_{Aj})}}{e^{(\beta_0 + \sum_{j=1}^{m} \beta_j X_{Bj})}} = e^{\sum_{j=1}^{m} \beta_j (X_{Aj} - X_{Bj})} \qquad (13.5)$$

For example, if X_A and X_B are specifications of the three variables smoking status (X_1, 1 = smoker, 0 = non-smoker), age (X_2, continuous), and gender (X_3, 1 = male, 0 = female), so that $X_A = (1, 45, 1)$ and $X_B = (0, 45, 1)$, then

$$OR_{X_A \text{ vs. } X_B} = e^{(1-0)\beta_1 + (45-45)\beta_2 + (1-1)\beta_3} = e^{\beta_1}$$

In this example, the smoking status variable changes from 1 in Group A to 0 in Group B, whereas the other variables remain the same for group—namely, age is 45 and gender is 1. In general, whenever only one variable (e.g. smoking) changes, while the other variables are fixed, we say that the odds ratio comparing two categories of the changing variable (e.g. smokers versus non-smokers) is an adjusted odds ratio that controls the other variables (i.e. those that are fixed at specific values) in the model. The variable of interest—in this case, smoking status—is often referred to as the exposure (or study) variable; the other variables in the model are called the control (or confounder) variables.

13.4 Parameter Estimation

The maximum likelihood (ML) method is often used in parameter estimation of logistic regression. A likelihood function or logarithmic likelihood function is set up first, and then the values of parameters that maximize the likelihood function or logarithmic likelihood function are found. ML estimates of the regression coefficients are typically obtained by using standard computer packages for logistic regression. These estimates can be used in appropriate odds ratio formulae based on Formula (13.3) to obtain numerical values for adjusted odds ratios. Since these are point estimates, researchers typically carry out statistical inferences about the odds ratios that are being estimated. For example, if the adjusted odds ratio is given by the simple expression e^{β_1}, involving a single coefficient, then the null hypothesis that this odds ratio equals 1 can be stated equivalently as $H_0: \beta_1 = 0$, since, under $H_0: e^{\beta_1} = e^0 = 1$. The test for this null hypothesis can be carried out by using the Wald test or the likelihood ratio test described below on ML estimation methods. A CI for the adjusted odds ratio can be obtained by the formula:

$$\exp(\hat{\beta}_1 \pm Z_{\frac{\alpha}{2}} S_{\hat{\beta}_1}) \qquad (13.6)$$

where $\hat{\beta}_1$ is the ML estimate of β_1, $S_{\hat{\beta}_1}$ is the standard error of $\hat{\beta}_1$, and the confidence level is $1-\alpha$.

Example 13.1   In a case-control study of risk factors related to cancer of the esophagus, the data of two risk factors are listed in Table 13.1.

Table 13.1   A Case-Control Study Data of Risk Factors Related to Cancer of the Esophagus

Smoking status (X_1)	Alcohol use (X_2)	Case $(Y=1)$	Control $(Y=0)$
Smoking	Drinking $(X_2=1)$	265	151
$(X_1=1)$	Non-drinking $(X_2=0)$	44	57
Non-smoking	Drinking $(X_2=1)$	63	107
$(X_1=0)$	Non-drinking $(X_2=0)$	63	136

Figure 13.2 of computer output comes from fitting SPSS's binary logistic regression procedure for a logistic regression model that regresses the dependent variable case-control on the covariates smoking status and alcohol use.

Variables in the Equation

		B	SE	$Wald$	df	$sig.$	$\exp(B)$	95% CI for $\exp(B)$ Lower bound	95% CI for $\exp(B)$ Upper bound
Step 1[a]	X_1	0.886	0.150	34.862	1	0.000	2.424	1.807	3.253
	X_2	0.526	0.157	11.207	1	0.001	1.692	1.244	2.303
	Constant	−0.910	0.136	44.870	1	0.000	0.403	—	—

a. Variable(s) entered on step 1: X_1, X_2.

Figure 13.2   The Results of Coefficients (B), Wald Test $(Wald)$, OR $(\exp(B))$, and 95% CI for OR

From Figure 13.2, we can see that the ML coefficients obtained for the fitted model are:

$$\hat{\beta}_1 = 0.886, \hat{\beta}_2 = 0.526,$$
$$S_{\hat{\beta}_1} = 0.150, S_{\hat{\beta}_2} = 0.157$$

So the fitted model is given (in logit form) by

$$\text{logit}(P) = -0.910 + 0.886X_1 + 0.526X_2$$

Based on this fitted model and the information provided in the computer output, we then obtain the following value for the adjusted odds ratio:

$$\hat{OR}_{(X_1=1 \text{ vs. } X_1=0|X_2)} = e^{0.886} = 2.424$$
$$\hat{OR}_{(X_2=1 \text{ vs. } X_2=0|X_1)} = e^{0.526} = 1.692$$

A 95% CI for e^{β_1} and e^{β_2} can be obtained respectively.

$$\exp(0.886 \pm 1.96 \times 0.150) = (1.807, 3.253)$$
$$\exp(0.526 \pm 1.96 \times 0.157) = (1.244, 2.303)$$

13.5   Hypothesis Test of Coefficients

Once we have fitted a multiple logistic regression model and obtained estimates for the various parameters of interest, we want to answer questions about the contributions of various factors to the prediction of the binary response variable. There are three types of such questions:

(a) Overall test. Taken collectively, does the entire set of explanatory or independent variables contribute significantly to the prediction of response?

(b) Test for the value of a single factor. Does the addition of one particular variable of interest add significantly to the prediction of response over and above that which was achieved by other independent variables?

(c) Test for the contribution of a group of variables. Does the addition of a group of variables add significantly to the prediction of response over and above that which was achieved by other independent variables?

Here we discuss the second question: After the estimation of regression coefficients, is the population coefficient zero-hypothesis test of coefficients?

Usually, there are three methods for a hypothesis test of coefficients, which are the Wald test, likelihood ratio test, and score test.

(a) Wald test. The hypothesis being tested is:

$$H_0: \beta_i = 0$$
$$H_1: \beta_i \neq 0$$

The test statistic, which is called Wald χ^2, is

$$\chi_i^2 = \left[\frac{\hat{\beta}_i}{SE(\hat{\beta}_i)}\right]^2$$

where $\hat{\beta}_i$ is an estimated value of the regression coefficient β_i, and SE is the standard error of $\hat{\beta}_i$. When H_0 is true, if the sample size is large enough, then the statistic approximately follows a chi-square distribution with one degree of freedom. Based on the information provided in the computer output (Figure 13.2), we find that Wald chi-square statistic corresponding to the X_1 (smoking status) variable is 34.862, $P < 0.001$, and H_0 is rejected so that the population coefficient for X_1 is not equal to zero. Also, Wald chi-square statistic corresponding to the X_2 (alcohol use) variable is 11.207, $P = 0.001$, and H_0 is rejected so that the population coefficient for X_2 is not equal to zero.

(b) Likelihood ratio test. The likelihood ratio test of the same null hypothesis would require subtracting the log-likelihood statistic for model from the log-likelihood statistic for "reduced" model. Denote the maximum log-likelihood by the $\ln L$. The test statistics being used to describe the difference in terms of fitness between the two models is

$$G = 2(\ln L_1 - \ln L_0)$$

where $\ln L_1$ refers to model 1 with P variables, $\ln L_0$ refers to model 2 with l variables, $P > l$.

It can be proved, for large samples, when H_0 is true, G follows a chi-square distribution with degrees of freedom of $v=P-l$. Using SPSS, we can obtain

$$\ln L(X_1) = -585.326, \ln L(X_2) = -597.436, \ln L(X_1, X_2) = -579.711$$

For X_1:

$$H_0 : \beta_1 = 0$$
$$H_1 : \beta_1 \neq 0$$
$$G_1 = 2[\ln L(X_1, X_2) - \ln L(X_2)] = 2[-579.711 - (-597.436)] = 35.45$$
$$\chi_{0.05,1}^2 = 3.84, G_1 > 3.84, P < 0.05.$$

For X_2:

$$H_0 : \beta_1 = 0$$
$$H_1 : \beta_1 \neq 0$$
$$G_2 = 2[\ln L(X_1, X_2) - \ln L(X_1)] = 2[-579.711 - (-585.326)] = 11.23$$
$$\chi_{0.05,1}^2 = 3.84, G_2 > 3.84, P < 0.05.$$

The conclusion is the same as Wald test above.

(3) Score test. The score test would require calculating a statistic through a vector, which is called a score. Here we do not give the formula.

It can be proved, under H_0, the three test statistics of Wald test, likelihood ratio test, and score test are asymptotically equivalent. For large sample sizes, the values of the three test statistics tend to be close to each other.

13.6　Independent Variables Selection

We wish to identify from many available factors a small subset of factors that relate significantly to the outcome. Similar to the multiple linear regression, the methods of independent variable selection for logistic regression are forward selection, backward elimination, and stepwise regression, using test statistics being one of the likelihood ratio statistics, Wald statistics, and score statistics.

Example 13.2　In order to find the risk factors related to the occurrence of coronary heart disease, a case-control study was conducted on 26 patients with coronary heart disease and 28 controls. The description and data on various risk factors are shown in Table 13.2 and Table 13.3.

The computer output of Figure 13.2 comes from fitting SPSS's binary logistic regression procedure for a logistic regression model that regresses the dependent variable Y on the covariates $(X_1 - X_8)$, forward stepwise (Wald test), probability of entry = 0.05, probability of removal = 0.10.

From this information (Figure 13.3), we can see that four risk factors had been selected for the model. There are age (X_1), hyperlipidemia history (X_5), animal fat intake amount (X_6), and type A personality (X_8).

Variables in the Equation

		B	SE	Wald	df	sig.	exp(B)	95% CI for exp(B)	
								Lower bound	Upper bound
Step 4[a]	X_1	0.924	0.477	3.758	1	0.053	2.519	0.990	6.411
	X_5	1.496	0.744	4.044	1	0.044	4.464	1.039	19.181
	X_6	3.135	1.249	6.303	1	0.012	23.000	1.989	265.945
	X_8	1.947	0.847	5.289	1	0.021	7.008	1.333	36.834
	Constant	−4.705	1.543	9.295	1	0.002	0.009		

a. Variable(s) entered on step 4: X_1.

Figure 13.3　The Results of Coefficients (B), Wald Test ($Wald$), OR (exp (B)), and 95% CI for OR

Table 13.2　Eight Possible Risks Factors and Code for Coronary Heart Disease Study

Factors	Variable	Encoding
Age/years	X_1	<45=1, 45~54=2, 55~64=3, ≥65=4
Hypertension history	X_2	None=0, have=1
Hypertension family history	X_3	None=0, have=1
Smoking	X_4	Non-smoking=0, smoking=1
Hyperlipidemia history	X_5	None=0, have=1
Animal fat intake	X_6	Low=0, high=1
BMI	X_7	<24=1, 24~25=2, ≥26=3
Type A personality	X_8	No=0, yes=1
Coronary heart disease	Y	Control=0, case=1

Table 13.3　Data on Case-Control Study on Risk Factors of Coronary Heart Disease

No.	X_1	X_2	X_3	X_4	X_5	X_6	X_7	X_8	Y
1	3	1	0	1	0	0	1	1	0
2	2	0	1	1	0	0	1	0	0
3	2	1	0	1	0	0	1	0	0
4	2	0	0	1	0	0	1	0	0
5	3	0	0	1	0	1	1	1	0
6	3	0	1	1	0	0	2	1	0
7	2	0	1	0	0	0	1	0	0
8	3	0	1	1	1	0	1	0	0
9	2	0	0	0	0	0	1	1	0

Continued

No.	X_1	X_2	X_3	X_4	X_5	X_6	X_7	X_8	Y
10	1	0	0	1	0	0	1	0	0
11	1	0	1	0	0	0	1	1	0
12	1	0	0	0	0	0	2	1	0
13	2	0	0	0	0	0	1	0	0
14	4	1	0	1	0	0	1	0	0
15	3	0	1	1	0	0	1	1	0
16	1	0	0	1	0	0	3	1	0
17	2	0	0	1	0	0	1	0	0
18	1	0	0	1	0	0	1	1	0
19	3	1	1	1	1	0	1	0	0
20	2	1	1	1	1	0	2	0	0
21	3	1	0	1	0	0	1	0	0
22	2	1	1	0	1	0	3	1	0
23	2	0	0	1	1	0	1	1	0
24	2	0	0	0	0	0	1	0	0
25	2	0	1	0	0	0	1	0	0
26	2	0	0	1	1	0	1	1	0
27	2	0	0	0	0	0	1	0	0
28	2	0	0	0	0	0	2	1	0
29	2	1	1	1	0	1	2	1	1
30	3	0	0	1	1	1	2	1	1
31	2	0	0	1	1	1	1	0	1
32	3	1	1	1	1	1	3	1	1
33	2	0	0	1	0	0	1	1	1
34	2	0	1	0	1	1	1	1	1
35	2	0	0	1	0	1	1	0	1
36	2	1	1	1	1	0	1	1	1
37	3	1	1	1	1	0	1	1	1
38	3	1	1	1	0	1	1	1	1
39	3	1	1	1	1	0	1	1	1

Continued

No.	X_1	X_2	X_3	X_4	X_5	X_6	X_7	X_8	Y
40	3	0	1	0	0	0	1	0	1
41	2	1	1	1	1	0	2	1	1
42	3	1	0	1	0	1	2	1	1
43	3	1	0	1	0	0	1	1	1
44	3	1	1	1	1	1	2	0	1
45	4	0	0	1	1	0	3	1	1
46	3	1	1	1	1	0	3	1	1
47	4	1	1	1	1	0	3	0	1
48	3	0	1	1	1	0	1	1	1
49	4	0	0	1	0	0	2	1	1
50	1	0	1	1	1	0	2	1	1
51	2	0	1	1	0	1	2	1	1
52	2	1	1	1	0	0	2	1	1
53	2	1	0	1	0	0	1	1	1
54	3	1	1	0	1	0	3	1	1

13.7　Goodness-of-Fit for Model

Usually, the value of log-likelihood function shows goodness-of-fit for the model. The larger the value of log-likelihood function, the better the fit. It can be proved, for a large sample, when H_0 is true, $-2\ln L$ follows a chi-square distribution with degrees of freedom ($v = N - k - 1$). Here N is the sample size, k is the number of explanatory variables in model.

When $-2\ln L \approx \chi^2 > \chi^2_{\alpha,v}$, the null hypothesis ($H_0$: The model fits the data) is rejected. It means the model does not fit the observed data and is not suitable to be used for prediction.

There are several other indices, such as Cox-Snell R-square (R^2) and Nagelkerke max-rescaled R-square (R^2_{res}), which can be obtained from statistical software, in practical use. However, they are controversial and lack a method of statistical testing. Nevertheless, they are intuitive and convenient because they have similar formats as the concepts in OLS.

The formula can be expressed as

$$R^2 = 1 - \left\{ \frac{L_0}{L_1} \right\}^{\frac{2}{n}} \qquad 0 \leqslant R^2 < 1 \tag{13.7}$$

$$R^2_{res} = \frac{R^2}{R^2_{max}} \qquad 0 \leqslant R^2_{res} \leqslant 1 \tag{13.8}$$

The following Figure 13. 4 of computer output comes from fitting SPSS's binary logistic regression procedure for Example 13. 1.

Model Summary

Step	-2Log-likelihood	Cox & Snell R-Square	Nagelkerke R-Square
2	1159. 422[a]	0. 074	0. 099

a. Estimation terminated at iteration number 3 because parameter estimates changed by less than 0. 001.

Figure 13. 4   Model Summary

From Figure 13. 4: $-2\ln L=1,159.422$, $\upsilon=886-2-1=883$, $P>0.05$, H_0 cannot be rejected, which means the model fits the data. $R^2=0.074$, $R^2_{res}=0.099$.

13.8   Applications and Considerations

The applications of logistic regression model may be summarized as follows:

(a) Screening of disease-related risk factors. As discussed before, the logistic regression model has its advantage in multiple factor analysis of disease etiological study. It is suitable to screen disease-related risk factors from many potential factors, as well as to analyze the interaction between different risk factors.

(b) Adjustment of confounding factors. In the studies of clinical medicine and epidemiology, there are confounding impacts of some non-study-interest factors on study factors frequently. They may bias the evaluation of the treatment effect. It is very convenient to control the confounding factors and to estimate the odds ratio and the CI by using the logistic regression model.

(c) Prediction and discrimination. Same as other regression analysis, logistic regression may be used for prediction. Logistic regression is a probability model and the probability of an event occurrence under certain conditions can be calculated for discrimination.

In the logistic analysis, we should pay attention to the following situations:

(a) Sample size. As the number of independent variables increases, the number of cross categorized levels between variables will increase rapidly. Therefore, a large enough sample size is necessary to ensure the stability of parameter estimation. In practice, the sample size may be 20 times above the number of independent variables.

(b) Value of variable. The independent variable in a logistic regression model may be a continuous variable, category variable, and ordinal variable. If the independent variable is a multi-level categorical variable, we may use several dummy variables to replace it. If the independent variable is a continuous variable, it is often transformed into an ordinal variable in order to be more easily explained.

(c) When matching on potential confounders is carried out in the selection of a subject, the conditional logistic regression model is recommended. When the dependent variable is an ordinal variable or multi-level categorical variable, the ordinal logistic regression model (cumulative logistic regression model) or the multinomial logistic regression model is recommended, respectively.

(**Wang Lesan, Liao Qi, Minyao Ng Derry, Anny Mamuchashvili**)

Question Bank

Chapter 14　Survival Analysis

14.1　Introduction

As demonstrated in the previous chapter, a multiple logistic regression model is one of most commonly and widely used statistical methods in research. Usually, this model is applied to estimate the association between a specific exposure and the outcome of interest, with a focus on comparing the odds of the disease between the exposed population and unexposed controls; this model cannot answer whether the disease is really induced by the exposure. To solve this problem, investigators should apply a prospective longitudinal study in which a single baseline and several follow-up measurements on the outcome are collected. The data obtained in a longitudinal study is also called lifetime data. In statistics, lifetime data can be used to validate the causal relationship between the exposure and the outcome by fully investigating associations of the outcome with exposure as well as the exposed duration.

In this condition, a novel statistical approach known as survival analysis should be applied instead of a multiple logistic regression model. This chapter briefly introduces the basic concepts, principles, and practical applications of survival analysis, including the Kaplan-Meier survival curve, the log-rank test for comparing two groups, the hazard ratio for data summary, and the Cox proportional hazards regression model, which replaces linear regression when continuous outcome data are survival times with censored observation. We hope this approach will be helpful for readers to understand and grasp this method.

14.2　Survival Data

Many applications in biostatistics involve modeling lifetime data. In these applications the outcome of interest is the time, T, until some "critical event" occurs. This event may be death, the appearance of a tumor, the development of some disease, recurrence of a disease, conception, cessation of smoking, or others. Even when the final outcome is not actual survival time, the length of time from entering the study to when the critical event occurs is called the survival time, or failure time. Survival data includes complete data and censored data. In complete data, end point events can be observed throughout the follow-up study; in other words, the survival time for complete data spans the start point to the end point for observation. In censored data, observations of a patient's end point event did not occur or were censored for some reason during follow-up (Figure 14.1).

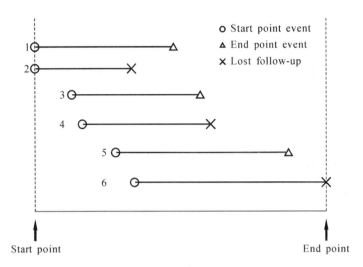

Figure 14. 1   A Schematic of Completed and Censored Data in Survival Analysis

There are three main reasons for censored data:

(a) Loss to follow-up. Contact with the patient is lost. For example, the patient does not reply to the questionnaires; the patient is absent from the house during home interviews; the patient does not respond to telephone interviews or moves to another place with an unknown address; and so forth.

(b) Dropping out. The patient withdraws from research. For example, accidental death, the patient died of other diseases or undergoes a temporary change of treatment plan, and so forth.

(c) Termination. The study period has expired and the observation is terminated. This is common in clinical trials and animal experiments. A distinguishing feature of survival data is the inevitable presence of "censored" observations. Censored observations arise in patients who are included in the study but for whom the critical event of interest has not yet been observed; instead, it is only known that this event is at least later than a given point in time. The techniques employed with such data are conventionally termed "survival" analysis methods.

Clinical follow-up data or survival data may have the following characteristics:

(a) Therapeutic indices include both outcome variable and time variables.

(b) Subjects in the follow-up study may be lost or die from other diseases.

(c) The study might be terminated prematurely due to research funding and time constraints.

In this situation, it is not possible to prolong the study until all the subjects have an outcome, inevitably resulting in incomplete information provided by some of the follow-up subjects. Disregarding the use of this data would result in loss of information.

14.3   Basic Concepts of Survival Analysis

14.3.1   Survival Time

Traditionally, survival time is defined as the duration between the two-time points of a participant's enrollment in a prospective cohort study. In modern usage, the meaning of "survival" is not restricted to being alive, and this term has been largely expanded to many other terminal events (e. g. surviving without the recurrence of cancer).

Example 14.1   Table 14.1 provides raw data on the postoperative recurrence of patients with breast cancer. This table is based on data collected from January 1, 1999 to March 31, 2009. Survival times are from the date of surgery to the date of recurrence of breast cancer.

Table 14.1   The Recurrence Data of Patients with Breast Cancer

from 1999 to 2009 (only 7 observations are shown)

Patient No.	Begin	End	Survival time	Outcome
1	2003-09-06	2004-05-19	8	Censored
2	2006-02-09	2008-02-01	24	Censored
3	2006-02-17	2009-04-24	38	Censored
4	2003-09-30	2009-04-25	67	Censored
5	2005-12-22	2008-07-01	30	Recurrent
6	2001-07-20	2003-07-21	24	Recurrent
7	2003-07-25	2004-11-15	15	Recurrent
...	...	...	...	...

14.3.2   Censored Data

Most survival data sets include some patients who are known to have survived up to a certain point in time, but whose survival status past that point is not known. Their data are designated as censored. Censored observations can arise in three ways:

(a) The patient is known to be alive when the trial analysis is carried out.

(b) The patient was known to be alive at some past follow-up, but the investigator has since lost track of him or her.

(c) The patient has died from causes totally unrelated to the disease in question.

Most survival time data are right-censored, because the true survival time interval, which is unknow in practice, has been cut off (i. e. censored) at the right side of the observed time interval, making an observed survival time shorter than the unknown true survival time. The event of interest is known to be later than a certain point in time, but we do not know the survival time exactly. In Table 14.1 these patients would be patient Nos. 1, 2, 3, and 4.

14.3.3 Survival Function

The basic quantity employed to describe time-to-event phenomena is the survival function. This function, also known as the cumulative survival rate, is the probability of an individual surviving from time 0 up to time t for each $t \geq 0$. It is defined as

$$S(t) = Pr(T \geq t) = \frac{\text{Number of subjects surviving at time }(t)}{\text{Total number of subjects}} \qquad (14.1)$$

Note that the survival function is a nonincreasing function with a value of 1 at the origin and 0 as t approaches infinity (the mortality rate is 100% if we wait long enough) (Figure 14.2).

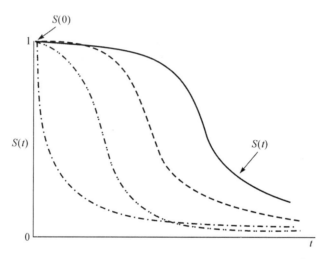

Figure 14.2 The General Shapes for Survival Functions

14.3.4 Median Survival Time

A useful summary of a survival data is the median survival time. Approximately 50% of the population under study could be expected to survive beyond the median. More formally, the median survival time is defined as

$$M = F^{-1}(0.5) \qquad (14.2)$$

where $F(t)$ is the probability of surviving less than or equal to time t. Note that the cumulative distribution function $F(t)$ is the complement of the survival function $S(t)$, that is, $F(t) = 1 - S(t)$. The median survival is used considerably more frequently than the mean as a summary statistic because of the difficulties in estimating means from heavily censored data. The estimated median survival time is $\hat{M} = \hat{F}^{-1}(0.5)$, which is the maximum observed event time where the estimated $\hat{F}(t)$ is not greater than 0.5.

14.3.5   Hazard Function

The hazard function, $h(t)$, also known as the hazard rate, is the instantaneous probability of having an event at time t, given that one has survived (i. e. has not had an event) up to time t. In particular,

$$h(t) = \frac{\left[\dfrac{S(t) - S(t+\Delta t)}{\Delta t}\right]}{S(t)} \text{ as } \Delta t \text{ approaches } 0 \tag{14.3}$$

The hazard function is particularly useful for describing the way in which the chance of experiencing critical event changes with time. The hazard rate can have many general shapes. Some generic types of hazard rates are increasing, decreasing, constant, bathtub-shaped, or hump-shaped (Figure 14.3).

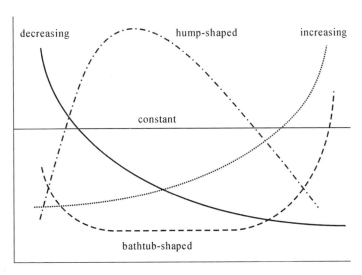

Figure 14.3   The General Shapes for Hazard Functions

Most population mortality data follow a bathtub-shaped hazard function: early in the process, deaths result primarily from infant diseases; then the death rate stabilizes; later, an increasing hazard rate sets in, due to the natural aging process. If the hazard rate increases early and eventually begins to decline, then the hazard is termed "hump-shaped." This type of hazard rate is often used to model survival after successful surgery where risk increases initially due to infection, hemorrhaging, or other complications just after the procedure, and then risk steadily decreases as the patient recovers.

Example 14.2   Based on US life table data in 1986, there were 100,000 men at age 0 of whom 80,908 survived to age 60, 79,539 survived to age 61, 34,789 survived to age 80, and 31,739 survived to age 81. Compute the approximate mortality hazard at ages 60 and 80, respectively, for US men in 1986.

Solution: there were 80,908 men who survived to age 60, and 79,539 men who survived to age 61. Therefore, the hazard at age 60 is approximately

$$h(60) = \frac{80,908 - 79,539}{80,908} = 0.017$$

Similarly, because 34,789 men survived to age 80, and 31,739 men survived to age 81, the hazard at age 80 is approximately given by

$$h(80) = \frac{34,789 - 31,739}{34,789} = 0.088$$

Thus, in words, the probability of dying in the next year is 1.7% for men who survived to age 60, and 8.8% for men who survived to age 80. The percentages 1.7% and 8.8% represent the approximate hazard at ages 60 and 80, respectively. To improve the approximation, time intervals shorter than 1 year must be considered.

14.4　Methods of Survival Analysis

For special survival data, it is easy to get the wrong statistical inference if using the classical statistical method to compare the curative effect. Although the survival time provided by censored data is incomplete, it indicates that the patient did not die during the period observed, and the true survival time can only be longer than the observed time. More importantly, it is difficult to handle incomplete data using classical statistical methods.

For survival data, the method of survival analysis is often used. This analysis method considers both the outcome and the survival time, and can make full use of incomplete data to form statistical description and statistical inference of the distribution characteristics of survival time. The main influencing factors of survival time can also be analyzed by the multi-factor model. Survival analysis is the only method that can comprehensively and accurately evaluate clinical follow-up data.

14.4.1　The Main Contents of Survival Analysis

(a) Describing the survival process. The survival analysis describes the survival process, studying the distribution characteristics of survival time, estimating survival rate and average survival time, and drawing survival curves. The survival rate at any point in time can be estimated, and the median survival time can be estimated according to the survival rate. Besides, survival characteristics can also be analyzed according to the survival curve.

(b) Comparative survival process. The survival process of a population can be explored by comparing the survival rate and its standard error to every sample. For example, comparing the positive and negative effects of bcl-2 and p53 protein expression on the breast cancer survival rate discovered important biomarkers that affect breast cancer survival.

(c) Analysis of factors affecting survival time. The emphasis is on exploring the factors that affect the survival time and outcome through the survival analysis model. Usually, survival time and outcome are dependent variables, and the factors affecting them are used as independent variables, such as age, gender, pathological type, lymph node metastasis, treatment plan, and whether the gene expression is positive. By fitting the survival analysis model, the protective factors and risk factors affecting survival time are screened, providing an important reference for clinical treatment.

14.4.2   The Basic Methods of Survival Analysis

(a) Non-parametric method. The main characteristic of the non-parametric method is that the survival rate is only estimated according to the sequential statistics provided by the sample, regardless of how the data are distributed. Common estimation methods are the Kaplan-Meier method and the life table method. When comparing the survival rates of two or more groups, it is not valid to assume that the distributions of two or more groups' survival times are the same; rather, specific distribution patterns and parameters should be inferred.

(b) Parametric method. The parametric method is characterized by assuming that the survival time obeys a specific parameter distribution, and then analyzing the time that affects survival according to the characteristics of the hypothetical distribution. The commonly used methods are the exponential distribution method, the Weibull distribution method, the log-normal regression analysis method, and logistic regression analysis. The parametric method obtains an estimation of the survival rate from the estimated parameters of the distributions, and can make statistical inferences based on the parameters.

(c) Semi-parametric method. The semi-parametric method combines the characteristics of the parametric and non-parametric methods. It is mainly used to analyze the factors affecting survival time and survival rate. It is a multi-factor analysis method and its typical method is the Cox proportional-hazards model.

14.5   The Estimation of Survival Curves: The Kaplan-Meier Estimator

The Kaplan-Meier (KM) estimator, which is also called the product-limit estimator, is a non-parametric estimator that may be used to estimate the survival function from survival data including censored observations.

Suppose individuals in the study population are assessed at times $t_1, \cdots, t_k$ where the times do not have to be equally spaced. If we want to compute the probability of surviving up to time t_i, we can write this probability in the form:

$$S(t_i) = Prob(\text{surviving to time } t_i) = Prob(\text{surviving to time } t_1)$$
$$\times Prob(\text{surviving to time } t_2 \mid \text{surviving to time } t_i)$$
$$\vdots$$
$$\times Prob(\text{surviving to time } t_j \mid \text{surviving to time } t_{j-1})$$
$$\vdots$$

$$\times Prob(\text{surviving to time } t_i \mid \text{surviving to time } t_{i-1})$$

$$(14.4)$$

Example 14.3 In the data set of SMOKE.DAT at www.cengagebrain.com, 234 smokers who expressed a willingness to quit smoking were followed for 1 year to estimate the cumulative incidence of recidivism (i. e. the proportion of smokers who quit for a time but then started smoking again). The data in Table 14.2 were obtained after subdividing the study population by age ($>40/\leqslant40$).

Table 14.2 Days without Smoking by Age Groups

Age/years	Days without smoking					
	$\leqslant91$	$91\sim180$	$181\sim270$	$271\sim364$	365	Total
>40	92	4	4	1	19	120
$\leqslant40$	88	7	3	2	14	114
Total	180	11	7	3	33	234
Percentage/%	76.9	4.7	3.0	1.3	14.1	—

Estimate the survival curve for people more than 40 years old and less than or equal to 40 years old for the participants depicted in Table 14.2.

Solution:

For persons more than 40 years old,

$$S(90)=1-\frac{92}{120}=0.233$$

$$S(180)=S(90)\times\left(1-\frac{4}{28}\right)=0.200$$

$$S(270)=S(180)\times\left(1-\frac{4}{24}\right)=0.167$$

$$S(365)=S(270)\times\left(1-\frac{1}{20}\right)=0.159$$

For persons younger than or equal to 40 years old,

$$S(90)=1-\frac{88}{114}=0.228$$

$$S(180)=S(90)\times\left(1-\frac{7}{26}\right)=0.167$$

$$S(270)=S(180)\times\left(1-\frac{3}{19}\right)=0.141$$

$$S(365)=S(270)\times\left(1-\frac{2}{16}\right)=0.123$$

These survival curves are plotted in Figure 14.4. Participants older than 40 years old have a slightly higher estimated survival probability (i. e. probability of remaining a quitter) after the first 90 days.

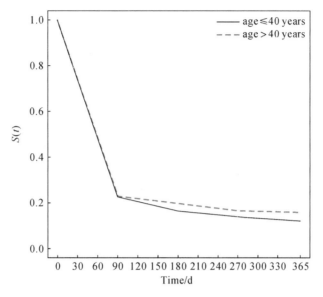

Figure 14. 4   The Survival Curves of Two Age Groups

In Example 14. 3, all individuals reach an end point during their period of follow-up. In other instances, some participants are not followed for the maximum period of follow-up but have not yet had an event. To estimate the survival function in the presence of censoring, suppose S_{t-1} patients have survived through time t_{i-1} and are not censored at time t_{i-1}. Among these patients, S_i patients survive, d_i patients fail, and l_i patients are censored at time t_i. Thus, $S_{t-1} = S_i + d_i + l_i$. We can estimate the probability of surviving to time t_i given that a patient has survived up to time t_{i-1} by $1 - \dfrac{d_i}{S_{t-1}} = 1 - \dfrac{d_i}{S_i + d_i + l_i}$. The l_i patients who are censored at time t_i do not contribute to the estimation of the survival function at time $> t_i$. However, these patients do contribute to the estimation of the survival function at time $\leqslant t_i$. The KM estimator of the survival probability at time t_i is

$$\hat{S}(t_i) = \left(1 - \frac{d_1}{S_0}\right) \times \left(1 - \frac{d_2}{S_1}\right) \times \cdots \times \left(1 - \frac{d_i}{S_{i-1}}\right), i = 1, \cdots, k \qquad (14.5)$$

Furthermore, the survival probability is assumed to remain constant between time t_{i-1} and t_i, i. e. at level $\hat{S}(t_{i-1})$.

Example 14. 4   A clinical trial was conducted to test the efficacy of different vitamin supplements in preventing visual loss in patients with retinitis pigmentosa (RP). Visual loss was measured by loss of retinal function as characterized by a 50% decline in the electroretinogram (ERG) 30 Hz amplitude, a measure of the electrical activity in the retina. In normal people, the normal range for ERG 30 Hz amplitude is $> 50 \mu$V. In patients with RP, ERG 30 Hz amplitude is usually $< 10 \mu$V and is often $< 1 \mu$V . Approximately 50% of patients with ERG 30 Hz amplitude near 0. 05 μV are legally blind compared with $< 10\%$ of patients whose ERG 30 Hz amplitude is near 1. 3 μV (the average ERG amplitude for patients in this clinical trial). Patients in the study were randomized to one of four treatment groups:

Group 1 received 15,000 IU of vitamin A and 3 IU (a trace amount) of vitamin E.

Group 2 received 75 IU (a trace amount) of vitamin A and 3 IU of vitamin E.

Group 3 received 15,000 IU of vitamin A and 400 IU of vitamin E.

Group 4 received 75 IU of vitamin A and 400 IU of vitamin E.

Let's call these four groups the A group, trace group, AE group, and E group, respectively. We want to compare the proportion of patients who fail (i.e. lose 50% of initial ERG 30 Hz amplitude) in different treatment groups. Patients were enrolled from 1984 to 1987, and follow-up was terminated in September 1991. Because follow-up was terminated at the same point in chronological time, the period of follow-up differed for each patient. Patients who entered the study early were followed for 6 years, whereas patients who enrolled in the study later were followed for 4 years. In addition, some patients dropped out of the study before September 1991 and had not failed. Dropouts were due to death, other diseases, side effects possibly due to the study medications, or unwillingness to comply (take study medications). Estimate the survival probability for each of six years for participants receiving 15,000 IU of vitamin A (i.e. groups A and AE combined) and participants receiving 75 IU of vitamin A (i.e. groups E and trace combined), respectively.

Solution: The calculations are given in Table 14.3. For example, for the participants receiving 15,000 IU of vitamin A, the survival probability at year 1 is 0.9826. The survival probability is assumed to remain constant between year 1 and year 2, i.e. $S(t) = 0.9826$ for $1 \leqslant t < 2$. The probability of surviving to year 2 given that one survived to year $1 = \frac{159}{165} = 0.9636$. Thus, the survival probability at year $2 = 0.9826 \times 0.9636 = 0.9468$, etc. These survival curves are plotted in Figure 14.5. The survival probabilities for the participants receiving 15,000 IU of vitamin A tend to be higher than that for the participants receiving 75 IU of vitamin A, particularly at year 6.

Table 14. 3   Survival Probabilities for Participants Receiving 15,000 IU
of Vitamin A and 75 IU of Vitamin A Daily, Respectively

Time	Fail	Censored	Survival	Total	Survival probability	$\hat{S}(t_i)$
15,000 IU daily						
1 year $= t_1$	3	4	165	172	0.9826	0.9826
2 years $= t_2$	6	0	159	165	0.9636	0.9468
3 years $= t_3$	15	1	143	159	0.9057	0.8575
4 years $= t_4$	21	26	96	143	0.8531	0.7316
5 years $= t_5$	15	35	46	96	0.8438	0.6173
6 years $= t_6$	5	41	0	46	0.8913	0.5502

Continued

Time	Fail	Censored	Survival	Total	Survival probability	$\hat{S}(t_i)$
75 IU daily						
1 year$=t_1$	8	0	174	182	0.9560	0.9560
2 years$=t_2$	13	3	158	174	0.9253	0.8846
3 years$=t_3$	21	2	135	158	0.8671	0.7670
4 years$=t_4$	21	28	86	135	0.8444	0.6477
5 years$=t_5$	13	31	42	86	0.8488	0.5498
6 years$=t_6$	13	29	0	42	0.6905	0.3796

Note: Survival probability $= \dfrac{\text{Number of subjects survived to time } t_i}{\text{Number of subjects survived up to time } t_{i-1}}$. A person fails if his or her ERG 30 Hz amplitude declines by at least 50% from baseline to any follow-up visit, regardless of any subsequent ERG values obtained after the visit where the failure occurs.

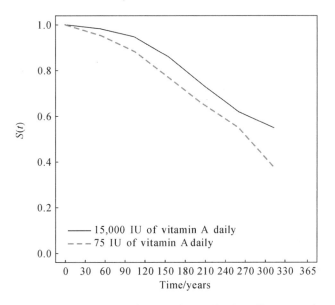

Figure 14. 5   The Survival Curves for Two Groups

Example 14. 5   The data for this example was derived from a study of the survival time of patients who underwent renal transplantation by two treatments. During the period of 1979—1982, 19 patients underwent renal transplantation to understand the survival time of kidney transplant recipients (Group 1). The starting time of follow-up is one day after operation, and the expected outcome is that the patient died of various causes related to kidney transplantation. From 1983 to 1986, another 14 cases were performed (Group 2). The data are as follows (Table 14. 5). The basic question of interest concerns describing the survival function of the two groups.

Table 14. 4　Survival Times for Two Groups of Patients with Renal Transplantation

Group	Survival times/d
Group 1	3　9　15　20　20　26　30　41　46　64+　64　135　223　365　450　596+　680+ 900+　900+
Group 2	10　70+　70+　120　225　366　390+　475+　518+　647+　801+　1001+ 1045+　1045+

"+" *indicates that the data were censored*

Of the 19 patients in Group 1, 14 failed during the study period and 5 were censored. In contrast, 4 failed and 10 were censored in Group 2. Ordered failure times are shown in Table 14. 5 for each group which provides the basic information for the computation of survival function curves.

Table 14. 5　The Survival Functions of Two Groups

Group	ID	Survival time/d	Failure	Mortality probability	Survival probability	Survival function
Group 1						
	1	3	1	$\frac{1}{19}$	$\frac{18}{19}$	0.947368
	2	9	1	$\frac{1}{18}$	$\frac{17}{18}$	0.894737
	3	15	1	$\frac{1}{17}$	$\frac{16}{17}$	0.842105
	4,5	20	1	$\frac{2}{16}$	$\frac{14}{16}$	0.736842
	6	26	1	$\frac{1}{14}$	$\frac{13}{14}$	0.684211
	7	30	1	$\frac{1}{13}$	$\frac{12}{13}$	0.631579
	8	41	1	$\frac{1}{12}$	$\frac{11}{12}$	0.578947
	9	46	1	$\frac{1}{11}$	$\frac{10}{11}$	0.526316
	10	64	1	$\frac{1}{10}$	$\frac{9}{10}$	0.473684
	11	64	0	0	1	0.473684
	12	135	1	$\frac{1}{8}$	$\frac{7}{8}$	0.414474
	13	223	1	$\frac{1}{7}$	$\frac{6}{7}$	0.355263
	14	365	1	$\frac{1}{6}$	$\frac{5}{6}$	0.296053
	15	450	1	$\frac{1}{5}$	$\frac{4}{5}$	0.236842
	16	596	0	0	1	0.236842
	17	680	0	0	1	0.236842

Continued

Group	ID	Survival time	Failure	Mortality probability	Survival probability	Survival function
	18,19	900	0	0	1	0.236842
Group 2						
	1	10	1	$\frac{1}{14}$	$\frac{13}{14}$	0.928571
	2,3	70	0	0	1	0.928571
	4	120	0	0	1	0.928571
	5	225	1	$\frac{1}{10}$	$\frac{9}{10}$	0.835714
	6	366	1	$\frac{1}{9}$	$\frac{8}{9}$	0.742857
	7	390	1	$\frac{1}{8}$	$\frac{7}{8}$	0.650000
	8	475	0	0	1	0.650000
	9	518	0	0	1	0.650000
	10	647	0	0	1	0.650000
	11	801	0	0	1	0.650000
	12	1,001	0	0	1	0.650000
	13,14	1,045	0	0	1	0.650000

Plots of the KM curves for Groups 1 and 2 using the KM method are shown in Figure 14.6. Notice that the KM curve for Group 2 is consistently higher than that for Group 1, indicating that group 2 has a better survival prognosis than Group 1. Moreover, as the number of days increases, the two curves appear to get farther apart, suggesting that the beneficial effects of Group 2 over Group 1 are greater the longer one stays in renal transplantation surgery.

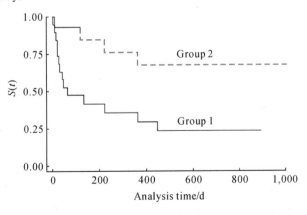

Figure 14.6   KM Plots for Example 14.5 Data

14.6   Log-Rank Test

The log-rank test, also known as the Mantel-Cox test, is based on the idea that when the null hypothesis is true, the theoretical deaths can be calculated based on the number of patients surviving and the actual number of deaths at each time, and then compared with the actual number of deaths in each group. The comparison of survival curves between two groups or multiple groups was generally performed by log-rank test. Two methods are used for comparing the survival rates of two groups: approximate method and precision method. Statistical software is often calculated using an accurate method.

In this section, we consider how to compare the two survival curves for participants receiving 15,000 IU of vitamin A with participants receiving 75 IU of vitamin A in Figure 14.5. We could compare survival rates at specific time points. However, a stronger comparison would consider the entire survival curve. We could also compare the mean survival time between groups. However, survival time distributions are often highly skewed and it is not clear how to treat censored observations in computing mean survival time. Suppose we want to compare the survival experience of two groups, the exposed and unexposed groups. Let $h_1(t)$ = hazard at time t for participants in the exposed group, and $h_2(t)$ = hazard at time t for participant in the unexposed group. We assume the hazard ratio is a constant = $\exp(\beta)$ over time, i.e.

$$\frac{h_1(t)}{h_2(t)} = \exp(\beta) \tag{14.6}$$

Note that the hazard function in each group can vary over time, but the hazard ratio is assumed to be constant.

We want to test the hypothesis $H_0: \beta = 0$ vs. $H_1: \beta \neq 0$. If $\beta = 0$, then the survival curves of the two groups are the same. If $\beta > 0$, then exposed participants are consistently at greater risk for disease than unexposed participants, or equivalently, the survival probability of the exposed group is less than that of the unexposed group at each time t. If $\beta < 0$, then the exposed participants are at lower risk than the unexposed participants and their survival probabilities are greater than those of the unexposed participants.

Consider the data in Table 14.3. These data could be analyzed in terms of cumulative incidence over 6 years; that is, the percentage of participants receiving 15,000 IU of vitamin A vs. participants receiving 75 IU of vitamin A whose ERG 30 Hz amplitude declined by at least 50% from baseline could be compared. However, if incidence changes greatly over time, this is not as powerful as the log-rank test described later. Using this procedure, when an event occurs rather than simply whether it occurs is taken into account.

To implement this procedure, the total period of follow-up is subdivided into shorter time periods over which incidence is relatively constant. In Example 14.4 time has been subdivided into 1-year intervals. For each time interval, the number of people who have not failed (his or her ERG 30 Hz amplitude declined by at least 50% from baseline) up to the beginning of the interval are identified. These people are at risk for failure during this time interval. This group is then categorized according to whether they survived or their ERG 30 Hz amplitude declined by at least 50% from baseline during the time interval. For each time interval, the data are displayed as a 2×2 contingency table relating treatment to incidence rates over the time interval. For the first time interval, $0 \sim 1$ year, 172 participants receiving 15,000 IU of vitamin A per day survived at time 0, of whom 3 failed during the 0- to 1-year period; similarly, of 182 participants receiving 75 IU of vitamin A, 8 failed during this period. These data are shown in a contingency table in Table 14.6. For the second time period, $1 \sim 2$ years, 165 participants receiving 15,000 IU of vitamin A daily survived at year 1, of whom 6 failed during the period from year 1 to year 2; similarly, 174 participants receiving 75 IU of vitamin A survived at year 1, of whom 13 failed from year 1 to year 2. Thus, the second contingency table would look like Table 14.7. Similarly, contingency tables for the time periods $2 \sim 3$ years, $3 \sim 4$ years, $4 \sim 5$ years, and $5 \sim 6$ years can be developed, as shown in Tables 14.8, 14.9, 14.10, and 14.11, respectively.

Table 14.6   Incidence Rates by Treatment for the 0- to 1-Year Period

Vitamin A dose	Fail	Survive	Total
15,000 IU	3	169	172
75 IU	8	174	182

Table 14.7   Incidence Rates by Treatment for the 1- to 2-Year Period

Vitamin A dose	Fail	Survive	Total
15,000 IU	6	159	165
75 IU	13	161	174

Table 14.8   Incidence Rates by Treatment for the 2- to 3-Year Period

Vitamin A dose	Fail	Survive	Total
15,000 IU	15	144	159
75 IU	21	137	158

Table 14.9   Incidence Rates by Treatment for the 3- to 4-Year Period

Vitamin A dose	Fail	Survive	Total
15,000 IU	21	122	143
75 IU	21	114	135

Table 14. 10   Incidence Rates by Treatment for the 4- to 5-Year Period

Vitamin A dose	Fail	Survive	Total
15,000 IU	15	81	96
75 IU	13	73	86

Table 14. 11   Incidence Rates by Treatment for the 5- to 6-Year Period

Vitamin A dose	Fail	Survive	Total
15,000 IU	5	41	46
75 IU	13	29	42

If vitamin A dose has no association with failure, then the incidence rate for failure for participants receiving 15,000 IU and 75 IU within each of the six time intervals should be the same. Conversely, if the survival rate for participants receiving 75 IU is less than participants receiving 15,000 IU, then the incidence rate should be consistently higher for participants receiving 75 IU within each of the six time intervals considered. Note that incidence is allowed to vary over different time intervals under either hypothesis. To accumulate evidence over the entire period of follow-up, the Mantel-Haenszel procedure, based on the 2×2 tables in Tables 14. 6 to 14. 11, is used. This procedure is called the log-rank test and is summarized as follows.

To compare incidence rates for an event between two exposure groups, where incidence varies over the period of follow-up (T), the following procedure is used:

(a) Subdivide T into k smaller time intervals, over which incidence is homogeneous.

(b) Compute a 2×2 contingency table corresponding to each time interval relating incidence over the time interval to exposure status ($+/-$). Consider censored subjects at a particular time as having a slightly longer follow-up time than subjects who fail at a given time. The ith table is displayed in Table 14. 12.

Table 14. 12   Relationship of Disease Incidence to Exposure Status over the ith Time Interval

Exposure	Event		Total
	$+$	$-$	
$+$	a_i	b_i	n_{i1}
$-$	c_i	d_i	n_{i2}
Total	$a_i + c_i$	$b_i + d_i$	n_i

In Table 14. 12, n_{i1} is the number of exposed people who have not yet had the event at the beginning of the ith time interval and were not censored at the beginning of the interval; n_{i2} is the number of unexposed people who have not yet had the event at the beginning of the ith time interval and were not censored at the beginning of the interval; a_i is the number of exposed people who had an event during the ith time interval; b_i is the number of exposed people who did not have an event during the ith time interval; and c_i, d_i are defined similarly for unexposed people.

(c) Perform the Mantel-Haenszel test over the collection of 2×2 tables defined in step b. Specifically, compute the test statistic

$$\chi_{LR}^2 = \frac{(|O-E|-0.5)^2}{Var_{LR}}$$

where

$$O = \sum_{i=1}^{k} a_i$$

$$E = \sum_{i=1}^{k} E_i = \sum_{i=1}^{k} \frac{(a_i+b_i)(a_i+c_i)}{n_i}$$

$$Var_{LR} = \sum_{i=1}^{k} V_i = \sum_{i=1}^{k} \frac{(a_i+b_i)(c_i+d_i)(a_i+c_i)(b_i+d_i)}{n_i^2(n_i-1)}$$

The statistic follows a chi-square distribution with one df under H_0.

(a) For a two-sided test with significant level α,

if $\chi_{LR}^2 > \chi_{1,1-\alpha}^2$, then reject H_0;

if $\chi_{LR}^2 \leqslant \chi_{1,1-\alpha}^2$, then do not reject H_0.

(b) The exact p-value for this test is given by

$$p\text{-value} = Pr(\chi_1^2 > \chi_{LR}^2)$$

(c) This test should be used only if $Var_{LR} \geqslant 5$.

The rejection regions for the log-rank test are shown in Figure 14.7. Computation of the exact p-value is given in Figure 14.8.

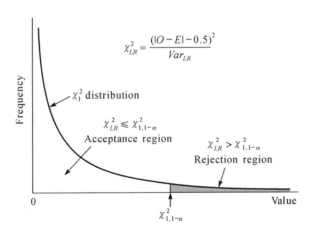

Figure 14.7　Rejection Regions for the Log-Rank Test

Refer to the six 2×2 tables (Tables 14.4—14.9) developed in Example 14.5. We have

$$O = 3+6+15+21+15+5 = 65$$

$$E = \frac{172 \times 11}{354} + \frac{165 \times 19}{339} + \frac{159 \times 36}{317} + \frac{143 \times 42}{278} + \frac{96 \times 28}{182} + \frac{46 \times 18}{88} = 78.432$$

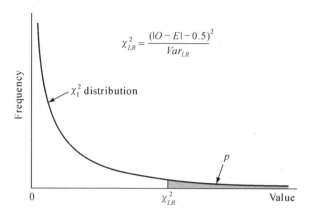

Figure 14.8   Computation of the p-Value for the Log-Rank Test

$$Var_{LR} = \frac{172 \times 182 \times 11 \times 343}{354^2 \times 353} + \frac{165 \times 174 \times 19 \times 320}{339^2 \times 338} + \frac{159 \times 158 \times 36 \times 281}{317^2 \times 316}$$

$$+ \frac{143 \times 135 \times 42 \times 236}{278^2 \times 277} + \frac{96 \times 86 \times 28 \times 154}{182^2 \times 181} + \frac{46 \times 42 \times 18 \times 70}{88^2 \times 87} = 33.649$$

Because $Var_{LR} \geqslant 5$, the log-rank test can be used. The test statistic is given by

$$\chi^2_{LR} = \frac{(|65 - 78.432| - 0.5)^2}{33.649} = 4.970, \ \chi^2_1 \text{ under } H_0$$

In this example, $\chi^2_{1, .095} = 3.84 < 4.970$, with p-value $= 0.026$. Therefore, there is a significant difference between the survival curves of the two groups. Because $O =$ observed number of events in the 15,000 IU group $= 65 < E =$ expected number of events in the 15,000 IU group $= 78.432$, it follows that the 15,000 IU group had a better survival experience than the 75 IU group. Stated another way, significantly fewer failures occurred in the 15,000 IU group compared to the 75 IU group.

The log-rank test compares the difference in survival curves between two or more groups to illustrate the effect of a factor on survival time. However, its outcome cannot replace the difference in survival rate or median survival time at some point specifically. The log-rank is a one-way analysis and does not take the effects of other factors into account. To accurately analyze the independent effects of a factor on the efficacy of a disease controlling other factors, the Cox regression model analysis is needed. When the log-rank test is used to compare the survival rate of samples, the survival curves of the two groups should not be crossed, and the crossover of the survival curve suggests some confounding factors are present. At this point, a layered approach or a multi-factor approach should be used to correct for confounding factors. In addition, when the hypothesis test is inferred to differ, the effects can be evaluated by indicators such as survival curve, median survival time, and relative risk.

14.7   Cox Proportional Hazards Model

The log-rank test is a very powerful method of analyzing data when the time to an event is important rather than simply whether or not the event occurs. The test can be used if variable periods of follow-up are available for each individual and/or if some data are censored. It can also be extended to allow one to look at the relationship between survival and a single primary exposure variable, while controlling for the effects of one or more covariate(s). This can be accomplished by stratifying the data according to the levels of the covariates; computing the observed number, expected number, and variance of the number of failures in each stratum; summing the respective values over all strata; and using the same test statistic as in section 14. 3. However, if there are many strata and/or if there are several risk factors of interest, a more convenient approach is to use a method of regression analysis for survival data.

Many different models can be used to relate survival to a collection of other risk factors. One of the most frequently used models, first proposed by D. R. Cox, is called the Cox proportional hazards (PH) model.

14.7.1   PH Model

Under a PH model, the hazard $h(t)$ is modeled as

$$h(t) = h_0(t)\exp(\beta_1 x_1 + \cdots + \beta_k x_k) \tag{14.7}$$

where $x_1, \cdots, x_k$ are a collection of independent variables, and $h_0(t)$ is the baseline hazard at time t, representing the hazard for a person with the value 0 for all the independent variables. By dividing both sides of Formula (14.7) by $h_0(t)$ and taking logarithms, a PH model can be written in the form

$$\ln\left[\frac{h(t)}{h_0(t)}\right]=\beta_1 x_1+\cdots+\beta_k x_k \tag{14.8}$$

This representation helps us interpret the coefficients of a PH model in a manner similar to that of a multiple logistic regression model. An important assumption of this method is that the hazard ratio (HR) of the primary exposure (and any other covariates in the model) remains constant over time.

The hypothesis $H_0:\beta_j=0$ vs. $H_1:\beta_j\neq0$ can be tested as follows:

(a) Compute the test statistic: $z=\dfrac{\hat{\beta}_j}{se(\hat{\beta}_j)}$, which follows standard normal distribution.

(b) To conduct a two-sided level α significance test,

if $z<z_{\frac{\alpha}{2}}$ or $z<z_{1-\frac{\alpha}{2}}$, then reject H_0;

if $z_{\frac{\alpha}{2}}\leqslant z\leqslant z_{1-\frac{\alpha}{2}}$, then do not reject H_0.

(c) The exact p-value is given by

if $z\geqslant0$, $P=2\times[1-\Phi(z)]$; if $z<0$, $P=2\times\Phi(z)$.

14.7.2   Estimation HR for Dichotomous Variables in PH Models

Suppose we have a dichotomous independent variable (x_j) that is coded as 1 if present and 0 if absent. For the PH model in Formula (14.7) the quantity $\exp(\beta_j)$ represents the ratio of hazards for two people, one with the risk factor present and the other with the risk factor absent, given that both people have the same values for all other covariates. The hazard ratio or relative hazard can be interpreted as the instantaneous relative risk of an event per unit time for a person with the risk factor present compared with a person with the risk factor absent, given that both individuals have survived to time t and are the same on all other covariates.

A two-sided $100\% \times (1-\alpha)$ CI for β_j is given by (e^{c_1}, e^{c_2}), where

$$c_1 = \hat{\beta}_j - z_{1-\frac{\alpha}{2}} se(\hat{\beta}_j)$$
$$c_2 = \hat{\beta}_j + z_{1-\frac{\alpha}{2}} se(\hat{\beta}_j)$$

14.7.3   Estimation HR for Continuous Variables in PH Models

Suppose there is a continuous independent variable (x_j). Consider two people who differ by the quantity Δ on the jth independent variable and are the same for all other independent variables. The quantity $\exp(\beta_j \Delta)$ represents the ratio of hazards between the two individuals. The hazard ratio can also be interpreted as the instantaneous relative risk of an event per unit time for an individual with risk factor level $x_j + \Delta$ compared with someone with risk factor level x_j, given that both people have survived to time t and are the same for all other covariates.

A two-sided $100 \times (1-\alpha)$ CI for β_j is given by (e^{c_1}, e^{c_2}) where

$$c_1 = \Delta[\hat{\beta}_j - z_{1-\frac{\alpha}{2}} se(\hat{\beta}_j)]$$
$$c_2 = \Delta[\hat{\beta}_j + z_{1-\frac{\alpha}{2}} se(\hat{\beta}_j)]$$

Note that the hazard $h(t)$ for a subject can vary over time, but the ratio of hazards between two subjects, one of whom has covariate values $(x_1, \cdots, x_k)$ and the other of whom has covariate values of 0 for all covariates is given by $\exp(\sum_{j=1}^{k} \beta_j x_j)$, which is the same for all t. The Cox PH model can also be thought of as an extension of multiple logistic regression where the time when an event occurs is taken into account, rather than simply whether an event occurs.

Example 14.5   Use the Cox PH model to compare the survival curves for subjects of different sex receiving a high dose (15,000 IU) vs. a low dose (75 IU) of vitamin A, based on the data in Table 14.3.

We have used the SPSS software to compare the survival curves. In this case, there is only a single binary covariate x defined by

$$x_1 = \begin{cases} 1, & \text{if high dose A} \\ 0, & \text{if low dose A} \end{cases} \qquad x_2 = \begin{cases} 1, & \text{if male} \\ 2, & \text{if female} \end{cases}$$

The output from the software is given in Table 14.13. We see that subjects on 15,000 IU of vitamin A have a significantly lower hazard than subjects on 75 IU of vitamin A (p-value=0.026, denoted by $sig.$). The hazard ratio is estimated by $e^{\beta} = e^{-0.365} = 0.694$ ($\hat{\beta}$ is denoted by B, and e^{β} is denoted by $\exp(B)$). Thus, the failure rate at any point in time is approximately 30% lower for patients on 15,000 IU of vitamin A than for patients on 75 IU of vitamin A. We can obtain 95% confidence limits for the hazard ratio by (e^{c_1}, e^{c_2}), where

$$c_1 = \hat{\beta} - 1.96se(\hat{\beta}) = -0.365 - 1.96(0.164) = -0.686$$
$$c_2 = \hat{\beta} + 1.96se(\hat{\beta}) = -0.365 + 1.96(0.164) = -0.044$$

Thus, the 95% CI = ($e^{-0.686}$, $e^{-0.044}$) = (0.504, 0.957). $se(\hat{\beta})$ is given in Table 14.13 and denoted by SE. The 95% confidence limits for β are given in the last two columns.

Table 14.13   Cox PH Model Run on the RP Data Set in Table 14.3

	B	SE	Wald	df	sig.	exp(B)	95% CI for exp(B) Lower bound	Upper bound
x_1	−0.365	0.164	4.970	1	0.026	0.694	0.504	0.957
x_2	−0.170	0.177	0.927	1	0.336	0.844	0.597	1.193

If there are no ties, that is, if all subjects have a unique failure time, then the Cox PH model with a single binary covariate and the log-rank test provide very similar results. In general, in the presence of ties, the Cox PH model and the log-rank test do not yield the same p-values, particularly in data sets with many tied observations. However, in this example the p-value from the Cox PH model (see Table 14.13, $P=0.026$) is similar to the p-value from the log-rank test (see section 14.3, $P=0.026$). The Cox PH model can also be used to control for the effects of other covariates as well as for other treatments.

14.8   Summary

In this chapter, we discussed how to analyze survival data using methods of survival analysis. We introduced the concept of a hazard function, which is a function characterizing how the instantaneous probability of having an event changes over time. We also introduced the concept of a survival curve, which is a function giving the cumulative probability of not having an event (i. e. surviving) as a function of time. The Kaplan-Meier estimator was introduced as a non-parametric method for estimating a survival curve. The log-rank test was then presented to help us statistically compare two survival curves (e. g. for an exposed vs. an unexposed group). If we want to study the effects of several risk factors on survival, then the Cox PH model can be used. This method is analogous to multiple logistic regression, where the time when an event occurs is considered rather than simply whether or not an event has occurred.

The important assumption of the Cox PH method is that the hazard ratio of the primary exposure (and any other covariates in the model) remains constant over time. This means the hazard for one individual is proportional to the hazard for any other individual, where the proportionality constant is independent of time. The PH assumption is not met if the graph of the hazards cross for two or more categories of a predictor of interest. However, it cannot be guaranteed by this method. Thus, we still use other approaches to evaluate the reasonableness of the PH assumption, such as log-log survival curves method, comparing observed versus expected survival curves, goodness-of-fit (GOF) testing approach, and the time-dependent covariates method.

(Ai Zisheng, Wu Ying, Yi Honggang)

Question Bank

Chapter 15　Foundations of Research Design

This chapter covers research designs and their methodology, including research procedures, observational designs, and experimental designs.

15.1　Overview

15.1.1　Definitions

The **research design** refers to the overall strategy employed to integrate the different components of the study in a coherent and logical way to address the research problems. The design should ensure the research hypotheses are well stated for the research question and appropriate data will be obtained in a way that permits an objective analysis, leading to valid inferences with respect to the stated problem. Medical research design is a systematic process of medical scientific research based on certain research purposes, with scientific, effective, and careful planning and arrangements to guarantee the rationality and sustainability of the study. It typically includes data collection, classification, analysis, and interpretation.

Generally, a good research design should be made from both professional and statistical perspectives and the organic union between them. The professional design ensures the advancement and practicability of the research topic, and the statistical design ensures the economy, stability, reliability, and repeatability of the research process. It must be emphasized that, without a proper research design, the accuracy and reliability of the results cannot be guaranteed. In addition, it is unscientific and detrimental to use statistical methods to try to make up for deficiencies in the research design.

There are many ways to classify research designs, but sometimes the distinction is artificial and other times different designs are combined. Medical research usually uses two categories: observational designs and experimental designs. Figure 15.1 illustrates two types of research designs: experiments and surveys.

Observational design represents one of the most common types of quantitative and social science research. The approximate area of this research encompasses any measurement procedures that involve asking questions of respondents. Surveys are one type of observational design. For example, in a survey study, the researcher selects a sample of respondents from a population and administers a standardized questionnaire to them. The purpose of the questionnaire is to describe the attitudes, opinions, behaviors, or

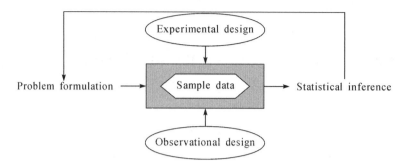

Figure 15. 1   Two Types of Research Designs Used in Scientific Investigations

characteristics of the population based on the sample data.

To determine why people prefer health intervention A to health intervention B, carry out investigations. You only need to ask different people about it, and you do not impose any intervention on them. You will get different reasons from different people. However, you will certainly find something common that makes health intervention A superior to health intervention B.

Experimental design is a research design that controls all factors influencing the outcome except for the cause being studied (independent variable). Usually, experimental design is conducted in situations in which researchers can manipulate the conditions of the experiment and can control the factors that are irrelevant to the research objectives. By noting how the manipulated independent variables affect a response variable, the researcher can test whether a causal relationship exists between the manipulated variables and the response variable. Experimental design consists of three basic elements: the experimental unit, the treatment, and the effect.

The most common way to design an experiment is to divide the participants into two groups—an experimental group and a control group, and then test the difference between the two groups.

For example, if you manage to uncover a drug for acquired immune deficiency syndrome (AIDS), then you need conduct experiments to investigate the effectiveness of the drug you discovered, compared with another drug. For that purpose, you should contact different people with AIDS and randomly allocate them to the drug-exposed group or the control group. If the drug works against the disease, then you can say that the experiment was successful and the drug can be made available on the market—but only after it gets approved by the Food and Drug Administration (FDA).

15.1.2 Objective of Research Designs

In scientific research, research design is not only an indispensable important issue, but also a crucial step to perform before conducting the research. The objective of the research design is to ensure that the evidence obtained enables the researchers to effectively address the research problem logically and as unambiguously as possible. It requires researchers to have a wealth of professional knowledge and a knowledge of statistics at the same time. The key to successful research lies in designing reasonable and scientific research to achieve the purpose of the study.

15.1.3   Basic Principles of Experimental Designs

The seminal ideas for experimental design can be traced to Sir Ronald A. Fisher who was the most famous statistician and geneticist of the 20th century. He had a profound influence on the development of modern statistical experimental design. During the 1920s and early 1930s, Fisher was responsible for statistics and data analysis at the Rothamsted Agricultural Experimental Station near London, England. Fisher systematically introduced statistical thinking and principles into designing experimental investigations. He first developed the insights that lead to the three basic principles of experimental design in his innovative books *The Arrangement of Field Experiments* (1926) and *The Design of Experiments* (1935).

For a research design to be considered sound, three basic principles must be present: control, randomization, and replication. These principles allow a valid test of significance. Each of the three basic principles is described briefly in the following subsections.

15.1.3.1   Control

(1) Definition

In addition to experimental factors, the experimental effect of interest is often influenced by other confounding factors. For example, the factors that affect the prognosis of diseases are diverse and complicated. There are significant differences between individuals, even between the same individual during different periods. These confounding factors cannot be removed by other methods, such as randomization and replication. In this situation, we must choose a design that controls all extraneous sources of variation. For this purpose, when researchers design their research, they are generally required to set up a control group, which is the basic step that controls various confounding factors.

A **control group** is a group of subjects or conditions that is matched as closely as possible with an experimental group but is not exposed to any of the conditions of the experiment, e. g. a group of experimental units does not receive any drug or pill of any kind.

(2) Objective

Control groups have one major purpose: they serve as a standard to which the treatment group is compared. They are usually used as reference points for experiments so that researchers can estimate the extent of the treatment's effectiveness. Figure 15. 2 illustrates the function of the control group.

(3) The conditions of the control group

In medical research, the control group must meet three conditions:

(a) Equity: Except for treatment factors, the control group must have the same

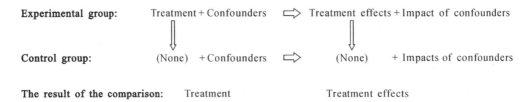

Figure 15. 2   The Function of the Control Group

confounding (nontreatment) factors as the treatment groups.

(b) Synchronization: The research process for both control and treatment groups should take place at the same time and in the same space.

(c) Specificity: The control group should be established exclusively for the relevant treatment groups in the study. Ideally, the experimental group is compared to current controls (rather than to historical controls).

(4) Category

Control groups in medical research can be classified into different types according to the research purpose and the specific questions.

According to time, control groups could be classified as a historical control group, a current control group, and a standard control group. A historical control group is a group of subjects who were observed at an earlier time or for whom data are available through records. This type of control group is not recommended. Current control groups are widely used. A standard control group is one kind of historical control group, in which standard values and normal values are used as reference values.

According to the study subjects, control groups could be classified as paired control groups and parallel control groups. A paired control study compares groups in which each subject is matched to a comparable subject in terms of confounding factors, such as age, sex, and any other measurable factor. A parallel control study is a type of study where two groups of treatments, A and B (the control group), are given so that one group receives only A while another group receives only B.

According to the study treatment, controls could be divided into blank controls, experimental controls, and mutual controls. No interventions are given to the blank control group. Experimental controls are experimental subjects not exposed to the treatments being investigated so that they can be compared with experimental groups that are exposed to the treatments.

15. 1. 3. 2   Randomization

(1) Definition

One principle of an experimental design is **randomization**, which is a random process of assigning treatments to the experimental units (Figure 15. 3).

The random process implies that every possible allotment of treatments has the same probability. Both the allocation of the experimental material and the order in which the

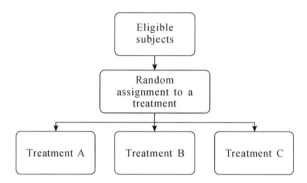

Figure 15. 3　A Visual Sketch Map of Random Allocation in Experimental Design

experiment's individual runs or trials are performed are randomly determined.

(2) Objective

The purpose of randomization is to remove bias and other sources of extraneous variation that are not controllable. It avoids systematic differences between groups with respect to known or unknown baseline variables that could affect the outcome. Another advantage of randomization (accompanied by replication) is that it forms the basis of any valid statistical test. It is the cornerstone underlying the use of statistical methods and provides a sound basis for statistical inference.

Randomization is usually performed using tables of random numbers, random number generation methods including hardware random number generators and pseudorandom numbers generated by computers.

We must stress that randomization does not mean that the groups are haphazardly chosen.

(3) Category

The three types of randomization are random sampling, random allocation, and random experimental order. Random sampling is a method of selecting a sample from a statistical population in such a way that every possible sample has a predetermined probability of being selected. Random allocation means that the experimental subjects ("units") should be assigned to the treatment groups at random. In random experimental order, experimental subjects receive the treatments in a random order.

15. 1. 3. 3　Replication

(1) Definition

The third principle of an experimental design is **replication** which is a repetition of the basic experiment. In replication, an experiment or test is conducted using three or more homogeneous experimental units subjected to the same treatment under similar conditions. Replication is essential, and each treatment should be repeated on a large enough number of units to allow systematic effects to be detected. Replication makes the significance tests possible.

(2) Objective

In all experiments, some variation is introduced because of the individual variation of the experimental units. This type of variation can be removed by using a number of experimental units. We therefore, perform the experiment more than once, i. e. we repeat the basic experiment.

The objectives of replication are as follows:

(a) To secure a more accurate estimate of the experimental error, a term that represents the differences that would be observed if the same treatments were applied several times to the same experimental units.

(b) To decrease the experimental error and thereby increase the precision, which is a measure of the variability in the experimental error.

(c) To attain a more reliable estimate of each treatment's effect by repeating each treatment on several subjects.

(3) Category

Replication includes the following:

(a) The whole study is repeated.

(b) Measurements of the same sample are repeated. It is important to control for errors in measurement.

(c) Measurements are taken from several independent subjects rather than from a single individual, which is important in the statistical inference of populations.

(4) Sample size estimation

During the planning stage of a medical study, the following questions are of particular interest to investigators: How many subjects are needed to adequately detect a clinically significant difference? To address this question, a statistical evaluation for sample size estimation is often performed. This evaluation plays an important role in assuring the validity, accuracy, reliability, and integrity of the intended study.

Sample size determination is the act of choosing the number of observations or replicates to include in a statistical sample. The sample size is an important feature of any empirical study in which the goal is to make inferences about a population from a sample. In practice, a study's sample size is determined based on the expense of data collection and the need to have enough statistical power.

The appropriate sample size for experimental design is largely determined by several factors:

(a) Study objectives;

(b) Primary study end point;

(c) Hypothesis;

(d) Study design;

(e) Clinically meaningful difference;

(f) Type I and type II errors;

(g) Standard deviation.

As shown above, many factors affect the sample size estimation. Some of the factors are under the control of the experimenter, whereas others are not. The following example will be used to illustrate the various factors.

Taking a two-sample parallel design as an example, we will introduce the methods of estimating sample size, for comparing two means or two rates.

Comparing two means

For an experimental design based on a two-sample parallel design sample, the objective is to test whether there is a difference between the two population means. Hence, the following hypotheses are considered:

$$H_0 : \mu_1 = \mu_2 ; \ H_1 : \mu_1 \neq \mu_2$$

The sample size required can be calculated according to the following formula:

$$N = \left(\frac{1}{Q_1} + \frac{1}{Q_2} \right) \frac{[\mu_\alpha + \mu_{\beta(1)}]^2 \sigma^2}{\delta^2} \tag{15.1}$$

where μ_α is the upper $\frac{\alpha}{2}$th quantile of the standard normal distribution; $\mu_{\beta(1)}$ is the upper βth quantile of the standard normal distribution; σ^2 is the variance of measurement variable; δ is the clinical difference between the two population means; $Q_i (i=1, 2)$ is the proportions of sample size of group i; and N is the of total sample size of n_i. $Q_1, Q_2 > 0$, $Q_1 + Q_2 = 1$.

If $Q_1 = Q_2$, Formula (15.1) leads to:

$$N = \frac{4[\mu_\alpha + \mu_{\beta(1)}]^2 \sigma^2}{\delta^2} \tag{15.2}$$

Example 15.1　Consider an example concerning a clinical trial for evaluating the effect of a test drug on a fibrinolytic system of patients with ischemic cerebrovascular disease. According to the literature, the value of fibrinogen reduced to $0.52 \pm 1.23 (g/l)$ in the experimental group ($n_1 = 109$), but 0.13 ± 0.86 in the control group ($n_2 = 114$). Please estimate the sample size.

At first, calculate the combined variance:

$$s_C^2 = \frac{(n_1 - 1)s_1^2 + (n_2 - 1)s_2^2}{n_1 + n_2 - 2} = \frac{(109 - 1) \times 1.23^2 + (114 - 1) \times 0.86^2}{109 + 114 - 2} = 1.1175$$

In this example, the sample size for achieving an 80% power at the 5% level of significance can be determined by:

$$N = 4 \times \frac{(1.96 + 1.282)^2 \times 1.1175}{(0.52 - 0.13)^2} = 309$$

Group sample sizes of 155 and 155 achieve 80% power to detect a difference of 0.4 between the null hypothesis that both group means are 0.52 and the alternative hypothesis that the mean of Group 2 is 0.13 with estimated group standard deviations of 1.23 and 0.86 and with a significant level of 0.05 using a two-sided two-sample t-test.

If $Q_1 : Q_2 = 3 : 1$, the sample size is:

$$N = \left(\frac{1}{0.75} + \frac{1}{0.25} \right) \frac{(1.96 + 1.282)^2 1.1175^2}{(0.52 - 0.13)^2} = 412$$

Comparing two proportions

Here our primary focus will be on comparing proportions between treatment groups with binary responses.

To test whether there is a difference between the mean response rates of the test group and the reference group, the following hypotheses are usually considered:

$$H_0 : \pi_1 = \pi_2 \; ; \; H_1 : \pi_1 \neq \pi_2$$

The sample size required can be calculated by:

$$N = \frac{\left[\mu_a \sqrt{2\bar{p}(1-\bar{p})} + \mu_{\beta(1)} \sqrt{Q_2 p_1 (1-p_1) + Q_2 p_2 (1-p_2)} \right]^2}{Q_1 Q_2 \delta^2} \tag{15.3}$$

where $\bar{p} = Q_1 p_1 + Q_2 p_2$ and $\delta = p_1 - p_2$.

15.1.4 Basic Types of Experimental Designs

Sir Ronald Fisher first developed the elements of experimental design at Rothamsted, Britain's oldest agricultural experiment station, in the 1920s (Figure 15.4). In 1935, Fisher published *The Design of Experiments*, a book that articulated the features of experimental research design that are still used today.

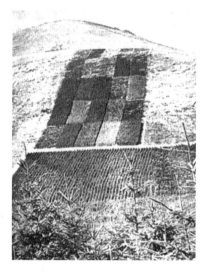

Figure 15.4   A Photo of an Experimental Design in an Agricultural Study

Here, we describe the three most common experimental designs: completely randomized design, paired design, and randomized block design.

15.1.4.1   Completely Randomized Design

(1) Definition

The completely randomized design is probably the simplest experimental design in terms of data analysis and convenience.

In a **completely randomized design**, treatments are assigned to each experimental unit completely at random, which means the randomization is performed without any restrictions.

In a completely randomized design, the subjects are assigned to treatments at random regardless of any characteristics or natural structure of the experimental material. As shown in Figure 15.5, there are a total of nine experimental units, all of which are of the same type. Any three experimental units may be assigned for each of the three treatments (G_1, G_2, and G_3).

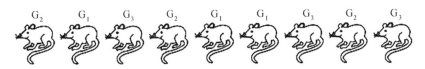

Figure 15.5   A Sketch Map of a Completely Randomized Design

A completely randomized design is considered to be more useful in situations where (a) the experimental units are homogeneous; (b) the experiments are small, such as laboratory experiments; and (c) some experimental units are likely to be destroyed or too impaired to respond.

A layout for a completely randomized design for a simulated experiment is shown in Table 15.1. In this design, the experimenter randomly assigned participants to one of two treatment conditions: the participants either received a placebo or received the test drug. The same number of participants (200) was assigned to each treatment condition.

Table 15.1   An Example of Completely Randomized Design

	Treatment	
	Test drug	Placebo
n	200	200

(2) Randomization method

Randomization is typically performed by a computer program. However, the randomization can also be generated from random number tables (Appendix 8) or by some physical mechanism.

An example of a randomization method using a random permutation table is shown below.

Step 1: Every mouse is numbered with M_1, M_2, M_3, M_4, ···, M_{15}.

Step 2: Select one row of random numbers from the random permutation table (Appendix 9). For example, select 15 random numbers that are less than 16, from left to right, on row 9.

Step 3: Based on a predetermined method, allocate all the mice into different groups (Table 15.2). For example, based on the value of the random number, mice with random numbers between 1 and 5 are allocated into Group A; mice with random numbers between 6 and 10 are allocated into Group B; and the rest are allocated into Group C.

Table 15.2　The Result of the Random Allocation of 15 Mice

Mice	M_1	M_2	M_3	M_4	M_5	M_6	M_7	M_8	M_9	M_{10}	M_{11}	M_{12}	M_{13}	M_{14}	M_{15}
Random number	3	6	14	13	10	5	1	9	12	11	15	7	8	4	2
Group	A	B	C	C	B	A	A	B	C	C	C	B	B	A	A

Finally, we obtain the result of random allocation for 15 mice:

Group A: 1　6　7　14　15

Group B: 2　5　8　12　13

Group C: 3　4　9　10　11

(3) Properties

The advantages of a completely randomized design are as follows:

(a) It is probably the simplest experimental design in terms of data analysis and convenience.

(b) It has one primary factor. The experiment compares the values of a response variable based on the different levels of the primary factor. This method is also called single-factor design.

(c) The design is completely flexible, i.e. any number of treatments and any number of units per treatment may be used. Usually, each treatment is applied (or replicated) an equal number of times. Moreover, the number of units per treatment need not be equal.

(d) It is easy to estimate the sample size.

(e) It relies on randomization to control for the effects of extraneous variables. The researcher assumes that, on average, extraneous factors will affect the treatment conditions equally, so any significant differences between conditions can be reasonably attributed to the independent variable.

(f) It is best used when the set of experimental units is homogenous with respect to the factors that may affect the results. A completely randomized design is not recommended when the experimental units display great variability.

15.1.4.2　Paired Design

(1) Definition

A paired design is an experimental design in which the experimental units are paired up. For a paired design, the participants are first grouped through the coupling of units from similar attributes such as age and sex. Then, within each pair, subjects are randomly assigned to different treatments. This design is a special case of randomized block design and can be used when the treatment has only two levels.

Figure 15.6 shows the sample layout of the paired design. Each column represents a level of the treatment (drug); each row represents a pair (weight). There are 3 pairs and 2 treatments (drugs A and B) in this sample.

Drug A　　Drug B

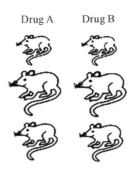

Figure 15. 6　A Sketch of the Paired Design

The two types of paired designs can be briefly described as follows:

(a) Two samples in which the members are clearly paired or are matched explicitly by the researcher. An example of this type is the measurement of drug effects on pairs of mice of the same sex and with the same weight.

(b) Two samples in which the same variable is measured twice for each subject under different circumstances. This type is commonly called repeated measures. An example of this type is the effects of a drug on patients before and after using a particular drug.

Here, we can see a simple example. Table 15. 3 shows a matched pairs design for a hypothetical medical experiment, in which 200 subjects each received one of two treatments: a placebo or the test drug. The 200 subjects are grouped into 100 matched pairs. Each pair is matched on sex and age. For example, Pair 1 might be two 40-year-old men; Pair 2 might be two 25-year-old women; Pair 3 might be two 35-year-old men; and so on.

Table 15. 3　An Example of a Paired Design

Pair	Treatment	
	Test drug	Placebo
1	1	1
2	1	1
3	1	1
⋮	⋮	⋮
99	1	1
100	1	1

For this hypothetical example, the matched pairs design is an improvement over a completely randomized design. Like the completely randomized design, the matched pairs design uses randomization to control for confounding. However, unlike the other design, the matched pairs design explicitly controls for two potential confounding variables: age and sex.

(2) Randomization method

The following example of the randomization procedure for the paired design presents 16 mice paired by sex and weight. Please allocate these mice into two groups.

The randomization procedure of the paired design follows these steps:

Step 1: Number every mouse. For example, mice in the first pair are numbered with 1. 1 and 1. 2, separately; mice in the second pair are numbered with 2. 1 and 2. 2, separately; and so on.

Step 2: Select one row of random numbers from the random permutation table (Appendix 9). For example, select eight random numbers that are less than 9, from left to right on row 2.

Step 3: Based on a predetermined method, allocate all the mice in every pair into a different group. For example, based on the even and odd random numbers, mouse 1. 1 with an even random number (4) is allocated to Group B, and another mouse (1. 2) in the same pair is then allocated to Group A. The details are shown in Table 15. 4.

Table 15. 4　The Results of the Random Allocation of 16 Mice in a Paired Design

Mice	1. 1	1. 2	2. 1	2. 2	3. 1	3. 2	4. 1	4. 2	5. 1	5. 2	6. 1	6. 2	7. 1	7. 2	8. 1	8. 2
Random number	4		5		7		1		8		2		3		6	
Group	B	A	A	B	A	B	A	B	B	A	B	A	A	B	B	A

Finally, we obtain the result of the random allocation of 16 mice in a paired design:

Group A: 1. 2　2. 1　3. 1　4. 1　5. 2　6. 2　7. 1　8. 2

Group B: 1. 1　2. 2　3. 2　4. 2　5. 1　6. 1　7. 2　8. 1

(3) Properties

A paired design offers the following advantages:

(a) Improved precision. Comparisons are made within matched pairs of experimental units, eliminating the possibility of differences between individuals that might affect the results.

(b) Reduced sampling errors. In general, if the paired samples are positively correlated (as they frequently will be), the paired design will lead to smaller sampling errors than the completely randomized design.

(c) The same material can be used twice.

(d) No order effects. Since each participant performs the task only once, temporal effects known as order effects, which can influence results, can be avoided.

The disadvantages of a paired design are as follows:

(a) Matching participants is very time consuming and difficult. In fact, it is impossible to match people on all characteristics, even if twins were used in the two groups.

(b) Variability will always exist, even with carefully matched pairs. While the design is an excellent compromise between reducing the order effects and smoothing out the variation between individuals, it is certainly not perfect.

(c) The researcher might be incorrect in their assumptions about which variables are the most important and miss a major confounding variable.

Despite these disadvantages, paired designs are useful, because they allow researchers to perform streamlined and focused research studies while maintaining a good degree of validity.

15.1.4.3   Randomized Block Design

(1) Definition

The randomized block design originates from the standard design for agricultural experiments. The field or orchard is divided into units to account for any variation in the area. Treatments are then assigned at random to the subjects in each block. As stated by Ronald A. Fisher, a randomized block design is the simplest design for comparative experiments using all three basic principles of experimental designs: randomization, replication, and local control.

The **randomized block design** refers to an experimental design in which experimental units are first divided into more or less homogeneous groups—called **blocks**—of plots, and the treatments are then randomly assigned to the experimental units in each block. It is used when the experimental units have varying characteristics that may affect the results of the experiment. It differs from the completely randomized designs in that the experimental units are grouped into blocks according to known or suspected variation, which is isolated by the blocks.

Within each block, the conditions are as homogeneous as possible, but between blocks, large differences may exist. Figure 15.7 shows the sample layout of the randomized block design. Different columns represent different levels of treatment (drug); each row represents a block (weight). This sample shows three blocks (Blocks 1 — 3) and four treatments (Drugs A—D).

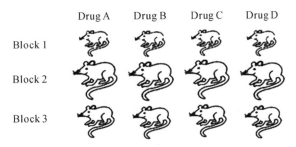

Figure 15.7   A Sketch of the Randomized Block Design

Blocking is the process of arranging experimental units into groups (blocks) that are similar to one another. Typically, a blocking factor is a source of variability that is not of primary interest to the experimenter. An example of a blocking factor might be a patient's sex; blocking on sex controls this source of variability, thus leading to greater accuracy.

For example, Table 15.5 shows a randomized block design for a simulation experiment. Participants are assigned to blocks based on gender. Then, within each block, participants are randomly assigned to treatments. For this design, 100 men receive the placebo, 100 men receive the test drug, 100 women receive the placebo, and 100 women receive the test drug.

Table 15.5   An Example of a Randomized Block Design

Gender	Treatment	
	Test drug	Placebo
Male	100	100
Female	100	100

Because men and women are physiologically different and react differently to medication, this design ensures that each treatment condition includes an equal proportion of men and women. As a result, differences between treatment conditions cannot be attributed to gender. This randomized block design removes gender as a potential source of variability and as a potential confounding variable.

In this example, the randomized block design is an improvement over the completely randomized design. Both designs use randomization to implicitly guard against confounding, but only the randomized block design explicitly controls for gender.

The randomized block design evaluates differences among more than two groups that contain matched samples or repeated measures placed in blocks. Blocking removes as much variability as possible from the random error so that the differences among the groups are more evident.

(2) Randomization method

The randomization procedure of the randomized block design must follow these basic requirements:

(a) Each replicate is randomized separately.

(b) Each treatment has the same probability of being assigned to a given experimental unit within a replicate.

(c) Each treatment must appear at least once per replicating.

Here is an example of the randomization procedure for a randomized block design. Based on weight, 24 mice are grouped into 6 blocks. Please allocate these mice into 4 groups with 6 blocks.

The randomization procedure of the randomized block design follows these steps:

Step 1: Number every mouse with $M_i (i=1, 2, \cdots, 24)$. For example, mice numbered with M_1, M_2, M_3, and M_4 are in block 1; mice numbered with M_{21}, M_{22}, M_{23}, and M_{24} are in block 6.

Step 2: Select six rows of random numbers from the random permutation table (Appendix 9). For example, select four random numbers less than 5, from left to right on row 4.

Step 3: Based on a predetermined method, allocate all mice in every block into different groups. For example, based on the value of the random number, mice with random number 1 are allocated into Group A, mice with random number 2 are allocated into Group B, mice with random number 3 are allocated into Group C, and mice with random number 4 are allocated into Group D. The details are shown in Table 15. 6.

Table 15. 6   The Result of Random Allocation of 24 Mice in the Randomized Block Design

Block	Mouse number				Random number				Allocation			
									Group A	Group B	Group C	Group D
1	M_1	M_2	M_3	M_4	2	1	4	3	M_2	M_1	M_4	M_3
2	M_5	M_6	M_7	M_8	4	2	3	1	M_8	M_6	M_7	M_5
3	M_9	M_{10}	M_{11}	M_{12}	4	1	2	3	M_{10}	M_{11}	M_{12}	M_9
4	M_{13}	M_{14}	M_{15}	M_{16}	1	3	4	2	M_{13}	M_{16}	M_{14}	M_{15}
5	M_{17}	M_{18}	M_{19}	M_{20}	2	4	3	1	M_{20}	M_{17}	M_{19}	M_{18}
6	M_{21}	M_{22}	M_{23}	M_{24}	3	1	4	2	M_{22}	M_{24}	M_{21}	M_{23}

(3) Properties

The randomized block design offers the following advantages:

(a) Complete flexibility. This design can accommodate any number of treatments and any number of blocks, but each treatment must be replicated the same number of times in each block.

(b) Accuracy. Grouping enables more accurate results than the completely randomized design.

(c) Calculation of unbiased error for specific treatments.

(d) Expanded scope. Placing blocks under different conditions broadens the scope of an experiment.

Disadvantages of the randomized block design are as follows:

(a) Not suitable for large numbers of treatments because blocks become too large.

(b) Not suitable when the complete block contains considerable variability.

(c) Interactions between the block and treatment effects increase error.

(d) Missing data can complicate the analysis and may be less efficient than the completely randomized design.

(e) The design is less efficient when there is more than one source of unwanted variation.

15. 2   Procedures

Preparing the research design is a problem-solving step, which includes following a detailed strategy to obtain the necessary data. The number of steps varies from one description to another, but a fairly standard outline of the scientific method consists of six steps, which are summarized in Figure 15. 8. Statistics should play a role in every step of a scientific study, from the initial problem formulation to the drawing of final conclusions.

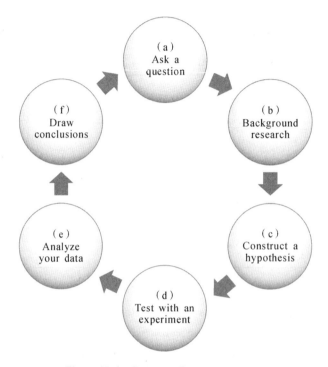

Figure 15. 8   Research Process Flowchart

15.2.1 Hypothesis Generation

(1) Definition of a hypothesis

A **hypothesis** is the stated explanation for an observation. Researchers create hypotheses when speculating on the outcome of a study or experiment, which typically focuses on the prediction of the relationship between two or more assessable variables. A hypothesis is generally based on both theoretical expectations about how things work and pre-existing scientific evidence.

A hypothesis transforms research questions into a format for testing or into a statement that predicts an expected outcome. It is written as a prediction of the experiment's outcome. A hypothesis can predict no relationship existing between two variables, in which case it is a null hypothesis (H_0); or it can predict the existence of a relationship between variables, which is known as an alternative hypothesis (H_1).

For example, when examining which factors influence the incidence rate of lung cancer in a certain area, existing evidence and theories recognize the connection between tobacco use and lung cancer. A researcher might ask the question: "Is there a relationship between tobacco use and lung cancer?" To answer this question, the null hypothesis might be stated as follows: "There is no relationship between tobacco use and lung cancer. " In contrast, the alternative hypothesis would be: "There is a relationship between tobacco use and lung cancer. "

(2) Formulating a hypothesis

The research hypothesis must serve as the core of every research design and guide the aim of the research. A hypothesis can be formulated at the very beginning of the research, or after some research is underway. It can be generated in many ways but is usually the result of inductive reasoning from observations towards the formation of a theory.

A hypothesis comes from a research problem and is usually framed as a question. It might ask what or why something is happening. For example, we might wonder "Why is the incidence rate of lung cancer in a metropolitan area increasing?" However, this question is too broad and is not testable by any reasonable scientific means. It is merely a tentative question arising from literature reviews and intuition. Many people would think that instinct and intuition are unscientific, but many of the greatest scientific leaps were a result of so-called hunches. The research hypothesis pares down the problem into something testable and falsifiable. In the above example, a researcher might speculate that the increase in the rate of lung cancer is due to more serious air pollution. The researchers must generate a realistic and testable hypothesis around which they can build the experiment.

A research question is a highly focused question that addresses one concept or component of the hypothesis; the hypothesis itself states the relationship between two variables.

The hypothesis should:

(a) Be clear and concise;

(b) Have both independent and dependent variables;

(c) Be falsifiable, i. e. whether it is possible to prove or disprove the statement;

(d) Make a prediction or speculate on an outcome;

(e) Be practicable, i. e. whether you can measure the variables in question;

(f) Hypothesize about a proposed relationship between two variables or an intervention into this relationship.

15.2.2 Protocol

15.2.2.1 Definition

The research protocol is an essential part of a research project. Every study has a protocol or action plan for conducting the research or experiment. The protocol describes what will be done in the study, how it will be conducted, and why each part of the research is necessary.

Research protocols are documents that describe the objectives, design, methodology, statistical analysis methods and aspects related to the organization of the whole study.

Protocols provide the background and rationale for conducting a study, highlight the specific research questions and hypotheses to be addressed, and consider ethical issues. For example, the protocol should describe the selection of subjects. Each study has its own inclusion criteria. Some studies require volunteers with a certain disease and healthy people as controls. However, some studies may require only healthy people.

15.2.2.2 Structure

The protocol should describe the research in as much detail as possible. A useful outline of a study protocol would include the following contents.

(1) Presentation

The presentation includes the study's formal title with a short, accurate, and concise summary. This section lists all the investigators as well as the main centers collaborated in the study.

(2) Background

This section includes the specific statement of the research problem and the justification for the study.

(3) Objectives

This section describes the study question and the research hypothesis briefly and clearly.

(4) Methods

The methods section describes, in specific detail, the procedures undertaken to achieve the study objectives, including the sampling design, study population, sample size estimation, data collection and management, and data analysis methods.

(5) Ethical considerations

This section explains all ethical considerations for performing the study.

(6) Project management

The participating institutions and people should be described in detail in this section, as well as their responsibilities and tasks.

(7) Timetable

All operational and practical issues can be described here, including the planning and organization of the study, and the time to complete milestones such as the questionnaire design, participant recruitment, and materials purchases.

Resources, references, and appendices would also be included in the protocol.

15.2.3 Quality Assurance and Quality Control

Quality assurance and quality control efforts endeavor to identify factors affecting the accuracy and reliability of research data. Their essential role is to prevent and correct errors in the study and provide feedback to the researchers. Quality assurance and quality control measures can minimize the chance of obtaining faulty data and drawing erroneous conclusions. They should be performed during all stages of the study, including the study design, sample collection, data processing and analysis, and conclusions.

There are many methods for controlling the quality of the research at different stages of the study.

In the pre-implementation or developmental stage:

(a) Design high-quality questionnaires and forms;

(b) Pretest all aspects of the research;

(c) Develop the operations manual;

(d) Design a good data management system and plan;

(e) Conduct staff training and certification.

During the implementation stage:

(a) Make periodic study- and data-monitoring reports;

(b) Conduct periodic research meetings;

(c) Complete interim staff training and performance reviews;

(d) Provide continuous supervision;

(e) Review all aspects related to implementation of the study.

15.2.4　Data Collection

Data collection is the process of gathering and measuring information on targeted variables from research subjects, which is then analyzed to test the research hypothesis. The methods of data collection include sampling, observations, interviews, questionnaires, and tests. In this step, the researcher must describe how the data will be collected and by whom, and what will be the tools for data collection (e. g. questionnaires or instruments). In the case of questionnaires, will they be self- or interviewer-administered, face-to-face or telephone interviews? While methods vary by study, the emphasis on ensuring accurate and honest collection remains the same. The goal for all data collection is to capture quality evidence that allows analysis to inform convincing and credible answers to the research questions.

15.2.5　Data Management

Data management refers to an organization's handling of data using a variety of different techniques that facilitate and ensure data flow from collection/generation to processing, utilization, and deletion. A data management plan (DMP) is a formal document that outlines how the data are to be handled both during a research project and after the project is completed. The goal of a data management plan is to consider the many aspects of data management, metadata generation, data preservation, and analysis before the project begins; this document ensures that data are well managed in the present and prepares for their preservation in the future.

Most DMPs have five basic components intended to address the major sections of research data management:

(a) A description of the types of data that will be collected or generated during the study;

(b) The standards that will be used for those data and their associated metadata;

(c) A description of the policies pertaining to the data that will be collected or generated;

(d) Plans for archiving and preserving the data generated;

(e) A description of the resources that will be needed to accomplish data management, including personnel, hardware, software, and budgetary requirements.

15.2.6 Data Analysis

Data analysis is the active and interactive process of organizing, providing structure, and eliciting meaning. The analysis plan should describe which statistical tests will be used to check the significance of the research question/hypothesis, with appropriate references. The names of the variables that will be used in the analyses and the name of statistical analysis methods that will be performed to assess the outcome should be listed.

If computer programs are to be applied, it is important to mention the software used and its version.

A statistical analysis plan (SAP) describes the planned analysis for a study. In contrast to the protocol, which outlines the analysis, the SAP is a technical document that describes in detail the statistical techniques for the study analysis. It provides relevant information on the scope of the planned analyses, the population definitions, and the methodology on how prospective decisions are to be made for constructing the analysis data sets and presenting the study results, including shell tables, figures, and listings (TFLs). The SAP and the annotated case report form (CRF) are the documents most often used by statistical programmers.

The following contents should be included in the SAP:

(a) The description of the study and the research purpose;

(b) The statistical methods;

(c) The definitions of the analysis populations;

(d) The data management methods, such as the imputation methods and descriptions of the derived variables;

(e) All shell TFLs to be produced by the statistical programmer.

15.2.7 Study Report

In medicine, a study report is typically very long and provides much detail about the methods and results of a study. For example, the structure and content of a clinical trial report should be well written and follow the International Council for Harmonization (ICH) E3 guidelines, which include a title page, a synopsis, a table of contents, a list of abbreviations and definitions of terms, ethics statements, the investigators and study administrative structure, an introduction, the study objectives, the investigational plan, the study patients, an efficacy and safety evaluation, a discussion and the overall conclusions, tables, figures and graphs, references, and appendices.

15.3   Observational Design

15.3.1   Definition

An **observational design** is a type of correlational (i. e. nonexperimental) study in which a researcher observes ongoing phenomena or behaviors. This research technique involves the direct observation of phenomena or study subjects' behaviors in natural contexts. This characteristic differentiates it from experimental research in which an artificial environment is created to control for spurious factors (confounding factors) and where at least one of the variables (treatments) is manipulated to determine the effect for the subjects as part of the experiment. In contrast, there is no attempt to manipulate or intervene in an observational study.

Consider, as an example, a study of the long-term effects of brain damage in children. Deliberately inflicting brain damage on an experimental group to measure their outcomes will never be feasible or desirable. Therefore, researchers must use patients with pre-existing brain damage or their medical records to make inferences from small samples to the general population.

15.3.2   Categories

Observational designs can take many forms, though they all share the common feature of not manipulating subjects. Observational designs can be classified into two categories: descriptive studies and analytical studies. A cross-sectional study is one type of descriptive study that involves collecting data on many subjects from a population or a representative subset at one specific point in time. It includes censuses, sampling surveys, and typical surveys. A longitudinal study is another type of descriptive study that involves repeated observations of the same variables over long periods of time. Analytical studies include case-control studies and cohort studies.

In this section, the three types of cross-sectional studies are summarized in detail.

15.3.2.1   Census

A well-organized procedure of gathering, recording, and analyzing information about every member of a population is called a **census** or a complete survey. By contrast, sampling obtains information from only a subset of a population. In a census, the enumeration is conducted by considering the entire population. Thus, censuses require much financing, time, and labor to gather information. This method is useful for determining the parameters of the population, such as determining a country's ratio of men to women from its national census.

15.3.2.2   Sampling Survey

A survey study is a kind of incomplete survey often used to assess thoughts, opinions, and feelings. A survey consists of a predetermined set of questions given to a sample. A sampling survey selects a representative sample of elements from a target population and then infers the characteristics of the population based on the sample information. With a representative sample (e. g. one that represents the larger population of interest), one can describe the attitudes of the population from which the sample was drawn. A good sample selection is key because it allows one to generalize the findings from the sample to the population, which is the whole purpose of survey research.

The sampling method refers to the way that observations are selected from a population to be included in the sampling survey. As a group, sampling methods fall into one of two categories: probability samples and nonprobability samples. With probability sampling methods, each population element has a known (nonzero) chance of being chosen for the sample. The four categories of probability sampling methods are described below. With nonprobability sampling methods, the probability that each population element will be chosen is unknown or unclear.

(1) Probability sampling

(a) Simple random sampling

The most widely known type of random sampling is the simple random sample (SRS). A sample of size n from a population of size N is obtained through simple random sampling if every possible sample of size n has an equally likely chance of occurring. The sample is then called a simple random sample. The most important characteristic of this method is that the probability of selection is the same for every case in the population.

Steps for obtaining a simple random sample include:

Step 1: Obtain a frame that lists all the individuals in the population of interest.

Step 2: Number the individuals in the frame from 1 to N.

Step 3: Use a random number table or statistical software to randomly generate n numbers where n is the desired sample size.

Figure 15. 9 illustrates a simple random sampling strategy.

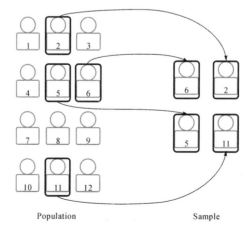

Population   Sample

Figure 15. 9   A Visual Sketch Map of the Simple Random Sampling Strategy

(b) Systematic sampling

At first glance, this method of sampling is very different from SRS. In practice, it is a variant of simple random sampling that involves listing the elements: every nth record is selected from a list of population members for inclusion in the sample. Suppose you have a list of 1,000 people and you want a sample of 100.

Creating such a sample includes three steps:

Step 1: Divide the number of cases in the population by the desired sample size. In this example, dividing 1,000 by 100 gives a value of 10.

Step 2: Select a random number between one and the value attained in step 1. In this example, we choose a number between 1 and 10. For example, suppose we pick 5.

Step 3: Starting with the case number chosen in step 2, take every tenth record (5, 15, 25, etc.).

Figure 15. 10 illustrates the systematic sampling strategy.

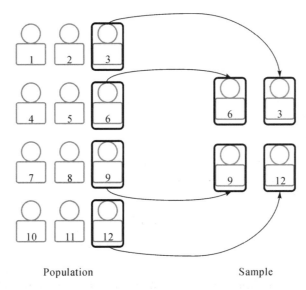

Population　　　　　　　　　　　　Sample

Figure 15. 10　A Visual Sketch Map of the Systematic Sampling Strategy

(c) Stratified random sampling

Stratified sampling is designed to organize the population into strata before sampling and then draw a random sample within each stratum. A stratum is a subset of the population that shares at least one common characteristic. Examples of strata might be sex or race. Strata are nonoverlapping, and together, they compose the entire population.

The researcher first identifies the relevant strata and their actual representation in the population. Random sampling is then used to select a sufficient (i. e. a sample size large enough for the researcher to be reasonably confident that the stratum represents the population) number of subjects from each stratum. Stratified sampling is often used when one or more of the population strata have a low incidence relative to the other strata. This commonly used probability method is superior to random sampling because it reduces the sampling error.

Figure 15. 11 illustrates the stratified sampling strategy.

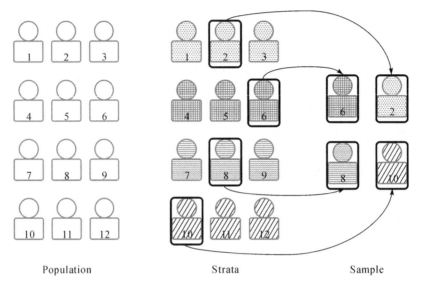

Population   Strata   Sample

Figure 15. 11   A Visual Sketch Map of the Stratified Sampling Strategy

(d) Cluster sampling

Cluster sampling is used when "natural" but relatively homogeneous groupings are evident in a statistical population. In this technique, the total population is divided into these groups (or clusters), and a simple random sample of the groups is selected. Then, the required information is collected from a simple random sample of the elements within each selected group.

Cluster sampling has the following properties.

• The population is divided into N groups, called clusters.

• The researcher randomly selects n clusters to include in the sample.

• The number of observations within each cluster M_i is known, and $M = M_1 + M_2 + M_3 + \cdots + M_{N-1} + M_N$.

• Each element of the population can be assigned to one, and only one, cluster.

Although strata and clusters are both nonoverlapping subsets of the population, they differ in several ways.

• The sample represents all strata but only a subset of the clusters.

• With stratified sampling, the best survey results occur when elements within each stratum are internally homogeneous. However, with cluster sampling, the best results occur when elements within clusters are internally heterogeneous.

Figure 15. 12 illustrates the cluster sampling strategy.

(e) Multistage sampling

Multistage sampling is a complex form of cluster sampling that is useful when using all the sample elements in all the selected clusters is prohibitively expensive or unnecessary.

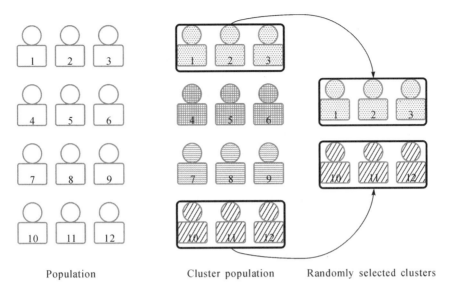

Population   Cluster population   Randomly selected clusters

Figure 15. 12 A Visual Sketch Map of the Cluster Sampling Strategy

With multistage sampling, the researcher randomly selects elements from each cluster, rather than using all the elements contained in the selected clusters. Constructing the clusters is the first stage. Deciding which elements within the cluster to use is the second stage. This technique is frequently used when a complete list of all the members of the population does not exist and is inappropriate.

Consider a population with a total of N clusters. In the first stage, n clusters are selected using the ordinary cluster sampling method. In the second stage, simple random sampling is primarily used. It is used separately in every cluster, and the numbers of elements selected from different clusters are not necessarily equal. The survey designer must predetermine the total number of clusters (N), the number of clusters selected (n), and the number of elements from the selected clusters.

(2) Nonprobability sampling

In some studies, probability sampling is difficult or impossible to achieve, and it is often necessary to employ another sampling technique: nonprobability sampling methods. With nonprobability sampling, the sample gathering process does not give all population individuals an equal chance of being selected. In contrast, with probability sampling, a nonprobability sample is not a product of a randomized selection process.

In these methods, the sample may or may not accurately represent the entire population. Therefore, the results of the study cannot be used to generalize the entire population.

(a) Convenience sampling

With convenience sampling, samples are composed of subjects who are accessible to the researcher. Subjects are chosen simply because they are easy to recruit. Because convenience sampling is considered the easiest, cheapest, and least time-consuming method, convenience sampling is probably the most common of all sampling techniques.

(b) Judgmental sampling

With judgmental sampling, subjects are chosen based on the researcher's knowledge and professional judgment. The researcher believes that some subjects are more suitable for the study compared to other individuals, therefore they are purposively chosen as subjects.

(c) Quota sampling

Quota sampling is a nonprobability sampling method wherein the researcher ensures equal or proportionate representation of subjects depending on which trait is considered the basis of the quota. In quota sampling, a population is first segmented into mutually exclusive subgroups. Then, the researcher uses his or her judgment to select the subjects or units from each segment based on a specified proportion.

(d) Snowball sampling

Snowball sampling is a nonprobability sampling method in which existing subjects recruit future subjects from among their acquaintances. In this type of sampling, the researcher asks the initial subject to identify another potential subject who also meets the criteria of the research. This type of sampling is usually performed when the population size is very small.

15.3.2.3　Typical Survey

A typical survey is also called a case survey. On the basis of a complete event analysis, researchers choose typical people or units and then conduct a survey. In this method, only a few subjects are observed who well reflect the main characteristics of the subject group. It is advantageous to further study its characteristics. If consistent with the overall survey, the results can be interpreted from the depth and span. However, there is no ground for any statistical inference.

15.3.2.4　Comparison of Three Types of Observational Design

The paramount differences among censuses, sampling surveys, and typical surveys are discussed in detail in the following table (Table 15.7).

Table 15.7　Comparison of Censuses, Sampling Surveys, and Typical Surveys

Basis for comparison	Census	Sampling survey	Typical survey
Meaning	A method that collects and records the data about all members of the population	A portion of the population is selected to represent the entire group in terms of all its characteristics	Only a few typical subjects are selected to reflect the characteristics of same kind of subjects
Enumeration	Complete	Partial	Partial
Subjects	Each and every subject of the population	Only a handful of subjects of the population	Only a few typical subjects of the population
Time required	Time-consuming process	Fast process	Fast process

Continued

Basis for comparison	Census	Sampling survey	Typical survey
Cost	Expensive method	Economical method	Economical method
Results	Reliable and accurate	Less reliable and accurate, due to the margin of error in the data collected	Unsuitable for statistical inference
Sampling Error	Not present	Dependent on the size of the population	Cannot be estimated
Appropriate for	Heterogeneous populations	Homogeneous populations	Further study

15.3.3　Characteristics

In the fields of epidemiology, medicine, and others, observational designs are an essential tool. Observational methods entail merely observing phenomena already in progress. The researchers observe the subjects and measure the variables of interest instead of assigning treatments to the subjects.

However, in an experiment, the researchers apply treatments to experimental units (people, animals, plots of land, etc.) and then proceed to observe the effect of the treatments on the experimental units.

15.3.4　Advantages and Disadvantages

Each type of observational design has both advantages and disadvantages. One of the main disadvantages of observational studies is that the researcher has no control over the composition of the control groups and cannot randomize the allocation of subjects. Therefore, the researcher has no way of determining whether other factors are involved in the results, which can create bias and can also mask causal relationships or, alternatively, suggest correlations where none exist (errors in research). Randomization is assumed to even out external causal effects, but this method is impossible in an observational design.

Another disadvantage of observational designs is the difficulty in isolating what the independent variable actually is, making it tricky to identify causal relationships. Lack of clarity and control around variables can lead to misunderstandings.

Despite its disadvantages, an observational design is sometimes the most appropriate approach. Taking a step back allows useful insight into a "real-world" phenomenon and eliminates all the problems associated with researcher manipulation or bias.

Sometimes, researchers simply do not have the legal or bureaucratic power to apply treatments on subjects, so observational designs allow them to investigate phenomena that they otherwise could not. Lastly, observational designs sidestep the many possible ethical and practical difficulties of setting up a large and cumbersome medical study.

In conclusion, observational designs are a key part of the research. They can help investigate relationships that cannot be tested under an experimental design, provide insight and develop hypotheses on what subsequent evidence is needed for future research, and provide an understanding of how phenomena work in practice.

15.4　Experimental Design

15.4.1　Definition

An **experimental design** is a research design that eliminates all factors that influence the outcome except for the causal variable of interest (independent variable). Usually, an experimental design is used in situations in which researchers can manipulate the conditions of the experiment and can control the factors that are irrelevant to the research objectives. By noting how the manipulated independent variables affect a response variable, the researcher can test whether a causal relationship exists between the manipulated variables and the response variable. Experimental designs consist of three basic elements: the treatment, the subjects, and the treatment effect.

The most common way to design an experiment is to divide the participants into two groups, the experimental group and the control group, and then test the difference between the experimental group and the control group.

For example, if you manage to find a cure for HIV/AIDS, then you will have to do experiments to check the effectiveness of the drug you discovered compared with another drug. For that purpose, you should randomly contact different people with positive HIV reports and allocate them to the drug-exposed group or the control group. If the drug works against the disease, then you can say that the experiment was successful and the drug can be made available on the market—but only after it gets approved by the FDA.

15.4.2　Basic Elements

All experiments have three **basic elements**: experimental units, treatments, and effects.

Suppose that in a hypothetical experiment, the researcher will assess the possible effects of vitamin C and vitamin E on general health conditions. Table 15.8 below shows the factors, levels, and treatments for the experimental units of the hypothetical experiment. The details of the three experimental design elements will be explained below using this hypothetical experiment.

Table 15.8   Factors, Levels, and Treatments for a Hypothetical Experiment

	Level	Vitamin C (Factor B)	
		0 mg	200 mg
Vitamin E	0 mg	Treatment 1	Treatment 2
(Factor A)	200 mg	Treatment 3	Treatment 4

15.4.2.1   Experimental Units

An **experimental unit**, also referred to as the experimental subject, is the person or object upon which the treatment is applied. The experimental units in an experiment could be anything—genes, proteins, animals, patients, or a healthy population that is subject to one or more treatments—and is, therefore, the source of observations or data. In the hypothetical experiment above, the experimental units would probably be people (or lab animals). When the experimental units are people, they are often called participants; when the experimental units are animals, they are often called subjects. The experimental units should be clearly defined and homogeneous in the study.

15.4.2.2   Treatments

A factor (also called an independent variable) is an explanatory variable manipulated by the researcher. The specific values that the researcher chooses for a factor are called the factor's levels. Each factor has two or more levels (i.e. different values of the factor). For one-factor experiments, the treatments are the levels of a single factor. For multi-factor experiments, the combination of specific levels from all the factors that an experimental unit receives is called a **treatment**. In experiments, treatments are often administered to experimental units by level, where "level" implies the factor's amount or magnitude. The treatments are the unique feature of experimental research that set this design apart from all other research methods.

The hypothetical experiment above includes two factors: the dosage of vitamin E and the dosage of vitamin C. Each factor has two levels: 0 mg per day and 200 mg per day. The experiment includes four treatments. Treatment 1 is 0 mg of vitamin E and 0 mg of vitamin C, treatment 2 is 0 mg of vitamin E and 200 mg of vitamin C, and so on. Researchers then divide the participants into four treatment groups, and each group is treated with different treatments to see which is the most effective. If the participants were given 0 mg or 200 mg of vitamin E, those amounts would be two levels of the factor.

15.4.2.3   Effects

The **effect** is what results after the treatment has acted on the subjects and is expressed by the relevant variables (also called the response variables or dependent variables). In the hypothetical experiment above, the researcher is studying the effect of vitamins on health. In this experiment, the dependent variable would be some measure of health (annual doctor bills, number of colds caught in a year, number of days hospitalized, etc.). The selection of a response variable to measure the effect of treatment has a great influence on the study's validity. The requirements include objectivity, validity, precision, and sensitivity.

The relationships between elements are depicted in Figure 15.13. For instance, in an experiment to evaluate the effect of a new hypoglycemic drug, using the new drug or not for the subjects is the treatment, the patients with the diabetes mellitus participating in the study are the experimental units, and the amount of decrease in glycosylated hemoglobin is the effect variable.

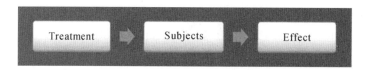

Figure 15.13　The Three Elements of an Experimental Design

15.4.3　Categories

Experimental designs can be categorized according to their objectives and the way they are organized. Designs might be distinguished based on whether they are aimed at assessing preventive interventions or evaluating new treatments for existing disease.

15.4.3.1　Prevention Trials

Prevention trials look at whether a particular treatment can help prevent particular medical conditions or prevent them from reoccurring in people already afflicted. For example, some studies have assessed whether exercise or a low-fat diet can reduce the risk of heart disease or cancer. These trials can be performed for the general population or for people who have a higher than normal risk of developing a certain disease.

15.4.3.2　Therapeutic Trials

Therapeutic trials enroll patients and provide a specific treatment to the patients to study their impact on a disease. They are often used to test new treatments, new combinations of drugs, or new approaches to surgery or radiation therapy. The treatment under investigation is believed to benefit participants in some way (at least those receiving the experimental drug in the case of drug trials).

15.4.4　Characteristics

Experimental designs and observational designs are the two major types of research studies. The main differences are their methodology and ability to manipulate conditions. Table 15.9 distinguishes the characteristics of the two types of research.

Experimental researchers are capable of performing experiments on experimental units and manipulating the variables of interest. These variables can often be controlled and fixed at predetermined values for each test run in the experiment. Therefore, the study is "controlled" in the sense that the researcher controls (a) how subjects are assigned to groups and (b) which treatments each group receives.

In an observational design, many of the variables of interest cannot be controlled, but they can be recorded and analyzed. Like experiments, observational design is also used to understand causal relationships. However, unlike experiments, the researcher is not able to control (a) how subjects are assigned to groups and/or (b) which treatments each group receives.

Table 15.9 The Difference between an Experimental Design and an Observational Design

Type	Characteristics
Experimental design	• During planning and implementing an experiment, the researcher has control over some of the conditions, such as where the study takes place and some aspects of the independent variable(s) (a presumed cause or a variable used to predict another variable) • Factor levels are manipulated to create treatments • Subjects are randomly assigned to these treatment levels • The responses of the subject groups across treatment levels are compared
Observational design	• No experiment or human intervention is conducted • Phenomena are described as they exist • Descriptive studies generally take raw data and summarize the data in a useable form • Also qualitative in nature if the sample size is small and the data are collected from questionnaires, interviews, or observations • Including complete surveys and sampling studies

15.4.5 Advantages and Disadvantages

Experimental research focuses mainly on the relationships between known variables. This type of research provides strong causally interpretable evidence. Knowing the advantages and disadvantages of experimental research can help determine whether this type of research is suitable for the researcher's needs.

The advantages of experimental research are presented below:

(a) Controlling over variables. This type of research aids in controlling an experiment's independent variables. It is less susceptible to confounding because the researcher determines who is exposed and who is not exposed. Therefore, the control over the irrelevant variables is higher compared to other research types or methods.

(b) Easily assessing the treatment and its causal relationship. An experimental design includes manipulating independent variables to easily assess the treatment and its causal relationship. In particular, if treatments are allocated randomly and the number of groups or individuals randomized is large, then even unrecognized confounding effects become statistically unlikely.

(c) Better results. Due to the experiments' controlled variables and strict conditions, biases can be controlled or reduced, and better results can be achieved. Furthermore, the experiments can be repeated, and the results can be checked again, which also gives researchers more confidence regarding the results.

The disadvantages of experimental research are presented below:

(a) Ethical constraints. One of the disadvantages of experimental research is that you may not be able to do experiments because you cannot manipulate the independent variables due to either ethical or practical reasons. In some situations, it is not acceptable to expose subjects deliberately to potentially serious hazards. This limits the application of experimental designs in the investigation of disease etiologies, although it may be possible to evaluate preventive strategies experimentally.

(b) Creating artificial conditions. Another disadvantage of experimental research is that this controls irrelevant variables at times, which also means creating conditions that are somehow artificial.

(c) Not being generalized to real-life situations. The results from experimental designs may not be generalizable to real-life situations. Experimental designs are frequently contrived scenarios that do not often mimic phenomena that occur in the real world. Thus, the degree to which results can be generalized across situations and real-world applications is limited.

（**Yi Honggang, Wu Siying**）

Question Bank

Chapter 16　Sample Size and Power Estimation

16.1　Introduction

For smart users and consumers of medical statistics, sample size and power estimating is a critical procedure when designing a new study. In this chapter, we outline the reasons that physicians, medical students, and others in the health care field should know about sample size and power estimation, and discuss some major considerations that should be fully taken into account in both observational and experimental studies. Though more and more novel study designs are developed nowadays, we limit our discussion to some frequently used cases. Furthermore, as the power can be deduced from the sample size, we mainly focus on the estimation of sample size in this chapter. In addition, the majority of sample size estimations will be presented with appropriate formulae. Associated codes for the required sample size calculation are presented based on SAS 9.4 (SAS Institute Inc., Cary, North Carolina, USA) when no available appropriate equations can be found. Readers of course can conduct their sample size estimation by means of other software such as R package, power analysis and sample size (PASS), SPSS, and others.

16.1.1　Basic Concepts

Although readers may be familiar with terminologies including homogeneity, population, randomization, sample, statistical inference, type I error and type II error from the former chapters, it is necessary to briefly repeat these basic concepts again before we delve into this chapter. Readers will benefit from a better understanding of sample size, power, and its associated knowledge.

In brief, **homogeneity** means similarity. In statistics, homogeneity is described as participants having the same or very similar characteristics or states. **Population** is a collection of participants with high homogeneity, which indicates that only those having very similar features can be included in a population, based on the aim of the study. In practice, population is described as the total number of persons inhabiting a country, city, or any district or area. **Randomization** represents the process of selecting the sample from a specific population randomly, or assigning participants enrolled in the sample to different intervention groups in a random manner, or treating all subjects in a random sequence, in which the features of the sample compared with those of the population, or participants' characteristics are very similar. In other words, randomization is usually defined as all participants in a population having the same chance to be selected when generating the sample, which is called randomized selection in an observational study, or all persons in your sample can obtain the same chance to be assigned into different groups, which is called randomized allocation in an experimental study. As one of the important approaches to reduce the impacts of random errors or bias caused by irrelevant variables, randomization has been widely accepted as a major principle followed with control, replication, and blindness in a study design; use of randomization become increasingly common in a large number of scientific research. The importance of randomization cannot be overestimated at any circumstance, especially in clinical trials. In the past several decades, an important advancement in medical studies is the acceptance and wide usage of randomization as the optimal study design. In statistics, a **sample** is a chosen subset of the population, which is also defined as the collection of participants selected from a study's population. The sample is usually, but not always, selected randomly in a population. However, only a randomized sample can be utilized to make reasonable inferences about a population. **Statistical inference** is a series of estimations on a specific population based on a randomized sample selected from the population. It is a major and most commonly used component of data analysis. Both **type I error** and **type II error** are important components in making statistical inference and should be well considered in a study design. As the number of participants in a population is usually huge in many conditions, conducting a census (systematically acquiring the information of all individuals directly) is quite difficult. To solve this problem, statisticians perform a well-designed sampling study instead of the census. This is the reason why most current researches are sampling studies, even though their goals are to know the features of a population rather than those of the samples they used. In fact, statistical inference has become the most commonly used strategy to estimate features about a population based on a randomized sample, though we may find some inevitable errors including type I error and type II error in the process. **Type I error** is presented to be α and defined as the error in which the null hypothesis is erroneously rejected when it is really true in a hypothesis test. It is also known as the "significant level" of hypothesis testing and conventionally set at 0.05. Meanwhile, we define the **type II error** to be β, which represents the chance to find no difference or association when there is one. It is usually recommended to be less than 0.2 to obtain an appropriate power in a study. Abundant evidence from previous studies reveal that a close relationship exists between type I and type II errors. Techniques that simply aim to minimize one kind of error can unwittingly increase the value of the other. Fortunately, the two types of error can be simultaneous reduced by enlarging your sample size.

The number of participants enrolled in a specific sample is called **sample size**. In general, when making an inference about a population, the researcher should estimate whether participants' features significantly differ among several groups or whether specific variables are significantly associated with others based on the sample. Differences or associations may exist that investigators cannot or do not observe, and this is highly affected by the power. In statistics, **power** is defined as the probability of rejecting the null hypothesis when it is indeed false or, equivalently, concluding that the alternative hypothesis is true when it really is true. It can be best described as the chance or ability of finding a significant effect in your data, if there is a real effect including the above-mentioned differences or associations. Obviously, high power is a valuable attribute for a study, because all investigators want to detect a significant result if it is present. Power is calculated as $1 - \beta$ and is intimately related to the sample size used in the study. The importance of addressing the power of a study cannot be overemphasized.

16.1.2   The Value of Estimating Sample Size and Power

Both sample size and power are fundamental considerations, which should be carefully considered when designing an observational or experimental study in which the goal is to make inferences about a population based on a randomized sample. In principle, sample size is significantly related to satisfied power. The larger the sample size, the more accurate estimations we will achieve, leading to higher precision when making statistical inference. Any study protocol should include an evaluation of the statistical power or sample size estimation. In general, only a statistical power equal to 80% or higher will be considered reasonable to achieve a study's objective and demonstrate that the conclusion is credible. Let's assess the influence of sample size on estimation with the following example. Suppose we have a population including 500,000 male teenagers whose height (centimeter, cm) follows a normal distribution [height $\sim N(149.99, 9.00^2)$]. If we select 5,000 boys from this population randomly, the mean height equals to 149.87 cm. At the same time, the mean height of a sample including 500 boys randomly selected from the same population is 150.29 cm. As the sample size is increased, the sample mean is close to the population mean, which reveals that the sampling error will decrease. This clearly demonstrates that the estimation accuracy will be greatly affected by sample size, and a larger sample would generally have a more precise estimate as compared to a smaller one (Figure 16.1).

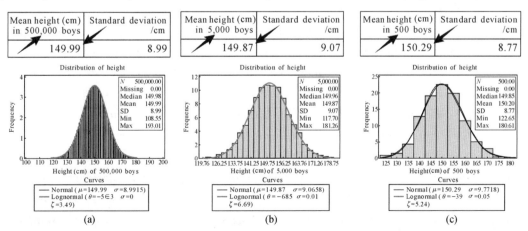

Figure 16.1   The Influence of Sample Size on the Precision of Parameter Estimation

Sample size and power estimation can optimize the study design, efficiently improve chances of obtaining a reasonable conclusion that might otherwise have be ignored, save money and time, and even minimize the risks to participants. Unfortunately, larger sample size will not only induce higher power, but also inevitably increase the difficulties of your study including increased costs and time, more chances of various systematic errors, and increased complexity of the research. However, insufficient sample size will dramatically decrease the precision of your findings. Therefore, obtaining appropriate sample size and power, which should be carefully estimated based on statistical principles, is both important and necessary to balance the impacts from the factors mentioned above. Investigators must plan appropriate sample size and power for their study prior to beginning research. The objective of sample size estimation is to achieve the minimum number of required observations while maintaining the accuracy and efficiency of the statistical inference.

16.2　How to Estimate Sample Size and Power

In general, conducting a census is the best way to know the features of a population, which is the goal in almost all studies. In a census, data are collected on the entire population; hence, the sample size is equal to the size of a population. Although obtaining information about a population without incurring random errors is valuable, conducting a census is cost-prohibitive and generally not feasible since the number of subjects to be investigated is great or boundless. To overcome this problem, statisticians developed an alternative method based on a well-designed random sampling study in which all sample participants are randomly selected from the population.

Under many conditions, larger sample size will necessarily induce higher power; however, this is not universally true. In some situations, a larger sample size may yield a limited increase in precision. Several factors will affect the sample size: greater variability of the measurements, smaller difference among groups, the presence of systematic errors (bias), a heavy-tailed distribution of data, weaker associations between variables, and others all require a larger sample size as compared to their counterparts. Alternatively, the significant level and power of a hypothesis test will also affect the sample size.

Sample size is usually based on an expected statistical power of 80% or higher to observe a positive result. Investigators trying to obtain higher power should pay attention to determining how many participants must be included in the study during the study design period. Investigators can obtain appropriate sample size by means of sample size estimation, which is the act of determining the number of observations or replicates to be included in a sample. In practice, the sample size used in a study is conventionally determined based on the expense of data collection, and the need to have sufficient statistical power. In complicated studies, several different sample sizes may be involved. For example, a stratified survey would include different sample sizes for each stratum. In an experimental study in which individuals will usually be divided into different treatment groups, each group may include different sample sizes.

16.2.1 Observational Study

16.2.1.1 Cross-sectional Study

As a major component of epidemiology, observational study, especially cross-sectional study, is a leading study type for researchers and has been widely conducted in almost all fields including epidemiology, social sciences, psychology, statistics, and others. In general, the goal of a descriptive study, such as a case report, cases series, cross-sectional study, or ecological study, is to describe the features of diseases, injuries, and others in different groups, locations, or time points; estimate the parameters of a specified population; and infer the differences in a subpopulation or the relationships among variables. In short, the goals of descriptive and analytical studies are to generate a reasonable hypothesis and test whether the hypothesis is true or not, respectively, based on individual findings. In practice, an observational study usually draws conclusions from a randomly selected sample to a population in which the predictors, also called independent variables, are not under the control of the investigator because of ethical concerns or logistical restrictions. In contrast with an experimental study, a descriptive study is a prevailing study, such as case report, cases series, cross-sectional study, ecological study, case-control study, and cohort study, in which the investigator provides no specific intervention to the participants and the subjects are assigned into different groups, outside the investigator's control. This does not mean that participants do not receive any interventions at all; in fact, subjects enrolled in an observational study often receive interventions beforehand, which were presented by people other than the associated investigator. In medical statistics, researchers only want to know the distribution and associated determinants of health-related status or events in a specific population based on an observational study.

Let's briefly introduce the principle of a completely randomized design (CRD). As the simplest and non-restricted study design, CRD has been globally accepted as the most commonly used approach for exploring the differences among several parallel groups or effects of a specific factor on another without considering the influences of other potential confounding factors. All subjects in a sample are randomly selected from a population or randomly assigned into different groups without considering the influences from other factors on the response variable.

In a cross-sectional study, at least four questions should be answered before determining power and sample size: (a) What is the significant level (α) or reliability ($1-\alpha$) of the statistical analysis? (b) What is the value or estimation of the standard deviation in a population (σ)? (c) What is the tolerable error (δ), which is defined as an accepted range of the maximum difference between sample statistic ($\bar{X}$ or p) and population parameters (μ or

π)? (d) How about the type II error (β)? In addition, a one-sided or two-sided test, which is far more common than a one-sided test, will also affect the final sample size. After this, we can determine the sample size by means of the formula presented below.

(1) Complete random sampling

(a) Suppose you want to estimate a population rate based on a sample randomly selected from an infinite population; Formula (16.1) can help you to determine the minimum sample size. Meanwhile, if your sample would be selected from a finite population, you can use Formula (16.2), which is revised from Formula (16.1):

$$n = \frac{U_{\frac{\alpha}{2}}^2 \pi (1-\pi)}{\delta^2} \qquad (16.1)$$

where n indicates the desired sample size; α means the significant level, which is usually set as 0.05 or 0.01; $U_{\frac{\alpha}{2}}$ is the critical value of the hypothesis test and is commonly equal to 1.96 if $\alpha = 0.05$ and a two-sided test; π is the estimated population rate, which is usually set as 0.5 if we have no idea of the real population rate; and δ is the tolerable error in your study. Formula (16.2) is expressed as

$$n_a = \frac{n}{1 + \frac{n}{N}} \qquad (16.2)$$

where n indicates the desired sample size based on an infinite population; n_a means the sample size based on a finite population; and N is the total number of participants of the finite population. If the ratio of $\frac{n}{N}$ is very small(e.g. less than 0.05), Formula (16.1) can also be used to calculate the sample size from a finite population.

(b) To estimate population mean for an infinite population, Formula (16.3) is a good option for obtaining the appropriate sample size. If your sample is selected from a finite population, Formula (16.2) should be used to adjust for some potential minor error induced by Formula (16.3):

$$n = (\frac{U_{\frac{\alpha}{2}} \sigma}{\delta})^2 \qquad (16.3)$$

where n is the desired sample size; α means the significant level, which is usually set as 0.05 or 0.01; $U_{\frac{\alpha}{2}}$ is the critical value of the hypothesis test and is commonly equal to 1.96 if $\alpha = 0.05$ and a two-sided test; σ is the estimated standard deviation of the population; and δ is the study's tolerable error.

(2) Stratified random sampling

The formulae that have been discussed earlier are known as simple random sampling, which is widely accepted as the basis of other sampling procedures. In more complex designs, particularly in large surveys or multicenter randomized double-blind clinical trials, investigators usually like to perform stratified random samples in which the population or enrolled participants are first classified into different subgroups (commonly based on some important confounding factors such as age, gender, race, a specific clinical characteristic or geographic location), and then construct simple random samples within each subgroup (strata), in which each member's chance of being selected is the same as in a simple random sample. This method is often applied when obvious variations exist in the number of people, demographic, and clinical characteristics in the different subpopulations. To obtain an appropriate sample and the desired precision in the results, stratification is a better option than a simple random sample and can also reduce data collection costs. Though the procedure of stratification is somewhat complicated and difficult, the chance of random error is much lower than other sampling strategies.

(a) To calculate the minimum sample size for estimating the rate of a finite population based on a stratified random sampling study by Neyman's optimum allocation, investigators can use Formula (16.4) to achieve their goal. This formula can be used for the calculation if your sample is randomly selected from an infinite population:

$$n = \frac{(\sum W_i \sqrt{p_i q_i})^2}{V + \sum \dfrac{W_i p_i q_i}{N}} \tag{16.4}$$

$$n_i = nW_i = \frac{nN_i \sqrt{p_i q_i}}{\sum N_i \sqrt{p_i q_i}}, W_i = \frac{N_i \sqrt{p_i q_i}}{\sum N_i \sqrt{p_i q_i}} \tag{16.5}$$

where n is the needed sample size; $W_i = \dfrac{N_i}{N}$, which reveals the importance of each stratum in a population; N_i, p_i, and q_i represent the frequency, positive rate, and negative rate in the ith stratum, respectively; N means the total number of observations in the population; and V is the estimated variance of the population rate, which is usually determined as $V = (\dfrac{\delta}{U_{\frac{a}{2}}})^2$. The number of observations in the ith stratum can be calculated with the following equation. The meaning of each parameter in Formula (16.5) is the same as that in Formula (16.4).

(b) The desired minimum sample size for estimation of population mean can be determined with Formula (16.6):

$$n - \frac{\sum \dfrac{W_i^2 S_i^2}{W_i}}{V + \sum \dfrac{W_i S_i^2}{N}} \tag{16.6}$$

where $W_i = \dfrac{N_i}{N}$; $W_i = \dfrac{N_i S_i}{\sum N_i S_i}$; N_i and S_i indicate the number of observations and standard deviation of the ith stratum, respectively; N is the total number of participants in the population; and V is the estimated population variance, which is usually equal to $\left(\dfrac{\delta}{U_{\frac{a}{2}}}\right)^2$;

and $n_i = \dfrac{nN_i S_i}{\sum N_i S_i} = nW_i$.

(3) Cluster random sampling

Cluster random sampling is used when the internally heterogeneous are evident in the subpopulation and an obvious homogeneity among the groups can be observed. In this sampling plan, the population is first divided into groups or clusters. Then one or several clusters will be randomly selected in a simple random sampling manner. Individuals in each selected cluster are then sampled. A major motivation of the cluster random sampling is to largely reduce the total amount of sampling and the costs. However, this method will lead to a larger chance of random error as compared to the completely random sampling and stratified sampling.

Unlike the former two sampling plans, the result for estimation of the sample size in a cluster random sampling is the number of selected clusters instead of the number of enrolled participants in the sample.

(a) To estimate the overall rate in an infinite population, we can use Formula (16.7). If the sample will be selected from a countable population, Formula (16.7) should be adjusted for using Formula (16.8):

$$k_0 = U_{\frac{a}{2}}^2 \sum \frac{m_i^2 (p_i - p)^2}{(k_y - 1)\overline{m}^2 \delta^2} \tag{16.7}$$

$$k_1 = k_0 (1 - \frac{k_0}{k}) \tag{16.8}$$

where k_0 is the number of clusters in the boundless population; k_y is the number of clusters to be investigated; m_i and p_i are the total number of participants and proportion of the events in the ith cluster to be investigated; $\overline{m}$ and p represent the average number of participants and rate in the k_y cluster; δ indicates the tolerable error; and K is the total number of the clusters in the finite population.

(b) To calculate the overall mean of an infinite population, Formula (16.9) can be used. If the sample is selected from a countable population, Formula (16.9) should be additionally adjusted with Formula (16.8):

$$k_0 = U_{\frac{a}{2}}^2 \sum \frac{m_i^2 (\overline{X}_i - \overline{X})^2}{(k_y - 1)\overline{m}^2 \delta^2} \tag{16.9}$$

where $\overline{X}_i$ is the mean of the examined variables in the ith cluster; $\overline{X}$ is the mean of the variables in all participants from the k_y clusters. The others are denoted as in Formula (16.7).

16.2.1.2   Case-Control Study

A case-control study is a type of observational study to identify factors that may contribute to an outcome by comparing participants who are patients(cases) with non-patients but are otherwise similar (controls). Case-control studies are a major component of an analytical studies that mainly aim to detect the association between the outcome and some potential determinants, assess the potential impacts due to the determinants on the outcome, and provide some potential effective suggestions on preventing and controlling the outcome. The case-control study has become embedded as a standard epidemiological tool, which is applied in a wide range of human disease research. However, a case-control study only provides odds ratio (OR), which is a weaker measure of association strength compared to relative risk (RR). In general, a case-control study can be performed based on either completely random samples (cases and controls) or paired samples in which the cases and controls may be matched by several major confounding factors of the specific outcome.

The desired minimum sample size of a case-control study is highly linked to the following items: (a) the proportion of the exposure in the controls or a general population (P_0); (b) OR; (c) the significant level of the statistical inference (α), which is usually determined as 0.05; (d) the desired power ($1-\beta$), which is usually suggested to be more than 80%.

(1) Non-paired design

Calculating the sample size for a non-paired (also known as completely random sampling) design can be achieved with Formula (16.10):

$$n = \frac{[U_{1-\frac{\alpha}{2}} \sqrt{2\,\overline{P}(1-\overline{P})} + U_\beta \sqrt{P_1(1-P_1)+P_0(1-P_0)}]^2}{(P_1 - P_0)^2} \qquad (16.10)$$

where $U_{1-\frac{\alpha}{2}}$ and U_β are the critical values at probability of $(1-\frac{\alpha}{2})\%$ and $\beta\%$ in a two-sided standard normal distribution, respectively. P_0 indicates the proportion of exposure in the controls. P_1 is the exposure ratio in the cases, which can be estimated by means of the equation: $P_1 = \frac{OR \times P_0}{1-P_0+OR \times P_0}$ if P_1 is unknown; $\overline{P} = \frac{P_0+P_1}{2}$.

(2) Paired design

The procedure of non-paired design is known as a simply randomized design. In more complex designs such as a paired design, investigators sometimes use a matching strategy, in which some major widely accepted confounding factors such as gender, race, geographic location, or important demographic and clinical characteristics, are matched to make the cases and controls more comparable. As compared to a simply randomized design, conclusions based on paired design will be more credible and reasonable because the impacts due to these potential confounding factors have been avoided by means of a well-designed matching procedure. Formulae (16.11) and (16.12) can be used to achieve the desired minimum sample size in paired case-control studies where the cases and controls are matched by a 1 : 1 ratio:

$$m = \frac{\left[\dfrac{U_{1-\frac{\alpha}{2}}}{2} + U_\beta \sqrt{P(1-P)}\right]^2}{(P-0.5)^2} \qquad (16.11)$$

$$M = \frac{m}{P_0(1-P_1)+P_1(1-P_0)} \qquad (16.12)$$

where m indicates the unmatched pairs of the exposure in the cases and controls; $U_{1-\frac{\alpha}{2}}$ and U_β are the critical values at probability of $(1-\frac{\alpha}{2})\%$ and $\beta\%$ in a two-sided standard normal distribution, respectively. $P = \frac{OR}{1+OR}$; P_0 indicates the proportion of exposure in the controls.

P_1 is the exposure ratio in the cases, which can be estimated by means of the equation: $P_1 = \dfrac{OR \times P_0}{1 - P_0 + OR \times P_0}$ if P_1 is unknown; M represents the pairs wanted in the study.

To obtain the desired sample size in a paired case-control study in which the cases and controls are matched by $\dfrac{1}{r}$ ratio, Formula (16.13) can be used. Previous evidence reveals that a study will be dramatically more difficult to carry out if the r-value is more than 4; in general, r should not exceed 4 to ensure the study is feasible to conduct. Formula (16.13) is expressed as

$$n = \frac{\left[U_{1-\frac{\alpha}{2}} \sqrt{(1+\frac{1}{r})\overline{P}(1-\overline{P})} + U_{\beta} \sqrt{\frac{P_1(1-P_1)}{r} + P_0(1-P_0)} \right]^2}{(P_1 - P_0)^2} \qquad (16.13)$$

where n indicates the number of participants in the cases and the sample size in the controls is equal to $n \times r$ in which r is the reciprocal of the ratio. For example, r is equal to 4 if the matched ratio is $\dfrac{1}{4}$; $U_{1-\frac{\alpha}{2}}$ and U_{β} are the critical values at a probability of $(1-\frac{\alpha}{2})\%$ and $\beta\%$ in a two-sided standard normal distribution, respectively. P_0 indicates the proportion of exposure in the controls. P_1 is the exposure ratio in the cases, which can be estimated by means of the equation: $P_1 = \dfrac{OR \times P_0}{1 - P_0 + OR \times P_0}$ if P_1 is unknown; $\overline{P} = \dfrac{P_1 + r \times P_0}{1 + r}$.

16.2.1.3　Cohort Study

In contrast to the case-control study, a cohort study is a specific form of longitudinal study based on a cohort, in which a large amount of people share a defined exposure or characteristic, typically those who experienced a common event in a selected period. In a cohort study, including retrospective, prospective, and bidirectional cohort study, the exposures, which are detected as participants' pre-existing characteristics, are known and the outcome is unknown at the beginning of the study. All participants in both the exposures and controls (non-exposure) are measured at baseline and then subsequently followed over time to observe the incidence of the outcome in question. The cohort study represents one of the fundamental designs of epidemiology, which are increasingly used in a wide range of fields. In medicine, a cohort study is often used to identify the causes of diseases and can reveal how risk factors affect their incidences. The multiple Cox proportional hazards regression model is commonly used to evaluate the extent to which the exposure variable contributes to the incidence of the disease.

Similar to a case-control study, the desired minimum sample size of a cohort study is highly affected by the following items: (a) the incidence in the controls or a general population (P_0); (b) the difference of the incidence between the exposed population and the controls (d); (c) the significant level of the statistical inference (α), which is usually determined as 0.05; (d) the desired power ($1-\beta$), which is usually suggested to be more than 80%, commonly equals 90%.

Formula (16. 14) can be used to calculate the desired sample size of the exposure and control groups in a cohort study. Furthermore, in general, the sample size in the control group will not be less than that of the exposure group. In addition, failure to follow-up in a cohort study is common, so the missing rate should also be considered during the estimation of the sample size. Because the missing rate in a cohort study should be less than 10%, an additional 10% or more of the number of participants in each group should be added in the sample size determined by Formula (16. 14):

$$n = \frac{(U_{1-\frac{\alpha}{2}} \sqrt{2 \overline{pq}} + U_{\beta} \sqrt{P_0 Q_0 + P_1 Q_1})^2}{(P_1 - P_0)^2} \qquad (16. 14)$$

where n indicates the number of participants in the exposure and the sample size in the controls is equal to $n \times r$ in which r is the reciprocal of the ratio. For example, r is equal to 4 if the matched ratio is $\frac{1}{4}$; $U_{1-\frac{\alpha}{2}}$ and U_{β} are the critical values at a probability of $(1-\frac{\alpha}{2})\%$ and $\beta\%$ in a two-sided standard normal distribution, respectively; and P_0 indicates the proportion of exposure in the controls. P_1 is the exposure ratio in the cases, which can be estimated by means of the equation $P_1 = \frac{OR \times P_0}{1 - P_0 + OR \times P_0}$ if P_1 is unknown; $\overline{P} = \frac{P_1 + r \times P_0}{1 + r}$.

16.2.2 Experimental Study

Another major component of epidemiology is experimental study, which is widely performed in various fields such as medicine, social sciences, psychology, and statistics, and is generally easier to identify than observational study in the medical literature. Experimental study includes randomized clinical trials (RCT) involving humans and tends to draw conclusions about a particular procedure or treatment; these studies should strictly follow the guidelines of good clinical practice (GCP). The objective of an experimental study is to confirm whether the intervention is effective and safe on specific subjects, who are enrolled from a population that meets the criteria of inclusion and exclusion, randomly assigned into different groups. The study type includes parallel design, crossover design, factorial design, repeated measures design, superiority or equivalence or non-inferiority test design, and others that will be explicitly stated compared to an observational study. In medicine, especially in an epidemiological study, investigators can illustrate the characteristics of the outcome of interest including diseases and injuries in different populations, locations, or time points (the major contents of observational study), estimate the parameters of a specific population (parameter estimation), and determine the differences in several subpopulations or the relationships between or among different variables (hypothesis test) based on the experimental study's baseline data.

Furthermore, the comparison between or among the intervention and control groups can be applied to assess the efficacy and safety of the intervention. In short, experimental studies may be considered the steps in advance of an observational study. In fact, the findings of a descriptive study can help investigators to generate a reasonable hypothesis. Subsequently, they can then conduct an analytical study, either a case-control study or cohort study, to test whether the hypothesis is true or false.

Finally, a well-designed experimental study can be used to confirm the accuracy of the findings of the analytical study, to efficiently discover the potential mechanism of the initiation or development of the disease, or to validate the causal relationships between the outcomes and exposures. This is why more and more experimental studies including RCT have been conducted in many fields, especially in medical research. The most important element to be considered in an experimental study is randomization, which will lead to accurate results and credible findings because of a reduced risk of being biased.

In practice, experimental studies can be classified into two categories: with specially designed control (more than 95%) or without specially designed control. In general, a specified intervention is compared with the control to determine whether the intervention makes a difference in the controlled experimental study. While in an uncontrolled experimental study, no specified control is used. Controlled experimental studies are believed to have far greater validity than those without controls because they are much more likely to identify whether the observed differences between groups are really due to the intervention or other factors as compared to the counterparts.

16.2.2.1　Parallel Design

A parallel designed study is a type of clinical study where two or more groups of specified interventions and a control are provided to the subjects in a random manner (Figure 16.2). It is the basis of other experimental studies and has previously been the most commonly used type of all experimental studies in the past. A parallel study is beneficial to confirm the effects in question. The interventions in a parallel study can consist of several completely separate treatments, such as different drugs or simply different doses of a specified drug, while the control group may be a placebo (mainly in animal experiments) or another previously accepted treatment (often in human studies). Because the subjects enrolled in the majority of trials are patients, a placebo is no longer permitted to be used as the control in any epidemiological intervention trial due to ethical considerations.

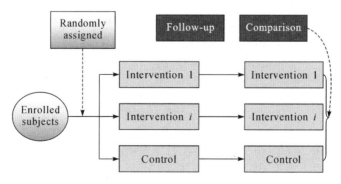

Figure 16.2　Parallel Design

(a) Comparison of the rates between a sample and a known population is shown in Formula (16.15):

$$n = \pi_0 (1 - \pi_0) \left(\frac{U_{\frac{\alpha}{2}} + U_{\beta}}{\delta} \right)^2 \tag{16.15}$$

where π is the known population rate; n is the desired sample size; α means the significant level, which is usually set as 0.05 or 0.01; $U_{\frac{\alpha}{2}}$ is the critical value of the hypothesis test, commonly equal to 1.96 if $\alpha = 0.05$ and a two-sided test; and δ is the tolerable error in your study ($\delta = \pi_1 - \pi_0$).

(b) Comparison between the rates of an intervention and a control group is shown in Formula (16.16):

$$N = \frac{(U_{\frac{\alpha}{2}} + U_{\beta})^2 + (1 + \frac{1}{k}) p(1 - p)}{(p_t + p_c)^2} \tag{16.16}$$

where N is the sample size of the intervention group; U indicates that the sample size estimation will be based on standard normal distribution; α and β represent type I and type II error; p_t and p_c are defined as the rates of the intervention and control groups, respectively; k is the ratio of the numbers of participants between control and intervention groups; p is the combined rates of the intervention and control groups, which can be achieved with the equation $p = \frac{p_t + k p_c}{1 + k}$.

For example, an investigator wants to know whether the efficacy is significantly different between treatments A and B in type 2 diabetes mellitus patients. He knows the population rates of the treatments A and B would be 60% and 85% based on previous literature. How many subjects should be enrolled? Suppose that the ratio of participants in the intervention and control groups are 1 : 1, and the significant level and power will be set as 0.05 and 0.9, respectively.

$$N = \frac{(1.96 + 1.28)^2 (1 + \frac{1}{1}) \frac{0.6 + 0.85}{2} (1 - \frac{0.6 + 0.85}{2})}{(0.6 + 0.85)^2} = 67.1 \approx 68$$

So, the desired sample size of this example would be 136 (68 for each treatment) participants.

(c) Comparison of the rates among several interventions and a control group is shown in Formula (16.17):

$$n = \frac{1,641.4\lambda}{(\sin^{-1} \sqrt{\pi_{\max}} - \sin^{-1} \sqrt{\pi_{\min}})^2} \tag{16.17}$$

where n is the sample size of each group; λ represents the value from the λ critical value table with the degree of freedom (df) equal to the number of groups (g) minus 1 at the level of $\alpha = 0.05$ and $\beta = 0.1$ (usually). $\pi_{\max}$ and $\pi_{\min}$ are the maximum and minimum of the known population rates, which can also be replaced with the observed sample rates if we have no information on π.

(d) Comparison of the means between a sample and known population is shown in Formula (16. 18):

$$n = \left(\frac{U_{\frac{\alpha}{2}} + U_{\beta}}{\frac{\delta}{\sigma}} \right)^2 \tag{16.18}$$

where n is the desired sample size; α is the significant level; β is the type II error; σ indicates the population standard deviation, which can be replaced with the sample standard deviation in many conditions; U represents that the sample size estimation is based on a standard normal distribution; δ is the tolerable error, which is often defined as the difference between the two population means ($\mu - \mu_0$). In general, we can define the value of $\frac{\delta}{\sigma}$ as 0. 1 if we do not know the values of δ and σ.

(e) Comparison of the means between two independent samples is shown in Formula (16. 19):

$$n = 2 \left(\frac{U_{\frac{\alpha}{2}} + U_{\beta}}{\frac{\delta}{\sigma}} \right)^2 \tag{16.19}$$

where n is the desired sample sizes for each group; α is the significant level; β is the type II error; σ indicates the population standard deviation, which can be replaced with the sample standard deviation in many conditions; U represents that the sample size estimation is based on a standard normal distribution; δ is the tolerable error, which is often defined as the difference between the two population means ($\mu_1 - \mu_2$). In general, we can define the value of $\frac{\delta}{\sigma}$ as 0. 1 if we do not know the values of δ and σ.

(f) Comparison of the means between the two paired groups is shown in Formula (16. 20):

$$n = \left(\frac{U_{\frac{\alpha}{2}} + U_{\beta}}{\frac{\delta}{\sigma}} \right)^2 \tag{16.20}$$

where n is the pairs of desired sample size; α is the significant level; β is the type II error; σ indicates the population standard deviation, which can be replaced with the sample standard deviation in many conditions; U represents that the sample size estimation is based on a standard normal distribution; δ is the tolerable error, which is often defined as the difference between the two population means ($\mu - \mu_0$). In general, we can define the value of $\frac{\delta}{\sigma}$ as 0. 1 if we do not know the values of δ and σ.

(g) Comparison of the means among multiple groups is shown in Formula (16. 21):

$$n = \frac{\Psi^2 \dfrac{\sum \sigma_i^2}{g}}{\dfrac{\sum (\mu_i - \mu)^2}{g - 1}} \tag{16.21}$$

where n is the desired sample size of each group; g represents the number of groups; μ_i is the population mean of the ith group, which can be replaced with the $\overline{X}_i$ when we can achieve no information about the μ_i; $\mu = \dfrac{\sum \mu_i}{g}$, which can be replaced with $\overline{X} = \dfrac{\sum \overline{X}_i}{g}$ in many conditions; ψ can be found from the critical value table for the comparisons of multiple means at the level of $\alpha=0.05$, $\beta=0.1$.

(h) Inference of the relationship between two continuous variables is shown in Formula (16.22):

$$n = 4\left[\frac{U_{\frac{\alpha}{2}}+U_{\beta}}{\ln(\frac{1+r}{1-r})}\right]^2 + 3 \tag{16.22}$$

where n is the desired sample size; α is the significant level which is usually equal to 0.05; β is the type II error, which is usually equal to 0.1; U represents that the sample size estimation is based on a standard normal distribution; r represents Pearson coefficient of correlation, which indicates that the two continuous variables should both meet normal or similar normal distribution.

16.2.2.2　Crossover Design

As we know, participants in the appropriate control group should be provided a placebo, a substance having no pharmacological effect but administered as a control in an experimental study, to accurately assess the efficacy of a specific intervention. However, subjects enrolled in a clinical study, especially in an RCT, are more often designed as a parallel study and are usually specified patients. All of them should obtain timely, efficient treatments. Although placebo is greatly beneficial on precisely examining the "real" efficacy of the intervention as compared to other controls, it cannot be presented to subjects as a control in an RCT because of ethical considerations. To overcome this limitation of a parallel study design, scientists developed a crossover study design. In medicine, a crossover study is a longitudinal study in which subjects receive a sequence of different treatments (or exposures). Though crossover studies can be observational studies, the majority of important crossover studies are experimental studies. In fact, crossover designs are quite common for experiments in many scientific disciplines including psychology, pharmaceutical science, and medicine. In nearly all crossover designed studies, subjects will receive the same number of treatments, participate for the same number of periods, and receive all treatments.

As compared to a parallel study design, crossover experiments are especially important in health care. Nearly all crossover is designed to make each subject receive the same treatments in a random order and participate for the same number of periods. In practice, all patients in a crossover trial are assigned to a sequence of two or more treatments, and the control can be determined as a placebo, which is not permitted in a classical parallel designed clinical trial due to ethical considerations, even though placebo has been widely accepted as the better control. In statistics, statisticians suggest that the study should have at least three periods (Figure 16. 3). In the first period, enrolled subjects are randomly assigned into different groups, and then each group is given a specific intervention or placebo in a random manner. During the second period (usually more than 2 weeks), all subjects receive neither intervention nor placebo. In the third period, the intervention or placebo given in the first period is exchanged; that is, the intervention or placebo given to one group is now given to another and vice versa. Because no widely accepted specific formulae are available, it is suggested that the above-mentioned Formulae (16. 15) to (16. 22) are also suitable for estimating the appropriate sample size of each kind of crossover designed study, respectively.

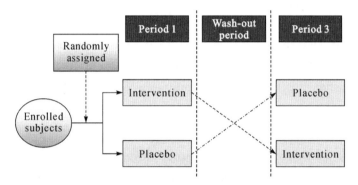

Figure 16. 3   The Principle of Crossover Design

16. 2. 2. 3   Factorial Design

As can be observed in the previous chapters, the above-mentioned parallel designed experiments or crossover designed studies are more commonly used and highly suitable for exploring the effects of a single intervention. However, the combined usage of two or more treatments is also common to achieve better efficacy and higher safety in clinical practice. To comprehensively assess the main and independent effects of each treatment as well as their interactions on the outcome in the same time, these two study designs have obvious limitations and no longer be used. To overcome this problem, statisticians developed a novel study design—factorial design, which has been commonly used over the years and is widely accepted as a more appropriate study design suitable for exploring the effects of two or more interventions in a study.

In statistics, a factorial design study usually includes two or more factors, each with discrete levels, and takes on all possible combinations of these levels across all factors. So, the researcher can investigate each factor's main effect and the independent effect on the outcome, as well as their interactions among factors. The simplest factorial experiment is called a 2×2 factorial design, which includes two factors, each with only two levels, and four combined interventions as neither A nor B, A alone, B alone, and both A and B. If the number of the intervention combinations in a full factorial design is too high to be feasibly conducted, investigators can apply an orthogonal design, which is a simplified factorial design, mainly focusing on some of the most important combinations of factors and omitting other combinations, instead of a full factorial design.

Because no widely accepted formula is available, the sample size and power estimation in a full factorial design is usually conducted by means of some statistical specific software including SAS, power analysis and sample size (PASS), and others. In this chapter, we provide the following codes to estimate the sample size and power estimation for a 2×2 factorial design study. Suppose a researcher wanted to examine the impacts of two different treatments (A and B) on the fasting plasma glucose (FPG) reduction using a 2×2 factorial designed study. He enrolled 80 type 2 diabetes patients in a pilot study and classified them into four subgroups with neither A nor B, A alone, B alone, as well as both A and B. Firstly, he can calculate the mean and standard deviation of the decrease of FPG for each group (Table 16. 1).

(a) SAS codes for the sample size and power estimation for a 2×2 factorial designed study

proc means mean std data = tmpp1 maxdec = 1; * to calculate the mean and standard deviation of the decrease of FPG (the results are presented in Table 16. 1)

    var dfpg; * dfpg indicates the decrease of FPG;

    class a b;

    ods output summary = tmp1; * to output the results into a dataset named tmp1;

run;

Table 16. 1   Summary of the Decrease of FPG (mmol/L) for Each Group

Treatment A	Treatment B	n	Mean	Std. dev.
No	No	20	-0.4	1.7
No	Yes	20	4.8	1.2
Yes	No	20	8.4	1.2
Yes	Yes	20	12.9	1.2

(b) To estimate the desired sample size for each combination of treatments

```
proc glmpower data = tmp1;
    class a b;
    model dfpg_mean = a | b;
    power
    stddev = 1. 2 1. 2 1. 2 1. 7
    ntotal = .
    power = 0. 80;
run;
```

Computed N Total

Index	Source	Std. dev.	Test df	Error df	Actual power	N Total
1	a	1.2	1	4	>0.999	8
2	a	1.2	1	4	>0.999	8
3	a	1.2	1	4	>0.999	8
4	a	1.7	1	4	0.999	8
5	b	1.2	1	4	0.984	8
6	b	1.2	1	4	0.984	8
7	b	1.2	1	4	0.984	8
8	b	1.7	1	4	0.845	8
9	$a \times b$	1.2	1	412	0.803	416
10	$a \times b$	1.2	1	412	0.803	416
11	$a \times b$	1.2	1	412	0.803	416
12	$a \times b$	1.7	1	824	0.801	828

Figure 16.4　The Results of the Sample Size Estimation of a 2×2 Factorial Designed Study

Figure 16.4 clearly reveals the desired sample size in different combinations of the two treatments. It shows that the power is more than 0.999 to observe the reduction of FPG in both treatments A and B when the sample size is equal to 8. Furthermore, if the investigator wants to obtain the power of 0.8 to detect the significant interaction between treatments A and B, the minimum total sample size should be equal to or greater than 416 (104 patients per subgroup) to 828 (207 subjects per subgroup).

(c) To estimate the power of a 2×2 factorial designed study

```
proc glmpower data = tmp1;
    class a b;
    model x_mean = a | b;
    power
    stddev = 1.2 1.2 1.2 1.7
    power = .
    ntotal = 828;
run;
```

Computed Power

Index	Source	Std. dev.	Test df	Power
1	a	1.2	1	>0.999
2	a	1.2	1	>0.999
3	a	1.2	1	>0.999

| | | | | Continued |
Index	Source	Std. dev.	Test df	Power
4	a	1. 7	1	>0. 999
5	b	1. 2	1	>0. 999
6	b	1. 2	1	>0. 999
7	b	1. 2	1	>0. 999
8	b	1. 7	1	>0. 999
9	$a \times b$	1. 2	1	0. 978
10	$a \times b$	1. 2	1	0. 978
11	$a \times b$	1. 2	1	0. 978
12	$a \times b$	1. 7	1	0. 801

Figure 16. 5   The Results of Power Estimation of a 2×2 Factorial Designed Study Based on the Sample Size of 828

16. 2. 2. 4   Repeated Measures Design

In the past several decades, many longitudinal studies have been performed to compare the differences between a specific intervention and control, or explore the relationships among variables. Compared to a cross-sectional study, longitudinal data enable the investigator to efficiently detect the individual effects of a specified intervention, as well as the changes of the intervention over time and their joint effect. A longitudinal study usually involves multiple measures of the same variable, more commonly repeated measurements of a continuous variable. Information on variables within the same subject is collected several times, strictly following the project's protocol or its specified standard operation procedure (SOP). Therefore, this type of study is also called repeated measures design, because it takes on the same participants over several time points.

In practice, a repeated measures design study is very common for experiments in many scientific fields such as psychology, education, pharmaceutical science, and health-care, especially in randomized, controlled clinical trials (RCT). In an RCT, the enrolled subjects are first randomly assigned into different groups. Subjects then receive a sequence of different interventions including at least two treatments, where one may be a standard treatment or a placebo, and the outcomes are measured repeatedly over several time points. As described in the previous section of this chapter, a crossover study is an example of repeated measures design. In fact, a crossover study is also a longitudinal study in which a sequence of different interventions or exposures is provided to all subjects. Many crossover studies are repeated measure, controlled experiments though they can also be observational studies. However, the majority of repeated measures studies are not crossover designs, because the longitudinal study of the sequential effects of repeated treatments does not cross over.

Compared to cross-sectional design, a repeated measures design has several advantages. First, collecting repeated measurements of key variables allows researchers to examine the within-person changes over time. Moreover, compared to non-repetitive measurement designs, a repeated measures design can simultaneously increase the statistical power for detecting changes while reducing the costs, when conducting a study based on collecting repeated measurements. Fewer participants are needed since the repeated measures design can obviously reduce the variance estimating treatment-effects, enabling the related statistical inference with fewer subjects. Higher efficiency is achieved because fewer investigators need to be trained to complete an entire experiment, therefore allowing several experiments to be completed more quickly. Furthermore, the repeated measures design allows investigators to watch carefully how subjects change during the whole study period and longitudinal analysis can be used to perform the estimations of population characteristics. In summary, a repeated measures designed study can efficiently reduce the costs and efforts required to conduct a study compared to its counterparts. However, unlike studies with independent observations, repeated measurements taken from the same participant may be highly correlated, and the correlations must be accounted for in calculating the appropriate sample size. Therefore, estimating the sample size for a repeated measures designed study is very complicated and requires profound statistical knowledge and programming skills that are beyond the resources available to many researchers. Some current software packages used for sample size calculations are based on oversimplified assumptions about correlation patterns, which can give investigators false confidence in the chosen sample size. The following section discusses how to calculate the sample size, in brief.

(1) Comparison of means in one sample using repeated measure design

In general, a random effect model is commonly conducted to estimate the required sample size of a repeated measures design study. The required sample size for one sample repeated measures design can be estimated using the following formula:

$$M = [1 + (k-1)\rho] \frac{\sigma^2 (U_{\frac{\alpha}{2}} + U_{\beta})^2}{k\delta^2} \tag{16.23}$$

where M is the minimum required sample size; U indicates that the sample size estimation will be based on standard normal distribution; α and β represent type I error and type II error; ρ is the coefficient of correlation between two adjacent measurements; k is the times of measurements; σ^2 is the mean of the variances for each participant's repeated measurements in a pilot study; δ is the tolerable error which is also defined as the smallest detectable difference between pre- and post-treatment.

Because a single sample of repeated measures design is the extension of a self-pairing design in which the times of the measurements is equal to 2, its required sample size is highly correlated to that of a paired design study. The relationship between them can be described with the following equation:

$$M = \frac{1 + (k-1)\rho}{k} N \qquad (16.24)$$

where N indicates the required sample size of a single sample in a self-pairing design study.

(2) Comparison of two survival curves

Suppose you are planning a prospective, repeated measures design clinical trial to compare the survival rates for proposed and standard cancer treatments, based on a log-rank test with non-parametrically compared overall survival curves for the two treatments. It needs to determine an appropriate sample size to achieve a power of 0.8 for a two-sided test with $\alpha = 0.05$. The survival curve for patients on the standard treatment is known to be approximately exponential with a median survival time of five years. The team conjectures that the new proposed treatment will yield a non-exponential survival curve with the survival rate as 0.95, 0.9, 0.75, 0.7, and 0.6 for the 1st, 2nd, 3rd, 4th, and 5th year, respectively. Patients will be enrolled in one year and then followed for an additional four years. Some loss to follow-up is expected, with roughly exponential rates that would result in about 50% loss with the standard treatment at the end of the 5th year. Although the loss to follow-up with the proposed treatment is difficult to predict, it is estimated that no more than 50% loss would be expected. As no widely accepted equation is available, you can use the TWOSAMPLESURVIVAL statement in SAS with the TEST = LOGRANK option to compute the required sample size for the log-rank test. Figure 16.6 clearly reveals that at least 474 (237 for each group) subjects should be enrolled in this study.

```
proc power;
    twosamplesurvival test = logrank
    curve("Standard") = 5 : 0.5
    curve("Proposed") = (1 to 5 by 1) : (0.95 0.9 0.75 0.7 0.6)
    groupsurvival = "Standard" | "Proposed"
    accrualtime = 1
    followuptime = 4
    groupmedlosstimes = 5 | 5 5
    power = 0.8
    npergroup = . ;
run;
```

(3) Comparison of means for a repeated measures design

The first step in computing a sample size should be selecting an appropriate power analysis method that adequately aligns with the data analysis approach. Suppose a researcher is interested in testing whether males and females respond similarly to a specific exposure. He plans to control for age, health status, etc. based on an analysis of covariance (ANCOVA) instead of a two independent samples t-test. A two-group t-test would be inappropriate for the sample size calculation because it will lead to unreasonable sample size and inconclusive findings. In the past several decades, statisticians have developed multiple

The POWER procedure log-rank test for two survival curves	
Fixed scenario elements	
Method	Lakatos normal approximation
Accrual time	1
Follow-up time	4
Group 1 survival curve	Standard
Form of survival curve 1	Exponential
Group 2 survival curve	Proposed
Form of survival curve 2	Piecewise linear
Group 1 median loss time	5
Nominal power	0.8
Number of sides	2
Number of time sub-intervals	12
α	0.05

Computed N per group			
Index	Median loss time 2	Actual power	N per group
1	5	0.801	237
2	5	0.801	237

Figure 16. 6　Sample Size Estimation for the Comparison of Two Survival Curves

mixed models, which have become the most popular method for analyzing repeated measures and longitudinal data.

In many cases, the planned data analysis has no published power analysis methods aligned with the data analysis. One possible method that we can perform to find reliable power or sample size when no power formulae are available is to use appropriate software that has been tested and validated whenever it is available. Several statistical software packages including SAS, R, SPSS, STATA, and others have the advantages of estimating the desired sample size. We therefore recommend that the sample size calculation be conducted using carefully built multiple mixed models since these will provide the best available power analysis. Another option is to compute sample sizes for studies with correlated observations based on the generalized estimating equation (GEE) approach.

For example, suppose you are interested in the long-term effect of a novel treatment (TrtA) on fasting plasma glucose (FPG) reduction, planning a pilot study to compare its efficacy to a standard treatment (TrtB) over a period of one year, assessing 40 (20 for each group) enrolled type 2 diabetes patients' baseline FPG and then again at the 1st, 4th, 13th, 26th, and 52nd week. The between-subject factor in your model is treatment, with two levels (TrtA versus TrtB), which is equally allocated for a balanced design. The within-subject factor is time, with six levels (0, 1, 4, 13, 26, and 52 weeks). You want to determine the number of patients required to achieve a power of 0. 9 at the significant level $\alpha=0. 05$ to test the interaction between time and treatment, where the contrast over time contains all pairwise comparisons. You also want to generate a plot of power versus sample size that covers the power range of 0. 1 to 1. The mean FPG for both treatments at each time point are presented in Table 16. 2.

Table 16. 2   The Mean of Fasting Plasma Glucose (mmol/L) by Treatments

Treatment	Baseline	1st week	4th week	13th week	26th week	52nd week
Novel	12. 40	10. 38	8. 05	7. 90	7. 02	6. 38
Standard	12. 41	10. 43	8. 36	8. 30	7. 86	7. 21

(a) You can use the following statements to create a data set named FPG which contains these means over the treatments and time.

```
Data FPG;
    input Treatment $ base wk1 wk4 wk13 wk26 wk52;
    datalines;
    Novel     12. 40   10. 38   8. 05   7. 90   7. 02   6. 38
    Standard  12. 41   10. 43   8. 36   8. 30   7. 86   7. 21
    ;
Run;
```

(b) You can specify a set of parameters that defines the entire covariance matrix of the residuals to characterize the variability. In this case, the standard deviation is estimated to be the same at all six-time points, with a value between 0. 92 and 1. 04. The uncertainty of the sample size analysis should include both the lower and upper ends of this range. You can assume that the correlation has a linear exponent autoregressive (LEAR) structure, with a correlation of about 0. 6 between measurements one week apart and a decrease rate of about 0. 8 over one-week intervals.

(c) You can use the following statements to perform the sample size analysis, and the associated results are presented in Figure 16. 8. It clearly reveals that at least 406 type 2 diabetes patients (203 subjects in each group) should be enrolled in this repeated measures designed study.

```
ods graphics on/border=no;
proc glmpower data=fpg;
    class Treatment;
    model base wk1 wk4 wk13 wk26 wk52=Treatment;
    repeated Time contrast;
    power
        mtest=hlt
        alpha=0. 05
        power=. 9
        ntotal=.
        stddev=0. 92 1. 64
        matrix ("PainCorr")=lear(0. 6, 0. 8, 6, 0 1 4 13 26 52)
        corrmat="PainCorr";
```

```
        plot y=power min=0. 1 max=1 yopts=(ref=0. 9 crossref=yes)
          vary (linestyle by stddev, symbol by dependent source);
  run;

  ods graphics off;
```

The SAS System

The GLMPOWER Procedure F Test for Multivariate Model

Fixed scenario elements	
Wilks/HLT/PT method	O'Brien-Shieh
F test	Hotelling-Lawley Trace
α	0.05
Correlation matrix	PainCorr
Nominal power	0.9

Computed N Total

Index	Transformation	Source	Std. dev.	Effect	Num df	Den df	Actual power	N total
1	Time	Intercept	0.92	Time	5	2	0.980	8
2	Time	Intercept	1.64	Time	5	4	0.999	10
3	Time	Treatment	0.92	Time×Treatment	5	56	0.906	62
4	Time	Treatment	1.64	Time×Treatment	5	176	0.902	182
5	Mean(Dep)	Intercept	0.92	Intercept	1	2	>0.999	4
6	Mean(Dep)	Intercept	1.64	Intercept	1	2	>0.999	4
7	Mean(Dep)	Treatment	0.92	Treatment	1	128	0.903	130
8	Mean(Dep)	Treatment	1.64	Treatment	1	404	0.901	406

Figure 16.7　Sample Size Estimation for Comparison of Means in Repeated Measures Design

16.2.2.5　Superiority, Equivalence, and Non-inferiority Test Design

The field of statistics is increasingly complex and difficult for most investigators to fully understand. In the past, a traditional randomized clinical trial (RCT) was always performed to investigate whether a new drug or therapy is effective to alleviate clinical symptoms of the enrolled subjects—a specified number of patients randomly assigned into two different groups in which patients in one group receive the drug or therapy and another group receives a placebo. However, because the subjects are specific disease patients in the majority of RCTs, a placebo will not be permitted because of ethical considerations. Nowadays, the control of most RCTs has been determined with a standard treatment in which no "real" efficacy of the novel therapy will be observed. Furthermore, with the continuous development of medical drugs, therapies, devices, and others, it is becoming increasingly difficult to develop new RCTs with significantly higher efficacy than the standard controls.

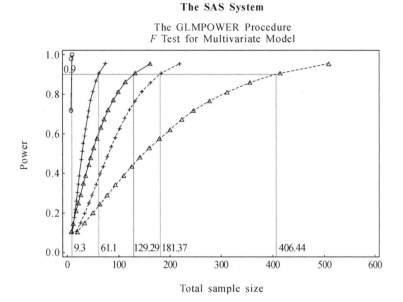

The SAS System

The GLMPOWER Procedure
F Test for Multivariate Model

Total sample size

Figure 16. 8   Plots of the Sample Size, and Power Estimation for Comparison of Means in Repeated Measures Design

This has led to the rapid development of other types of trials, including superiority, equivalence, and non-inferiority trials. In this case, investigators can only detect whether the novel therapy will be more effective than the standard treatment, which is defined as a superiority trial, and whether the novel therapy is similar to the control (equivalence trial) or not inferior to the control (non-inferiority trial).

In general, results are accepted if the magic p-values $<=0.05$. Because the p-value will be largely affected by the sample size, significant results may be achieved if the sample size is large enough—even if the effects are quite small in a specific study. This may be a limitation of modern statistics. For example, a researcher aims to assess the efficacy of a novel blood pressure medication. The decreased systolic blood pressure (SBP) of the intervention and control (standard treatment) groups are 5.4 ± 2.3 and 5.1 ± 2.0 mmHg, respectively, in an RCT with a sample size as 240 (120 for each). He cannot observe a significant difference between the intervention and control since the p-value associated with the comparison is 0.281. However, if 960 (480 for each) hypertensive patients are enrolled in the same study with the same decreased SBP between the two groups, the p-value would be 0.031. His conclusion may be that the novel treatment is more effective in reducing patients' SBP than the control. Such a result is hardly acceptable for reliable testing.

The major objectives of this section are to introduce superiority, equivalence, and non-inferiority testing as novel statistical approach to avoid the risk of statistically significant but clinically irrelevant results. As compared to a traditional RCT in which a significant efficacy of a new treatment is accepted if the null-hypothesis of no treatment effect is rejected at $P=0.05$, the superiority testing would be much better since it demonstrates the effects of the new treatment, based on a stricter criterion than a p-value of 0.05 as the cut-off criterion. In practice, researchers should define a priori clinically relevant boundary of superiority, equivalence, and non-inferiority of the new treatment. We do not have to worry about the p-values in either superiority, equivalence, or non-inferiority trials. Figure 16. 9 gives the principles of superiority, equivalence, and non-inferiority testing. In statistics, if the 95% CI of the study result is more than the upper boundary, superiority is accepted and the investigator may conclude that the novel therapy is more effective than the standard treatment. If the 95% CI of the effect is within the two boundaries and/or includes the null hypothesis (H_0), equivalence is achieved and the effect of novel therapy is considered similar to the control. Furthermore, if 95% CI of the effect of the new treatment includes the H_0, non-inferiority is observed and the novel treatment may be considered not inferior to the standard treatment. In brief, a superiority testing often assumes the effect of the novel therapy is better than the control. With an equivalence/non-inferiority testing, investigators usually have prior arguments to assume that little difference exists between the new treatment and the control, and are mainly interested in similarity and non-inferiority of the new treatment versus the control, rather than a statistically significant difference between the two treatments.

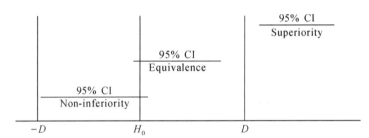

Figure 16. 9   Principles of Superiority, Equivalence, and Non-inferiority Study Design

(1) Superiority testing

(a) Comparison of the proportions based on two independent two samples is shown in Formula (16.25):

$$N = \left[\frac{U_\alpha \sqrt{\pi_C(1-\pi_C)(Q_1^{-1}+Q_2^{-1})} + U_\beta \sqrt{\dfrac{\pi_1(1-\pi_1)}{Q_1} + \dfrac{\pi_2(1-\pi_2)}{Q_2}}}{\delta - \Delta} \right]^2 \quad (16.25)$$

where n is a total of the required sample size of a superiority testing; U_α and U_β are the critical values of a standard normal distribution; π_1 and π_2 are the estimated positive rates for the novel therapy and standard treatment groups; π_C is the pooled positive rate of both groups ($\pi_C = Q_1\pi_1 + Q_2\pi_2$); Q_1 and Q_2 are the ratios of the sample size in each group ($Q_1 = \dfrac{n_1}{N}$, $Q_2 = \dfrac{n_2}{N}$); δ is the tolerable error ($\delta = \pi_1 - \pi_2$); and Δ is the boundary of a superiority testing, which should be greater than 0. If no previous literature can be cited, Δ can be set as 10%~15% of the effective rate of the standard treatment.

For example, an investigator is interested in assessing whether a novel treatment is more effective in improving a specific disease based on a superiority trial with a standard treatment as the control. Based on previous literature, he knows that the effective rate for the new therapy and control are 85% and 80%, respectively. Only an effective rates difference more than 0.15 will be accepted. How many subjects should be enrolled in this superiority designed RCT? Suppose the significant level is set as 0.05, the power should be 0.9 and $Q_1 = Q_2 = 0.5$.

$$N = \left[\frac{1.645 \sqrt{0.825(1-0.825)(2+2)} + 1.282 \sqrt{\dfrac{0.80(1-0.80)}{0.5} + \dfrac{0.85(1-0.85)}{0.5}}}{0.85 - 0.80 - 0.15} \right]^2 = 494$$

which means that at least 494 (247 for each group) subjects should be enrolled in this superiority designed RCT.

(b) Comparison of the means based on two independent two samples is shown in Formula (16.26):

$$N = \left[\frac{(U_\alpha + U_\beta)\sigma}{\delta - \Delta} \right]^2 (Q_1^{-1} + Q_2^{-1}) \tag{16.26}$$

where N is a total of the required sample size of a superiority testing; U_α and U_β are the critical values of a standard normal distribution; σ is the pooled standard deviation of both groups $\left(\sigma = \sqrt{\dfrac{(n-1)\sigma_1^2 + (n_2-1)\sigma_2^2}{n_1 + n_2 - 2}} \right)$; n_1 and n_2 represent the sample size for the intervention and control group; Q_1 and Q_2 are the ratios of the sample size in each group $\left(Q_1 = \dfrac{n_1}{N}, Q_2 = \dfrac{n_2}{N} \right)$; δ is the tolerable error $(\delta = \mu_1 - \mu_2)$; and Δ is the boundary of a superiority testing, which should be greater than 0. If no previous study can be found, Δ can be $10\% \sim 15\%$ of the mean of the standard treatment.

(2) Equivalence testing

(a) Comparison of the proportions based on two independent two samples is shown in Formula (16.27):

$$N = \left[\frac{U_{\frac{\alpha}{2}} \sqrt{\pi_C (1-\pi_C)(Q_1^{-1} + Q_2^{-1})} + U_{\frac{\beta}{2}} \sqrt{\dfrac{\pi_1(1-\pi_1)}{Q_1} + \dfrac{\pi_2(1-\pi_2)}{Q_2}}}{\delta - \Delta} \right]^2 \tag{16.27}$$

where N is a total of the required sample size of an equivalence testing; $U_{\frac{\alpha}{2}}$ and $U_{\frac{\beta}{2}}$ are the critical values of a two-sided standard normal distribution; π_1 and π_2 are the estimated positive rates for the novel therapy and standard treatment groups; π_C is the pooled positive rate of both groups $(\pi_C = Q_1 \pi_1 + Q_2 \pi_2)$; Q_1 and Q_2 are the ratios of the sample size in each group $\left(Q_1 = \dfrac{n_1}{N}, Q_2 = \dfrac{n_2}{N} \right)$; δ is the tolerable error $(\delta = \pi_1 - \pi_2)$; and Δ is the boundary of an equivalence testing. If no previous literature can be cited, Δ can be set as $10\% \sim 15\%$ of the effective rate of the standard treatment.

(b) Comparison of the means based on two independent two samples is shown in

Formula (16.28):

$$N = \left[\frac{(U_{\frac{a}{2}} + U_{\frac{\beta}{2}})\sigma}{\delta - \Delta}\right]^2 (Q_1^{-1} + Q_2^{-1}) \tag{16.28}$$

where N is a total of the required sample size of an equivalence testing; $U_{\frac{a}{2}}$ and $U_{\frac{\beta}{2}}$ are the critical values of a two-sided standard normal distribution; σ is the pooled standard deviation of both groups ($\sigma = \sqrt{\frac{(n_1-1)\sigma_1^2 + (n_2-1)\sigma_2^2}{n_1+n_2-2}}$); n_1 and n_2 represent the sample size for the intervention and control group; Q_1 and Q_2 are the ratios of the sample size in each group ($Q_1 = \frac{n_1}{N}$, $Q_2 = \frac{n_2}{N}$); δ is the tolerable error ($\delta = \mu_1 - \mu_2$); and Δ is the boundary of an equivalence testing. If no previous study can be found, Δ can be set as $10\% \sim 15\%$ of the mean of the standard treatment.

(2) Non-inferiority testing

(a) Comparison of the proportions based on two independent two samples is shown in Formula (16.29):

$$N = \left[\frac{U_a \sqrt{\pi_C(1-\pi_C)(Q_1^{-1}+Q_2^{-1})} + U_\beta \sqrt{\frac{\pi_1(1-\pi_1)}{Q_1} + \frac{\pi_2(1-\pi_2)}{Q_2}}}{\delta - |\Delta|}\right]^2 \tag{16.29}$$

where n is a total of the required sample size of a non-inferioring testing; U_a and U_β are the critical values of a two-sided standard normal distribution; π_1 and π_2 are the estimated positive rates for the novel therapy and standard treatment groups; π_C is the pooled positive rate of both groups ($\pi_C = Q_1\pi_1 + Q_2\pi_2$); Q_1 and Q_2 are the ratios of the sample size in each group ($Q_1 = \frac{n_1}{N}$, $Q_2 = \frac{n_2}{N}$); δ is the tolerable error ($\delta = \pi_1 - \pi_2$); and Δ is the boundary of a non-inferiority testing, which should be less than 0. If no previous literature can be cited, Δ can be set as $10\% \sim 15\%$ of the effective rate of the standard treatment.

(b) Comparison of the means based on two independent two samples is shown in Formula (16.30):

$$N = \left[\frac{(U_a + U_\beta)\sigma}{\delta - |\Delta|}\right]^2 (Q_1^{-1} + Q_2^{-1}) \tag{16.30}$$

where N is a total of the required sample size of a non-inferiority testing; U_a and U_β are the critical values of a one-sided standard normal distribution; σ is the pooled standard deviation of both groups ($\sigma = \sqrt{\frac{(n_1-1)\sigma_1^2 + (n_2-1)\sigma_2^2}{n_1+n_2-2}}$); n_1 and n_2 represent the sample size for the intervention and control group; Q_1 and Q_2 are the ratios of the sample size in each group ($Q_1 = \frac{n_1}{N}$, $Q_2 = \frac{n_2}{N}$); δ is the tolerable error ($\delta = \mu_1 - \mu_2$); and Δ is the boundary of a non-inferiority testing, which should be less than 0. If no previous study can be found, Δ can be set as $10\% \sim 15\%$ of the mean of the standard treatment.

Question Bank

(**Mao Guangyun, Li Jushuang, Yi Honggang**)

Chapter 17   Tutorial for SPSS

17.1   Introduction to SPSS

17.1.1   Introduction to SPSS Software

Statistical Product and Service Solutions (SPSS) is a powerful statistical tool to manage, edit, analyze, and present data, with a user-friendly, point-and-click interface. It can run descriptive statistics, parameter estimation, hypothesis testing, linear correlation and regression, multivariate analysis, and many more. The purpose of this chapter is to show students how to perform the statistical procedures discussed in the previous chapters using SPSS 23.0 for Windows.

17.1.2   Interface of SPSS Software

After SPSS is started, the cover and wizard interface of SPSS will appear. Click "Cancel" and the main interface window of SPSS will appear. SPSS has three main windows: Data Editor, Viewer, and Syntax Editor.

17.1.2.1   SPSS Data Editor

The entire data editor window is divided into the title bar, menu bar, toolbar, edit bar, storage bar, and status bar. SPSS is a large program with many commands and functions. In this instruction, 10 primary menu commands are introduced (as shown in Figure 17.1). Their main functions are as follows:

 (a) File (File management menu): file creation, open, save, display, printing, etc.

 (b) Edit: selection, copy, clip, search and replacement of text content, etc.

 (c) View: the display of toolbar, status bar, font selection, grid, etc.

 (d) Data (Data management menu): the increase or decrease, definition, sorting, weighting, and summary of relevant data variables and records.

 (e) Transform (Data transformation processing menu): assignment and recording of the relevant variable, missing value substitution, etc.

 (f) Analyze (Statistics menu): a series of statistical analysis functions.

 (g) Graphs: a series of statistical mapping functions.

 (h) Utilities (User options menu): command interpretation, definition of title, etc.

 (i) Windows: window arrangement, selection, display, etc.

 (j) Help: invoking, querying, and displaying of help files.

In the lower-left corner of the interface, you can see two buttons: "Data View" and "Variable View." By default, SPSS shows the data view for data entry. By clicking the "Variable View" button, you can switch to the variable view, which allows you to set variable attributes.

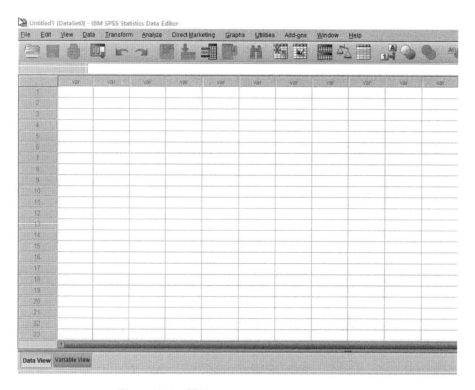

Figure 17. 1   SPSS 23. 0 Main Window Interface

17. 1. 2. 2   SPSS Output Window

The SPSS Output Window is used to display the statistical analysis results of SPSS. The menu is similar to the data edit window, except that a few menu items are reduced, and an Insert menu item is added. The new menu provides more functions: insert new titles, insert new text, insert charts, insert text files, insert objects, etc. In the graphics editing window, graphics conversion can be done (Figure 17. 2).

17. 1. 2. 3   SPSS Syntax Editor

In the Syntax Editor window, the SPSS procedure takes the form of command sentences. This window can edit commands for special procedures that the dialog box cannot implement. The function is rarely used at this stage, so we will not explain the Syntax Editor in detail in this section.

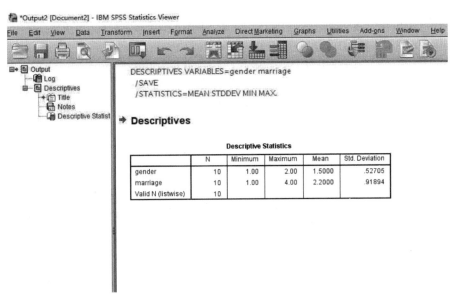

Figure 17. 2   SPSS Output Window

17.1.3   Creating an SPSS Data File

Example 17. 1   Data entry for a questionnaire on transportation options

---

Questionnaire

1. ID _____

2. Gender: _____   □male; □female

3. Birthday: (mm/dd/yyyy)

4. Age: _____

5. Marriage: _____   □unmarried; □married; □widowed; □divorced

6. Choice of daily transportation (multiple-choice): _____

   □walk; □public transport; □private cars; □other _____

7. The amount of time spent on transportation each day: _____ hours

8. Survey date: (mm/dd/yyyy)

Run SPSS program into the main window or open the File menu, "New"→"Data," and then create a new data file through the data editor. Creating a new data file includes defining the database structure (variable name, variable type, and width) and entering the data.

17.1.3.1   Variable Setting

Common attributes of SPSS variables are: Name, Type, Width, Decimals, Label, Value, etc.

(a) Variable name

Variable naming follows the rules: fewer than 8 characters; the first character is a letter, followed by letters or numbers or characters other than "?", "!", and " * "; you cannot use "_" or "." as the last character of a variable name.

(b) Variable type

As shown in Figure 17. 3, SPSS variables have three basic types: numeric, string, and date.

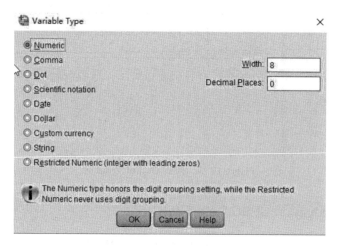

Figure 17. 3   Variable Type Options

(c) Variable label and values

The variable label is an additional comment on a variable name and is optional and may or may not be defined (Figure 17. 4). Values label is a further indication of the possible value of a variable. For a classification variable, you need to define the label for its value. The variable value label is also optional (Figure 17. 5).

	Name	Type	Width	Decimals	Label	Values	Missing	Columns	Align	Measure	Role
1	ID	Numeric	8	0		None	None	4	Right	Nominal	Input
2	Gender	Numeric	8	2		{1.00, male}...	None	6	Right	Nominal	Input
3	Birthday	Date	10	0		None	None	8	Right	Scale	Input
4	Marriage	Numeric	8	2		{1.00, Unma...	None	8	Right	Nominal	Input
5	Transportation1	Numeric	8	2	Walk	{1.00, yes}...	None	12	Right	Nominal	Input
6	Transportation2	Numeric	8	2	Public transport	{1.00, yes}...	None	11	Right	Nominal	Input
7	Transportation3	Numeric	8	2	Private cars	{1.00, yes}...	None	12	Right	Nominal	Input
8	Transportation4	Numeric	10	0	Other	None	None	10	Right	Nominal	Input
9	Time	Numeric	8	0		None	None	6	Right	Nominal	Input
10	Surveydate	Date	10	0		None	None	8	Right	Scale	Input
11	Age	Numeric	8	2		None	None	7	Right	Scale	Input
12											

Figure 17. 4   Variable View

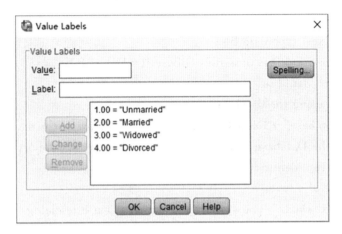

Figure 17. 5   Value Labels

17.1.3.2   Data Entry

After defining variables and variable attributes, click the label "Data View" to enter the data in the data management window (Figure 17.6).

	ID	Gender	Birthday	Marriage	Transportation1	Transportation2	Transportation3	Transportation4	Time	Surveydate	Age
1	1	1.00	10/20/1998	1.00	1.00	2.00	1.00	1	1	05/04/2019	20.00
2	2	1.00	05/06/1992	2.00	2.00	1.00	2.00	1	2	05/04/2019	26.00
3	3	2.00	07/03/1976	4.00	1.00	1.00	1.00	1	2	05/04/2019	42.00
4	4	2.00	04/21/1989	2.00	1.00	2.00	1.00	2	1	05/04/2019	30.00
5	5	1.00	10/15/1980	2.00	1.00	1.00	1.00	2	2	05/04/2019	38.00
6	6	2.00	11/12/1986	2.00	2.00	1.00	2.00	1	1	05/04/2019	32.00
7	7	2.00	02/06/1960	3.00	1.00	2.00	2.00	2	1	05/04/2019	59.00
8	8	1.00	07/08/1999	1.00	1.00	2.00	1.00	1	1	05/04/2019	19.00
9	9	2.00	06/08/1990	2.00	2.00	1.00	2.00	2	2	05/04/2019	28.00
10	10	1.00	01/02/1997	3.00	1.00	1.00	2.00	1	1	05/04/2019	22.00
11											

Figure 17. 6   Data View

17.1.3.3   Open and Save Data Files

(a) Open data file

For existing SPSS data files or other types of data files, open them by clicking "File"→ "Open"→"Data. " There are more than 10 types of data files that SPSS can directly call, for example:

SPSS (* . sav): SPSS type data file;

Excel (* . xls): Excel type data file;

dBase (* . dbf): Series dBase data files (dBase Ⅱ—Ⅳ);

Text (* . txt): text data file.

Open the data file using the database query:

"File"→"Open Database"→"New Query. " The first window of the database wizard pops up—Welcome to the Database Wizard. It lists the data types supported by all installed drivers that SPSS can identify.

Import a data type of a text:

"File"→"Read Text Data. " The system pops up an Open File dialog box. The file type automatically jumps to Text (* . txt).

(b) Data file storage

"File"→"Save," and then select save types and paths.

17. 1. 3. 4   Addition or Deletion of Data

(a) Insert a new variable

To insert a new variable column before a variable:

• In the "Data View," activate any cell in the column

• "Right-click"→"Insert Variable"

To insert a new row of data (A record):

• In the "Data View," activate any cell in the row

• "Right-click"→"Insert Cases"

(b) Delete a row

• Select the entire row

• Press the "Delete" key or click "Edit"→"Clear"

(c) Delete a variable column

• Select the entire column

• Press the "Delete" key or click "Edit"→"Clear"

17. 1. 3. 5   Collation of Data

(a) Data sorting

• Select "Data"→"Sort Cases"

• Select a sort variable in the variable list box

• Click "▣"

• Select "Ascending" or "Descending"

• Click "OK" (Figure 17. 7)

(b) Row and column transpose of data

Convert a database that was previously arranged in row (column) direction to collated data in column (row) direction.

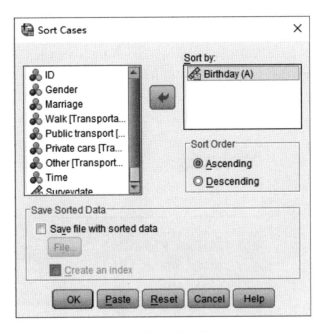

Figure 17. 7　Sort Cases

- Click "Data"→"Transpose"
- Select a transpose variable in the variable list box
- Click"▣"
- Select variable entry variable(s) box
- Name the new variable (Figure 17. 8)

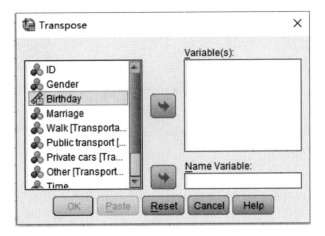

Figure 17. 8　Transpose

(c) Database splitting
- "Data"→"Split File"→"Organize output by groups"

(d) Selection of data
- "Data"→"Select Cases," and select data as needed

(e) The operation of data and the generation of new variables

• "Transform"→"Compute Variable"

For example, the age calculation in the questionnaire is shown in Figure 17. 9 using the "DATEDIFF" function that calculates the difference in years between a person's birthday and the survey date.

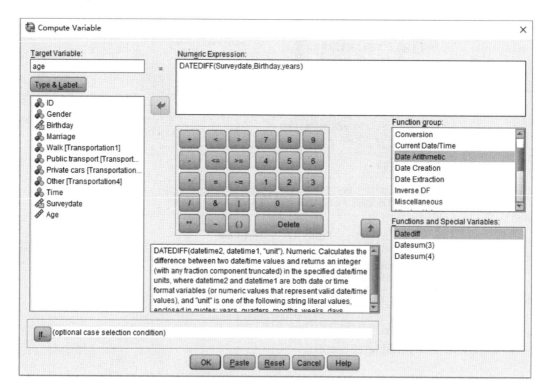

Figure 17. 9   Compute Variable

(f) Merge Files: add variables

Two or more data files with the same number of records can be linked horizontally together.

• "Data"→"Merge Files"→"Add Variables," and then "Read Files"→"Specify File Path, File Name"→"OK"

(g) Append vertical records

• "Data"→"Merge Files"→"Add Cases," and then "Read Files"→"Specify File Path, File Name"→"OK"

17. 2   SPSS for Descriptive Statistics for Continuous Data

Example 17. 2   Delayed treatment is an important risk factor of coronary artery lesions in patients with Kawasaki disease (KD). Consider the following treatment time, that is, the number of days before treatment, chosen randomly from a KD study. Please make a frequency distribution table and chart of the treatment time and calculate the indices of central tendency and dispersion tendency.

7	4	7	4	11	5	7	9	7	3	8	8	6	6	8	7	6	4	4	6
14	9	7	7	4	5	8	5	8	5	3	5	8	5	9	7	6	9	2	6
2	6	3	8	8	5	7	6	9	5	10	6	6	6	6	6	5	8	5	7
4	7	6	9	2	6	6	6	10	8	7	7	6	6	8	9	7	5	5	6
4	6	5	7	2	5	4	5	6	6	5	4	10	4	11	9	4	8	3	1

Open Example 17. 2. sav

(a) The SPSS procedure

• Click "Analyze"→"Descriptive Statistics"→"Frequencies"

• Highlight the "Treattime" variable and click the arrow button to move the variable into the right box

• Click the "Statistics" button

• Check the following options: "Mean," "Median," "Std. deviation," "Minimum," "Maximum," and "Quartiles"

• Click "Continue"

• Click "Charts"→"Histograms"→"Continue"→"OK"

(b) Read and explain the results

Figure 17. 10 shows the measures of central tendency and dispersion tendency. If the distribution of treatment time is normally distributed, Mean and Std. dev. are the best indices to describe the data sets. Otherwise, Median and Quartiles are better.

Statistics

Treattime		
N	Valid	100
	Missing	0
Mean		6. 22
Median		6. 00
Std. dev.		2. 195
Range		13
Minimum		1
Maximum		14
Percentiles	25	5. 00
	50	6. 00
	75	8. 00

Figure 17. 10   Descriptive Output of Treattime

Figures 17. 11 and 17. 12 show the frequency distribution table and chart of variable "Treattime. "

Treattime

		Frequency	Percent/%	Valid percent/%	Cumulative percent/%
Valid	1	1	1. 0	1. 0	1. 0
	2	4	4. 0	4. 0	5. 0
	3	4	4. 0	4. 0	9. 0
	4	11	11. 0	11. 0	20. 0
	5	16	16. 0	16. 0	36. 0
	6	23	23. 0	23. 0	59. 0
	7	15	15. 0	15. 0	74. 0
	8	12	12. 0	12. 0	86. 0
	9	8	8. 0	8. 0	94. 0
	10	3	3. 0	3. 0	97. 0
	11	2	2. 0	2. 0	99. 0
	14	1	1. 0	1. 0	100. 0
	Total	100	100. 0	100. 0	

Figure 17. 11   Frequency Distribution Table of Treattime

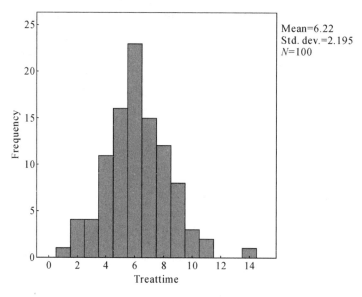

Figure 17. 12   Histogram for Treattime

Example 17.3   As part of a cross-sectional study of central obesity among male adults in a city, the waist circumference (cm) for 105 randomly chosen individuals was recorded. Please make a frequency distribution table and chart of the waist circumference (cm).

68.4	85.8	96.5	96.2	97.0	109.1	123.8
82.5	97.6	102.4	98.1	106.1	110.4	116.0
73.7	95.8	101.2	102.0	98.3	98.9	109.0
81.3	97.5	86.3	97.2	104.6	99.8	116.1
84.5	89.9	89.9	98.6	110.2	113.1	127.5
83.1	95.7	100.7	101.5	106.8	97.9	122.9
80.0	96.8	92.2	95.0	97.0	105.1	111.7
79.4	80.5	95.0	93.9	104.4	117.1	133.0
86.5	90.2	89.5	98.6	101.2	109.0	128.0
80.9	97.2	88.5	79.5	108.8	105.6	93.3
91.5	93.3	92.7	89.0	101.2	116.4	93.0
78.2	88.9	100.0	100.0	95.5	109.2	92.2
80.9	85.5	92.2	91.5	104.5	113.0	112.0
102.1	88.4	95.7	88.1	106.3	109.3	94.5
83.7	80.1	98.2	98.1	103.7	115.0	113.6

Open Example 17.3.sav

(a) Recode into different variables

- Click "Transform"→ "Recode into Different Variables"
- Highlight the "WC" variable and move it into the right box
- Name the new variable as "wcg5" and label it as "waist circumference (cm)"
- Click the "Change" button
- Click the "Old and New Values" button. Fills the two blanks of Range x_1 through x_2 with each lower limit and upper limit of each class in the "Old Value" blank and fills the numerical order of classes from lowest to highest into the "New Value" field (Figure 17.13).

(b) Frequency distribution table

- Click "Analyze"→"Descriptive Statistics"→"Frequencies"
- Highlight the "wcg5" variable and move it into the right box
- Click "OK"

Frequency distribution table (Figure 17.14) of waist circumference (cm) is shown as follows.

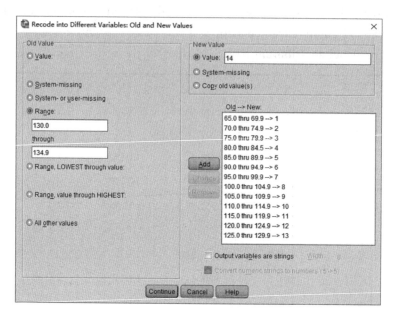

Figure 17. 13　Old and New Values

	Waist circumference /cm	Frequency	Percent/%	Valid percent/%	Cumulative percent/%
Valid	65. 0～69. 9	1	1. 0	1. 0	1. 0
	70. 0～74. 9	1	1. 0	1. 0	1. 9
	75. 0～79. 9	3	2. 9	2. 9	4. 8
	80. 0～84. 9	10	9. 5	9. 5	14. 3
	85. 0～89. 9	12	11. 4	11. 4	25. 7
	90. 0～94. 9	12	11. 4	11. 4	37. 1
	95. 0～99. 9	24	22. 9	22. 9	60. 0
	100. 0～104. 9	14	13. 3	13. 3	73. 3
	105. 0～109. 9	11	10. 5	10. 5	83. 8
	110. 0～114. 9	7	6. 7	6. 7	90. 5
	115. 0～119. 9	5	4. 8	4. 8	95. 2
	120. 0～124. 9	2	1. 9	1. 9	97. 1
	125. 0～129. 9	2	1. 9	1. 9	99. 0
	130. 0～134. 9	1	1. 0	1. 0	100. 0
	Total	105	100. 0	100. 0	

Figure 17. 14　Frequency Distribution Table of Waist Circumference (cm)

（c）Frequency distribution chart

• Click "Analyze"→"Descriptive Statistics"→"Frequencies"

- Highlight the "WC" variable and move it into the right box
- Choose "Charts"→"Histograms"
- Click "Continue"→"OK"

The result is as shown in Figure 17. 15.

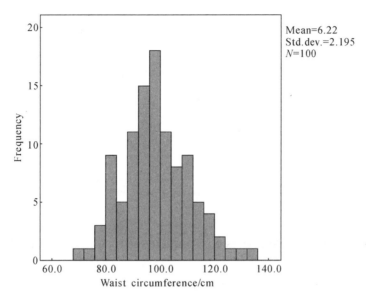

Figure 17. 15   Histogram of Waist Circumference Distribution

Example 17. 4   The Center for Disease Control and Prevention (CDC) of W city vaccinated 50 children using influenza vaccine. One month later, the antibody titers were measured, and the results were as follows. Please calculate the geometric mean of antibody titers.

Table 17. 1   Measurement Results of Antibody Titer

8	32	64	128	128
8	32	64	128	128
16	32	64	128	128
16	32	64	128	128
16	32	64	128	128
16	64	64	128	128
32	64	128	128	128
32	64	128	128	128
32	64	128	128	128
32	64	128	128	128

Open Example 17. 4. sav

Analysis procedure:

- Click "Analyze"→"Compare Means"→"Means"
- Highlight the "ANTI" variable and move it into the Dependent List box
- Click the "Options" button
- Highlight "Geometric Mean" and move it into the Cell Statistics box
- Click "Continue"→"OK"

The result of Geometric Mean of ANTI is shown in Figure 17. 16.

Report

ANTI

Mean	N	Std. dev.	Geometric mean
82. 8800	50	46. 33183	64. 8934

Figure 17. 16   Geometric Mean of ANTI

17. 3   SPSS for Descriptive Statistics for Categorical Data

Example 17. 5   This example is part of the questionnaire data from an actual survey, and the survey participants are coronary heart disease patients and the corresponding control population. The document is named Example 17. 8. The main survey content and the option code of the closed questions are displayed in Table 17. 2. We would like to know the distribution of variables X_1 ("agegroup") and X_7 ("bodytype").

Table 17. 2   Survey Content

Factors	Variable	Encoding
Age/years	X_1	$<45=1,\ 45\sim54=2,\ 55\sim64=3,\ \geqslant65=4$
Hypertension history	X_2	None=0, have=1
Hypertension family history	X_3	None=0, have=1
Smoking	X_4	Non-smoking=0, smoking=1
Hyperlipidemia history	X_5	None=0, have=1
Animal fat intake	X_6	Low=0, high=1
BMI	X_7	$<24=1,\ 24\sim25=2,\ \geqslant26=3$
Type A personality	X_8	No=0, yes=1
Coronary heart disease	Y	Control=0, case=1

(a) Analysis procedure

- Select "Analyze"→ "Descriptive Statistics" → "Frequencies" from the menu → "Variables frame: X_1, X_7"
- Click "OK"

(b) Read and explain the results

Figure 17. 17 shows the frequency table of variable "agegroup. " The "Percent" column shows the frequency of each group as a percent of total cases (including missing records). "Valid percent" column shows the effective percentage of each group when missing data are excluded from the calculations. The "Cumulative percent" column shows the cumulative percentage of each group. The distribution of age group and bodytype is shown in Figures 17. 17 and 17. 18.

Age Group

	Age/years	Frequency	Percent/%	Valid percent/%	Cumulative percent/%
Valid	<45	6	11. 1	11. 1	11. 1
	45~54	25	46. 3	46. 3	57. 4
	55~64	19	35. 2	35. 2	92. 6
	≥65	4	7. 4	7. 4	100. 0
	Total	54	100. 0	100. 0	—

Figure 17. 17   Age Frequency Table

Bodytype

	BMI	Frequency	Percent/%	Valid percent/%	Cumulative percent/%
Valid	<24	34	63. 0	63. 0	63. 0
	24~25	13	24. 1	24. 1	87. 0
	≥26	7	13. 0	13. 0	100. 0
	Total	54	100. 0	100. 0	—

Figure 17. 18   BMI Frequency Table

17. 4   SPSS for Statistical Tables and Graphs

Example 17. 6   Stem-and-leaf plot

The blood urea nitrogen levels (g/L) of 40 study subjects are as follows:

5. 7	3. 2	3. 6	4. 6	7. 1	5. 0	4. 3	3. 6	4. 3	3. 6
5. 0	3. 9	5. 4	6. 8	3. 9	3. 6	3. 6	2. 5	3. 9	8. 6
3. 2	4. 6	4. 6	3. 6	3. 9	5. 4	7. 5	3. 2	2. 9	4. 6
5. 4	2. 5	6. 8	5. 4	3. 9	2. 9	6. 4	5. 7	2. 9	5. 4

Open Example 17. 6. sav

(a) The SPSS steps for stem-and-leaf plot

• Select "Analyze"→"Descriptive Statistics"→"Explore"

- Select the variable "blood urea nitrogen levels" and move it into the "Dependent List" box
  - Click "Plots"→"Stem-and-Leaf"
  - Click "Continue"→"OK"

Figure 17. 19 shows the result of stem-and-leaf plot.

Frequency	Stem-and-Leaf	
0. 00	2.	
5. 00	2.	55999
3. 00	3.	222
11. 000	3.	66666699999
2. 00	4.	33
4. 00	4.	6666
7. 00	5.	0044444
2. 00	5.	77
1. 00	6.	4
2. 00	6.	88
1. 00	7.	1
1. 00	7.	5
1. 00 Extremes	(>=8. 6)	

Stem width: 100

Each leaf: 1 case(s)

Figure 17. 19   Stem-and-Leaf Plot of Blood Urea Nitrogen Levels

Stem-and-leaf plot is a device for presenting quantitative data in a graphical format, like a histogram, to assist in visualizing the shape of a distribution.

In the stem-and-leaf plot (Figure 17. 19), the data of the first column is the "Frequency," the observed number of records for each stem-and-leaf combination. The second column represents the "stem," the frequency of observed number divided by the "Stem width." The third column represents the "leaf"—a subgroup of stems. For example, the second group in Figure 17. 19 is 2 | 5 5 9 9 9, where 2 is the stem and 5, 5, 9, 9, 9 are the leaves, containing five values 2. 5, 2. 5, 2. 9, 2. 9, and 2. 9 in this group. The last third row shows the extreme numbers, and the second to last row shows the stem width, which is 1. 00 in this example. The last row shows that each of the leaves is 1 observed case.

There is an extreme number (>8. 6) in the stem-and-leaf plot. The stem number of the first row is 2, with a frequency of 0 and without any number in the leaf column, representing that there is no number less than 2. 5 in the data set.

Example 17. 7   Bar chart

Please draw a single-bar graph and a multiple-bar graph using data from Table 17. 3.

Table 17. 3   Numbers of Men and Women with Varying Degrees of Obesity

The degree of obesity	Men		Women	
	Cases	Percentage/%	Cases	Percentage/%
Overweight	1,398	58. 67	1,026	44. 55
Obesity class I	687	28. 83	719	31. 22
Obesity class II	237	9. 95	402	17. 46
Obesity class III	61	2. 55	156	6. 77
Total	2,383	100. 00	2,303	100. 00

Open Example 17. 7. sav

(a) Weighting cases

• Select "Data"→"Weight Cases"→"Weight cases by"

• Highlight the "Number" variable and move it into the "Frequency Variable" box

• Click "OK"

(b) Choose special character

If we only need to draw a bar chart for one of the genders, we can choose the gender in the "Select" box:

• Select "Data"→"Select Cases"→"If condition is satisfied"→"If"

• Highlight the "Gender" variable and move it into the blank field to the right, and then enter the formula "Gender=1 ("1" is the value of men)." If you want to select women, enter the formula "Gender=2"

• Click "Continue"→"OK"

You can find women were deleted in Variable View window of SPSS.

(c) Steps for bar charts

• Select "Graphs"→"Legacy Dialogs"→"Bar"→"Define"→"Simple"

• Highlight "Degree of obesity" and move it into the "Category Axis" box

• Click "OK"

The bar chart for numbers of men with varying degrees of obesity is shown in Figure 17. 20.

If you need to describe the number of men and women in the same bar chart, follow the steps:

• Select "Data"→"Choose Cases"→"All Cases," and click "OK"

• Select "Graphs"→"Legacy Dialogs"→"Bar"→"Cluster"

• Highlight the "Degree of Obesity" variable and move it into the "Category Axis" box, and move the "Gender" variable into the "Define Clusters By" box

• Click "OK"

The bar chart for numbers of individual with varying degrees of obesity is shown in Figure 17. 21.

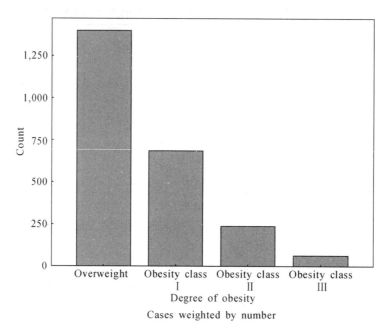

Figure 17. 20　Numbers of Men with Varying Degrees of Obesity

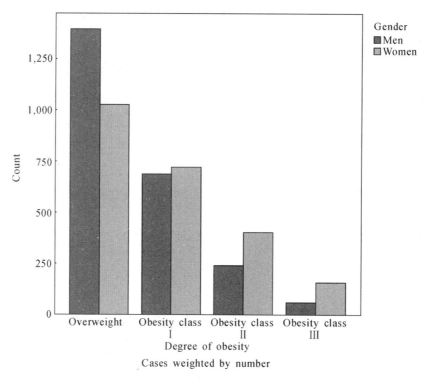

Figure 17. 21　Numbers of Men and Women with Varying Degrees of Obesity

Example 17. 8   Box plot

Open Example 17. 8. sav

Analysis procedure

● Select "Graphs"→"Legacy Dialogs"

● Select "Boxplot"→"Simple"→"Define"

● Move the "Plasma Glucose" variable into the "Variable" box, and move the "Gender" variable into the "Category Axis" box

● Click "OK"

The box plot of male and female plasma glucose concentrations is displayed in Figure 17. 22.

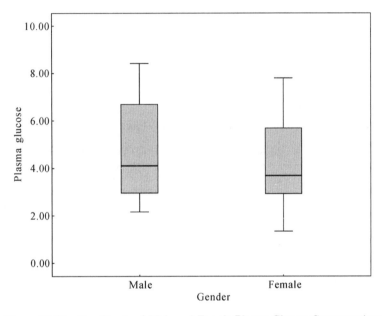

Figure 17. 22   Box Charts of Male and Female Plasma Glucose Concentrations

Example 17. 9   Pie chart

Please draw a pie chart according to Table 17. 3.

Open Example 17. 9. sav

The SPSS procedure:

● Select "Data"→"Weight Cases"→"Weight Cases By"

● Move the "Number" variable into the "Frequency Variable" box

● Click "OK"

● Select "Graphs"→"Legacy Dialogs"→"Pie"→"Define"

● Move the "Degree of Obesity" variable into the "Define Slice By" box

● Click "OK"

Figure 17. 23 shows the pie chart of different levels of obesity in men and women.

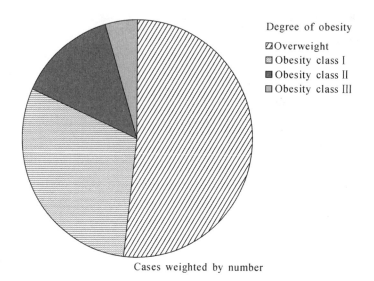

Cases weighted by number

Figure 17. 23   Different Levels of Obesity in All Participants

Example 17. 10   Percentage bar chart

Please draw a percentage bar chart according to Table 17. 4.

Table 17. 4   Male and Female Hypertension Monitoring Results

Gender	Subjects with normal blood pressure/%	Subjects with hypertension/%		
		Class I	Class II	Class III
Men	2,736 (79. 26)	546 (15. 82)	145 (4. 20)	25 (0. 72)
Women	2,813 (81. 23)	424 (12. 53)	198 (5. 72)	28 (0. 81)

Open Example 17. 10. sav

The SPSS procedure:

- Select "Data"→"Weight Cases"→"Weight Cases By"
- Move the "Number" variable into the "Frequency Variable" box
- Click "OK"
- "Graphs"→"Legacy Dialogs"→"Bar"→"Stacked"→"Define"
- Move the "Gender" variable into the "Category Axis" box, and then move the "Degree of Hypertension" variable into the "Define Stacks By" box
- Click "OK"

The bar chart for numbers of hypertension among men and women is shown in Figure 17. 24.

- Double-click the bar chart in the Output 1 window to open the Chart Editor box
- From the Chart Editor box, click the "Options" menu→"Transpose Charts"→"Scale to 100%"→"File"→"Close"

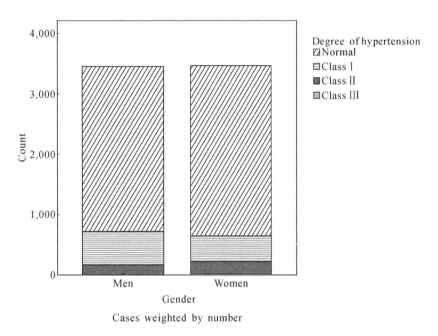

Figure 17. 24   Bar Chart for Numbers of Hypertension among Men and Women

The result is as show in Figure 17. 25.

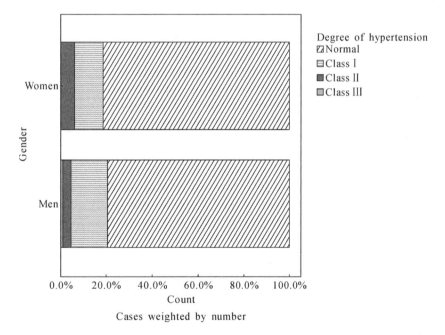

Figure 17. 25   Bar Charts of Hypertension among Men and Women

Example 17. 11   Scatter plot

Please draw a scatter plot according to Table 17. 5.

Table 17.5   Body Mass Index (BMI) and Waist Circumference (WC) of 30 Subjects

ID	BMI/(kg/m²)	WC/cm	ID	BMI/(kg/m²)	WC/cm
1	29.10	99.9	16	27.47	87.7
2	22.56	81.6	17	20.98	71.7
3	29.39	90.7	18	27.96	86.5
4	30.94	108.0	19	23.2	91.0
5	30.62	112.8	20	29.74	110.4
6	27.33	100.3	21	24.05	81.0
7	26.68	86.7	22	29.28	107.5
8	23.68	81.0	23	20.48	73.9
9	39.76	125.7	24	30.38	95.1
10	25.93	90.6	25	23.93	79.0
11	37.60	114.5	26	25.85	93.0
12	19.44	73.4	27	32.14	111.4
13	36.16	116.1	28	29.14	93.7
14	30.23	99.3	29	20.84	73.8
15	31.42	99.8	30	22.85	83.5

Open Example 17.11. sav

The SPSS procedure:

• Select "Graphs"→"Legacy Dialogs"→"Scatter/Dot"→"Simple Scatter"→"Define"

• Move the "BMI" and "WC" variables into the Y and X Axis, respectively

• Click "OK"

Scatter plot is shown in Figure 17.26.

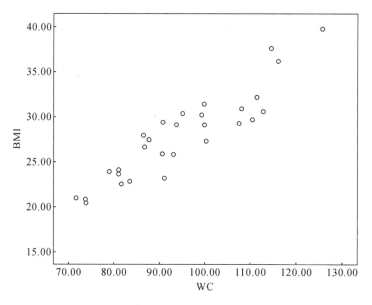

Figure 17.26   Simple Scatter Plot of BMI and WC

Example 17. 12   Line chart

Please draw a simple line graph according to Table 17. 6.

Table 17. 6   Serum Folate Levels at Different Ages

Age/years	Folate/(nmol/L)	Age/years	Folate/(nmol/L)
18	25. 31	23	27. 18
19	26. 50	24	26. 85
20	25. 73	25	27. 67
21	26. 38	26	27. 63
22	26. 25	27	28. 14

Open Example 17. 12. sav

The SPSS procedure

• Select "Graphs"→"Legacy Dialogs"→"Line"→"Simple"

• Click the "Define" button

• Select "Other statistic (e. g. mean)"

• Move the "Folate" variable into the "Variable" box

• Move the "Age" variable into the "Category Axis" box

• Click "OK"

The result of serum folate levels at different ages is as follows (Figure 17. 27).

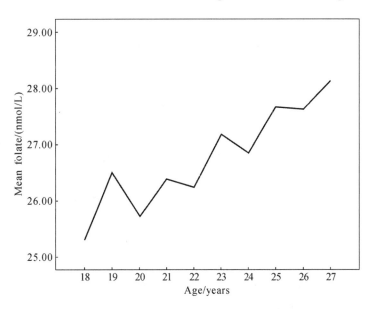

Figure 17. 27   Serum Folate Levels at Different Ages

17.5 SPSS for Parameter Estimation

Example 17.13 A doctor wanted to estimate the mean of the sagittal plane diameter of the spinal vertebral of all the patients, using a random sample of 20 patients. Please construct the 95% CI of the population mean based on Table 17.7.

Table 17.7 Sagittal Diameter of Spine in 20 Patients

14.80	14.80	15.00	14.30	14.20	12.50	15.30	12.55	12.90	12.80
13.80	13.70	16.20	14.35	13.50	15.00	13.10	15.05	12.60	14.20
13.20	13.55	17.40	16.60	16.00	14.45	15.80	13.00	15.20	15.40

Open Example 17.13. sav

(a) The SPSS procedure

- Select "Analyze"→"Descriptive Statistics"→"Explore"
- Move the "Diameter" variable from the variable list to the "Dependent List"→"Statistics"→"Descriptive"→"Confidence Interval" (95% in this case)
- Click "Continue"→"OK"

(b) Read and explain the results.

From the result (Figures 17.28 and 17.29), we find that the 95% CI is (13.89, 14.86).

Case processing summary

	Cases					
	Valid		Missing		Total	
	N	Percent/%	N	Percent/%	N	Percent/%
Diameter	30	100.0	0	0.0	30	100.0

Figure 17.28 Output 1 Window of Explore

Descriptives

			Statistic	SE
Diameter	Mean		14.3750	0.23524
	95% CI for mean	Lower bound	13.8939	
		Upper bound	14.8561	
	5% Trimmed mean		14.3250	
	Median		14.3250	
	Variance		1.660	

		Continued
	Statistic	SE
Std. dev.	1.28846	
Minimum	12.50	
Maximum	17.40	
Range	4.90	
IQR	2.05	
Skewness	0.379	0.427
Kurtosis	−0.458	0.833

Figure 17.29　Output 2 Window of Explore

17.6　SPSS for Foundations of Hypothesis Test

Example 17.14　A known population mean of pulses for the general healthy males is 72 times/min. A doctor randomly selected 20 healthy males in a mountainous area and measured their pulses, calculating the sample mean to be 75 times/min with a standard deviation of 6.3 times/min. The doctor thought that the mean of pulses for healthy males in the mountainous area was faster than that for the general healthy males. Is he right?

Open Example 17.14. sav

(a) Normality test

- Select "Analyze"→"Descriptive Statistics"→"Explore"
- Move "Pulse" variable into the "Dependent List" box
- Select "Plots"→"Normality Plots with Tests"
- Click "Continue"→"OK"

The results of normality tests are as shown in Figure 17.30.

Tests of normality

	Kolmogorov-Smirnov[a]			Shapiro-Wilk		
	Statistic	df	$sig.$	Statistic	df	$sig.$
Pulse of the healthy males in a mountainous area	0.186	20	0.067	0.914	20	0.077

a. Lilliefors Significance Correction

Figure 17.30　Results of Normality Tests

There are two sets of results of normality tests as shown in Figure 17.30, Kolmogorov-Smirnov test and Shapiro-Wilk test. We need to choose the suitable test according to the sample size: if the sample size is bigger than 5,000, we should choose the Kolmogorov-Smirnov test, but if the sample size is equal to or smaller than 5,000, we should choose the

Shapiro-Wilk test.

Because the sample size of the group is small, we choose the result of the Shapiro-Wilk test. Since the p-value is greater than 0.05, the data are normally distributed.

(b) One sample t-test

- Select "Analyze"→"Compare means"→"One-Sample t-Test"
- Move the "Pulse" variable into the "Test Variable(s)" box
- Fill in the "Test Value" blank with "72"
- Click "OK"

The results of one-sample t-test are as shown in Figures 17.31 and 17.32.

One-sample statistics

	N	Mean	Std. dev.	SE mean
Pulse of the healthy males in a mountainous area	20	75.00	6.300	1.409

Figure 17.31 Data Descriptions of One-Sample t-Test

Figure 17.32 shows the statistic of the one-sample t-test equals to 2.130. Since the p-value is greater than 0.05, there is significant difference between the pulses for healthy males in a mountainous area and that of the known population.

One-sample t-test (Test value=72)

	t	df	sig. (two-tailed)	Mean difference	95% CI of the difference	
					Lower bound	Upper bound
Pulse of the healthy males in a mountainous area	2.130	19	0.046	3.000	0.05	5.95

Figure 17.32 Result of One-Sample t-Test

Example 17.15

Please calculate the 95% CI for "Pulse" in Example 17.14.

Open Example 17.14. sav

Analysis procedure

- Select "Analyze"→"Compare means"→"One-Sample t-Test"
- Move the "Pulse" variable to the "Test Variable(s)" box
- Fill in the "Test Value" blank with "0"
- Click "OK"

The result of the 95% CI for μ is (72.05, 77.95) times/min (Figure 17.33).

One-sample test (Test value＝0)

	t	df	*sig.* (two-tailed)	Mean difference	95% CI of the difference	
					Lower bound	Upper bound
Pulse of the healthy males in a mountainous area	53.244	19	0.000	75.000	72.05	77.95

Figure 17.33   Result of 95% CI

17.7   SPSS for *t*-Test

17.7.1   Paired Design *t*-Test

Example 17.16   Serum folate concentrations of 12 women were measured by the Radioimmunoassay (RIA) and the ELISA method, with data shown in Table 17.8. The paired *t*-test helps determine whether there is a difference between the results of the two methods.

Table 17.8   Serum Folate Concentrations (nmol/L) of 12 Women Measured by Two Methods

Number of women (1)	RIA (2)	ELISA (3)
1	16.5	15.9
2	38.2	36.5
3	40.3	38.7
4	45.1	44.6
5	28.5	27.6
6	29.5	30.6
7	53.2	52.1
8	36.3	33.1
9	14.5	13.8
10	48.3	45.1
11	38.2	36.5
12	32.5	34.1
Total	—	—

This is a two-tailed, paired-designed study and the data belongs to measurement data. The paired samples *t*-test is used for inferential statistic. The procedures of paired samples *t*-test with SPSS are as follows.

Open Example 17. 16. sav

(a) The SPSS procedure

• Select "Analyze"→"Compare Means"→ "Paired-Samples *t*-Test"

• Select "RIA, ELISA" from the variable list and place it in the "Paired Variables"

• Select "Options" and change the "Confidence Interval Percentage" to 95%→"Exclude Cases Analysis by Analysis"

• Click "Continue"→"OK"

(b) Read the result

From the result (Figures 17. 34, 17. 35, and 17. 36), we find that the *t*-value is 2. 513 and the *p*-value is 0. 029, which is smaller than 0. 05. As a result, we can conclude that there is a statistically significant difference between the measurement of these two methods.

Paired-samples statistics

		Mean	N	Std. dev.	SE mean
Pair 1	RIA	35. 0917	12	11. 68351	3. 37274
	ELISA	34. 0500	12	11. 22793	3. 24122

Figure 17. 34 Output 1 Window of Paired-Samples *t*-Test

Paired samples correlations

		N	Correlation	Sig.
Pair 1	RIA & ELISA	12	0. 993	0. 000

Figure 17. 35 Output 2 Window of Paired-Samples *t*-Test

Paired samples test

	Mean	Std. dev.	SE mean	Lower bound	Upper bound	T	df	sig. (two-tailed)
Pair 1 RIA&ELISA	1. 04167	1. 43619	0. 41459	0. 12915	1. 95418	2. 513	11	0. 029

Figure 17. 36 Output 3 Window of Paired-Samples *t*-Test

Example 17. 17 In order to study the effects of different temperatures on blood sugar level in rabbits, one researcher matched 6 pairs of rabbits according to their nests. Two rabbits in each pair were randomly allocated to Group A with a temperature of 15°C and Group B with a temperature of 30°C, respectively. The blood sugar concentrations (mmol/L) of rabbits were measured and the result is shown in Table 17. 9. Can we determine if the blood sugar level of rabbits in Group B is higher than that of rabbits in Group A?

Table 17. 9　Blood Sugar Concentrations（mmol/L）of Rabbits between Two Groups

Nest	Group A	Group B
1	83. 21	112. 55
2	109. 10	139. 64
3	101. 15	121. 10
4	75. 20	109. 35
5	80. 23	102. 53
6	101. 75	137. 89
Total	—	—

The design of this example is allogeneic-pairing, where two rabbits in the same nest were paired and randomly assigned to two different temperature groups—the temperature of Group A is 15°C, and the temperature of Group B is 30°C. Since the data obtained is the paired quantitative data, we need to use the paired-samples t-test.

Open Example 17. 17. sav

(a) The SPSS procedure

• Select "Analyze"→"Compare Means"→"Paired-Samples t-Test"

• Select "Blood Sugar Concentrations（mmol/L）of Group A & Blood Sugar Concentrations（mmol/L）of Group B" from the variable list and place it in the "Paired Variables" area

• Click "Options" to open a new window to specify the "Confidence Interval Percentage" at 95%. Select "Exclude Cases Analysis by Analysis"

• Click the "Continue" button

• Click "OK"

(b) Read the result

From the result (Figures 17.37, 17.38, and 17.39), we can see that the t-value is −10.957 and the p-value is less than 0.001, which is a two-sided value. Since the one-sided p-value is smaller than 0.05, we conclude that there is a statistically significant and the blood sugar level of rabbits in Group B is higher than that of rabbits in Group A.

Paired-samples statistics

		Mean	N	Std. dev.	SE mean
Pair 1	Blood sugar concentrations (mmol/L) of Group A	91. 7733	6	13. 92066	5. 68309
	Blood sugar concentrations (mmol/L) of Group B	120. 5100	6	15. 35941	6. 27045

Figure 17. 37　Output 1 Window of Paired-Samples t-Test

Paired-samples correlations

		N	Correlation	*sig.*
Pair 1	Blood sugar concentrations(mmol/L) of Groups A & B	6	0.908	0.012

Figure 17.38   Output 2 Window of Paired-Samples *t*-Test

Paired-samples test

	Paired differences							
				95% CI of the difference		*t*	*df*	*sig.* (two-tailed)
	Mean	Std. dev.	SE mean	Lower bound	Upper bound			
Pair 1 Blood sugar concentrations (mmol/L) of Groups A & B	−28.73667	6.42442	2.62276	−35.47868	−21.99465	−10.957	5	0.000

Figure 17.39   Output 3 Window of Paired-Samples *t*-Test

17.7.2 Two Independent Samples *t*-test

Example 17.18   Table 17.10 shows the waist circumference between men and women aged over 60 years old. The question is whether the waist circumference is different from men and women aged over 60 years old.

Table 17.10   Waist Circumference (cm) for Adult Men and Women Aged over 60 Years Old

Men (X_1) ($n_1 = 11$)	106.5	89.5	112.2	113.0	95.0	84.8	87.5	99.9	108.0	112.8	100.3	—	—
Women (X_2) ($n_2 = 13$)	97.4	90.3	82.4	102.0	95.0	76.2	85.0	72.9	81.6	90.7	86.7	90.6	114.5

These are two independent-samples with two-tailed designed study, and the data belongs to quantitative data. The methods for inference we can use is the two independent-samples *t*-test.

Open Example 17.18. sav

(a) The SPSS procedure

● Select "Analyze"→"Compare Means"→"Independent-Samples *t*-Test"

● Select "Waist circumference (cm)" from the variable list and place it in the "Test Variable(s)"

● Select the "Group" variable as the "Grouping Variable"

● Click "Define Groups..."→"Use Specified Values"→Enter "1" and "2" in the "Group 1" and "Group 2" textbox

● Click "Continue"→"OK"

(b) Read the result

From the result (Figures 17. 40 and 17. 41), since the p-value of Levene's test is 0. 817, we can assume that the variances of two populations are the same, indicating that the result is from the "Equal variances assumed" section. With a p-value less than 0. 05 ($t = 2.534$), we can draw the conclusion that there is a statistically significant difference of the waist circumference between men and women aged over 60 years old.

Group statistics

	Gender	N	Mean	Std. dev.	SE mean
Waist circumstance/cm	Male	11	100. 864	10. 4994	3. 1657
	Female	13	89. 638	11. 0691	3. 0700

Figure 17. 40   Output 1 Window of Independent-Sample t-Test

Independent samples test

		Levene's test for equality of variances		t-Test for equality of means						
		F	*sig.*	t	df	*sig.* (two-tailed)	Mean differ-ence	SE differ-ence	95% CI of the difference Lower bound	95% CI of the difference Upper bound
Waist circumstance /cm	Equal variances assumed	0. 055	0. 817	2. 534	22	0. 019	11. 2252	4. 4302	2. 0376	20. 4128
	Equal variances not assumed	—	—	2. 545	21. 677	0. 019	11. 2252	4. 4098	2. 0718	20. 3785

Figure 17. 41   Output 2 Window of Independent-Sample t-Test

Example 17. 19   According to large-scale survey data, the statistics of serum cholesterol levels from male and female group are listed in Figure 17. 42. Please compare the difference in the serum cholesterol levels between males and females.

Open Example 17. 19. sav

(a) The SPSS procedure

- "Analyze"→"Compare Means"→"Independent-Samples t-Test"
- Move the "TC" variable into the "Test Variable(s)"
- Move the "Group" variable into the "Grouping Variable"
- Select "Define Groups"→"Use specified values"→Enter "1" and "2" in the "Group 1" and "Group 2" textbox
- Click "Continue"→"OK"

The basic situation description of the two groups of test variables is given in Figure 17. 41. From the result (Figure 17. 43), we find the Levene's Test for Equality of Variances is $F = 7.131$, $P = 0.008$, which means the variances of two populations are not equal.

	Gender	N	Mean	Std. dev.	SE mean
Serum cholesterol (mmol/L)	Male	4,050	4.9131	0.97121	0.01526
	Female	4,316	5.0288	1.01428	0.01544

Figure 17.42　Group Statistics

Independent samples test

		Levene's test for equality of variances		t-test for equality of means						
		F	sig.	T	df	sig. (two-tailed)	Mean difference	SE difference	95% CI of the difference Lower bound	Upper bound
Serum cholesterol (mmol/L)	Equal variances assumed	7.131	0.008	−5.319	8364	0.000	−0.11563	0.02174	−0.15824	−0.07301
	Equal variances not assumed			−5.326	8360.577	0.000	−0.11563	0.02171	−0.15818	−0.07307

Figure 17.43　Independent Samples Test

Since the variance of the two populations is not homogeneous, we need to select the result of the t-test correction, which is, the result of the second row. Since we find the $t = -5.326$ and $P < 0.05$, we can draw the conclusion that there is a statistically significant difference of the serum cholesterol levels between males and females.

Example 17.20　Homogeneity test of variances in Example 17.18.

Open Example 17.18. sav

(a) The SPSS procedure

- "Analyze"→"Descriptive Statistics"→"Explore"
- Select the "WC" variable from the variable list and place it in the "Dependent List"
- Select "Gender" from the variable list and place it in the "Factor List"
- "Statistics"→"Descriptive"
- Select "Options"→"Exclude Cases Listwise"
- Select "Plots"→"Normality Plots with Tests"
- Click "Continue"→"OK"

(b) Read the result

From the result (Figure 17.44), we get the two-sided critical values $F_{0.20}, (12,10) = 2.28$, $F < F_{0.20}, (12,10)$, $P > 0.20$ (exactly $P = 0.817$, which can be calculated by SPSS software), which indicates no significant statistical difference between the two variances. Therefore, we regard that the variances of the two populations are equal.

Test of homogeneity of variance

		Levene statistic	df_1	df_2	$sig.$
Waist circumstance/cm	Based on mean	0.055	1	22	0.817
	Based on median	0.053	1	22	0.820
	Based on median and with adjusted df	0.053	1	20.159	0.820
	Based on trimmed mean	0.053	1	22	0.820

Figure 17.44   Output of Test of Homogeneity of Variance

17.8   SPSS for Analysis of Variance

17.8.1   One-Way ANOVA for Completely Randomized Design

Example 17.21   In order to investigate the inhibition effect of the different treatments on the weight of the brain tumor, 40 tumor model mice were randomly assigned to be treated with four different drugs, and the weights of the tumors were measured. Is there a difference among the weights of four treatments?

Table 17.11   Inhibition Effect of 4 Kinds of Drugs on Tumor Weight (g)

ID	1	2	3	4
	Drug A	Drug B	Drug C	Drug D
1	3.6	3.0	0.6	3.3
2	4.6	2.5	1.7	1.2
3	4.2	2.4	2.3	0.4
4	4.4	1.1	4.5	2.7
5	3.7	4.0	3.6	3.0
6	5.7	3.7	1.3	3.2
7	7.0	2.7	3.2	0.6
8	4.1	1.9	3.0	1.4
9	5.2	2.6	2.1	1.2
10	4.5	1.3	2.5	2.1

Open Example 17.21.sav

(a) Normal distribution test

Methods and steps are the same as Example 17.14.

Because the sample size of the four groups are less than 5,000, we should choose the Shapiro-Wilk test. P-values of the four group are greater than 0.05. As a result, all four group's data are normally distributed.

(b) Homogeneity of variance and One-Way ANOVA test

● Select "Analyze"→"Compare Means"→"One Way ANOVA"

● Move the "Weight" variable to the "Dependent List" box

● Move the "Group" variable into the "Factor" box

● Click on the "Post Hoc" button, and tick the "SNK" checkbox

● Click "Continue"

● Click on the "Options" button, and tick the "Descriptive and Homogeneity of Variance Test" checkbox

● Click "Continue"→"OK"

The result of One-Way ANOVA is as shown in Figure 17. 45.

Descriptives

Weight

	N	Mean	Std. dev.	SE	95% CI for mean		Minimum	Maximum
					Lower bound	Upper bound		
Drug A	10	4. 7000	1. 02740	0. 32489	3. 9650	5. 4350	3. 60	7. 00
Drug B	10	2. 5200	0. 92832	0. 29356	1. 8559	3. 1841	1. 10	4. 00
Drug C	10	2. 4800	1. 14678	0. 36264	1. 6596	3. 3004	0. 60	4. 50
Drug D	10	1. 9100	1. 09082	0. 34495	1. 1297	2. 6903	0. 40	3. 30
Total	40	2. 9025	1. 47813	0. 23371	2. 4298	3. 3752	0. 40	7. 00

Figure 17. 45   Data Descriptions

Figure 17. 46 shows the variances are equal (the p-value of Levene's test of homogeneity of variances equals 0. 743, greater than 0. 05).

Test of homogeneity of variances

Weight

Levene statistic	df_1	df_2	$sig.$
0. 415	3	36	0. 743

Figure 17. 46   Levene's Test of Homogeneity of Variance

Figure 17. 47 shows the statistic of one-way ANOVA is equal to 13. 691, and the p-value is less than 0. 001, suggesting there is significant difference among the four groups.

ANOVA

Weight

	Sum of squares	df	Mean square	F	$sig.$
Between groups	45. 409	3	15. 136	13. 691	0. 000
Within groups	39. 801	36	1. 106	—	—
Total	85. 210	39	—	—	—

Figure 17. 47   ANOVA Table

Figure 17. 48 shows the means of groups, listed orderly in the column of subset. If two groups' means were not statistically different, they will be listed in the same column. Otherwise, they will be listed in different columns. Figure 17. 47 shows Drugs D, C, and B are listed in the same column, suggesting there is no difference among the means of three groups, while Drug A is listed in another column, suggesting the mean is different between Drug A and other groups, with the weight of Drug A group higher than the other three groups.

Weight

	Group	N	Subset for $\alpha=0.05$	
			1	2
Student-Newman-Keuls[a]	Drug D	10	1. 9100	—
	Drug C	10	2. 4800	—
	Drug B	10	2. 5200	—
	Drug A	10	—	4. 7000
	$sig.$	—	0. 406	1. 000

Means for groups in homogeneous subsets are displayed

a. Uses Harmonic Mean Sample Size=10. 000

Figure 17. 48   S-N-K Test for Multiple Comparisons

17.8.2 Two-Way ANOVA for Randomized Block Design

Example 17. 22   A doctor wanted to compare the changes in blood glucose of blood samples drawn from 8 pregnant women after leaving the samples in room temperature for 0, 45, 90, and 135 minutes. The blood glucose was tested after each time period for all samples in order to find out the influence of time on the concentration of blood glucose. The data were recorded and displayed in Table 17. 12.

Table 17. 12   Blood Glucose (mmol/L) in Different Times

Block	Time/min				Total	Mean
	0	45	90	135		
1	5. 24	5. 27	4. 94	4. 61	20. 06	5. 02
2	5. 24	5. 22	4. 88	4. 66	20. 00	5. 00
3	5. 88	5. 83	5. 38	5. 00	22. 09	5. 52
4	5. 44	5. 38	5. 27	5. 00	21. 09	5. 27
5	5. 66	5. 44	5. 38	4. 88	21. 36	5. 34
6	6. 22	6. 22	5. 61	5. 22	23. 27	5. 82
7	5. 83	5. 72	5. 38	4. 88	21. 81	5. 45
8	5. 27	5. 11	5. 00	4. 44	19. 82	4. 96
Total	44. 78	44. 19	41. 84	38. 69	169. 50	—
Mean	5. 60	5. 52	5. 23	4. 84	—	5. 30
$\sum_j X_{ij}^2$	251. 57	245. 07	219. 30	187. 56	903. 49	—

Open Example 17. 22. sav

(a) The SPSS procedure

• Select "Analyze"→"General Linear Model"→"Univariate"

• Move the "Glucose" variable into the "Dependent Variable" box

• Move the "Group" and "Block" variables into the "Fixed Factors" box

• Click the "Model" button→"Custom," choose main effects in the "Build Term(s)," and then highlight the "Group and Block" variable to the "Model" box

• Click "Continue"

• Click on the "Post Hoc" button and move the "Group and Block" variable to the "Post Hoc Test For" box

• Tick the "S-N-K" checkbox and click "Continue"

• "Options"→"Descriptive Statistics"→"OK"

(b) Read and explain the results

Figure 17. 49 shows that there is significant difference among the four groups ($F=74. 317$, $P<0. 001$) and eight blocks ($F=28. 123$, $P<0. 001$).

Tests of between-subject effects

Dependent variable: glucose

Source	Type III sum of squares	df	Mean square	F	$sig.$
Corrected model	5. 400[a]	10	0. 540	41. 981	0. 000
Intercept	897. 820	1	897. 820	69,794. 925	0. 000

Continued

Source	Type III sum of squares	df	Mean square	F	sig.
Group	2.868	3	0.956	74.317	0.000
Block	2.532	7	0.362	28.123	0.000
Error	0.270	21	0.013	—	—
Total	903.491	32	—	—	—
Corrected total	5.670	31	—	—	—

a. R-Squared$=0.952$ (Adjusted R-Squared$=0.930$)

Figure 17. 49   Result of Tests of Between-Subject Effects

Figure 17. 50 shows that the Blood Glucose of 0 minute and 45 minutes are higher than that of 90 minutes, and the Blood Glucose of 135 minutes is lower than that of the other three groups, while there is no significant difference of Blood Glucose between 0 minute and 45 minutes.

Glucose

Student-Newman-Keuls[a,b]

Group	N	Subset 1	Subset 2	Subset 3
135 minutes	8	4.8363	—	—
90 minutes	8	—	5.2300	—
45 minutes	8	—	—	5.5238
0 minute	8	—	—	5.5975
sig.	—	1.000	1.000	0.208

Means for groups in homogeneous subsets are displayed

Based on observed means

The error term is Mean Square (Error)$=0.013$

a. Uses Harmonic Mean Sample Size$=8.000$

b. $\alpha=0.05$

Figure 17. 50   Result of S-N-K Test for Four Groups

Figure 17. 51 shows that blood glucose of block 6 is the highest in the 8 blocks and blood glucose of blocks 1, 2, and 8 are among the lowest. Blood glucose of block 3 is higher than that of block 4, but there is no significant difference. At last, blocks 5 and 7 are not significantly different from block 4.

Glucose

Student-Newman-Keuls[a,b]

Block	N	Subset			
		1	2	3	4
8	4	4.9550	—	—	—
2	4	5.0000	—	—	—
1	4	5.0150	—	—	—
4	4	—	5.2725	—	—
5	4	—	5.3400	5.3400	—
7	4	—	5.4525	5.4525	—
3	4	—	—	5.5225	—
6	4	—	—	—	5.8175
sig.	—	0.738	0.087	0.082	1.000

Means for groups in homogeneous subsets are displayed

Based on observed means

The error term is Mean Square (Error)=0.013

a. Uses Harmonic Mean Sample Size=4.000

b. α=0.05

Figure 17.51   Result of S-N-K Test for Eight Blocks

17.8.3   Analysis of Variance for Repeated Measurement Data

Example 17.23   Six different subjects received a test about their fitness level before, during and after a fitness intervention that continued for 3 months. The detailed data can be found in Table 17.13.

Table 17.13   Three-Times Repeated Measurements of 6 Participants of Fitness Level

Participants/Subjects	Before	Middle	After 3 months
1	45	50	55
2	42	42	45
3	36	41	43
4	39	35	40
5	51	55	59
6	44	49	56

Open Example 17.23. sav

Repeat measurement data entry: analysis of variance of repeated measurement data is the measurement results of the same research object at multiple-time points, which need to be arranged in horizontal sequence.

- Click "Variable View"
- Enter the name of "Variable One" as "Participants," "Variable Two" as "Before," "Variable Three" as "Middle," "Variable Four" as "After," and input corresponding data seen from Example 17. 25. sav

(a) The SPSS procedure

- Click "Analyze"→"General Linear Model"→"Repeated Measures"
- Enter "3" in the "Number of Levels" box
- Click the "Add" button, and then the "Define" button
- Select "Before," "Middle," and "After," and move them into the "Within-Subject Variances" box
- Click "Model"→"Custom"→"Main Effects" in the "Build Term(s)," then highlight "Factorl," and move it into the "Within-Subject Model" box
- Click "Continue"
- Click the "Options" button, and move "Factor1" from "Factor(s) and Factor" interactions blank into the "Display Means For:" blank→"Compare Main Effects"→choose LSD method→"Descriptive Statistic"
- Click "Continue"→"OK"

(b) Read and explain the results

The spherical test results are shown in Figure 17. 52. The chi-square is 3. 343 and $P=0. 188>0. 05$, indicating that the spherical distribution is consistent, and the one-way variance result should be taken as the standard.

Mauchly's test of sphericity[a]

Measure: MEASURE_1

Within-subjects effect	Mauchly's W	Approx. chi-square	df	$sig.$	Epsilon[b]		
					Greenhouse-Geisser	Huynh-Feldt	Lower bound
Factor1	0. 434	3. 343	2	0. 188	0. 638	0. 760	0. 500

Tests the null hypothesis that the error covariance matrix of the orthonormalized transformed dependent variables is proportional to an identity matrix

a. Design: intercept

Within-Subjects Design: factor1

b. May be used to adjust the degrees of freedom for the averaged tests of significance. Corrected tests are displayed in the Tests of Within-Subject Effects table

Figure 17. 52　Result of Mauchly's Test of Sphericity

The results of within-subject variable effects are shown in Figure 17. 53, and sphericity assumed is the result of the spherical distribution assumption. In the test time factor 1 group, we can see $F=12. 534$ and $P<0. 01$, which means we can reject the null hypothesis and accept the alternative hypothesis. We conclude that there is a statistically significant effect of time on exercise-induced fitness.

Tests of within-subject effects

Measure: MEASURE_1

Source		Type III sum of squares	df	Mean square	F	sig.
Factor 1	Sphericity assumed	143.444	2	71.722	12.534	0.002
	Greenhouse-Geisser	143.444	1.277	112.350	12.534	0.009
	Huynh-Feldt	143.444	1.520	94.351	12.534	0.005
	Lower bound	143.444	1.000	143.444	12.534	0.017
Error (factor 1)	Sphericity assumed	57.222	10	5.722	—	—
	Greenhouse-Geisser	57.222	6.384	8.964	—	—
	Huynh-Feldt	57.222	7.602	7.528	—	—
	Lower bound	57.222	5.000	11.444	—	—

Figure 17.53   Result of Tests of Within-Subject Effects

Figure 17.54 shows that fitness levels of "Before" and "Middle" are significantly different with "After," suggesting that the fitness levels of participants generally improve 3 months after the program. While there is no significant difference between "Before" and "Middle."

Pairwise comparisons

Measure: MEASURE_1

(I) factor 1	(J) factor 1	Mean difference (I−J)	SE	sig.[b]	95% CI for difference[b]	
					Lower bound	Upper bound
1	2	−2.500	1.522	0.161	−6.413	1.413
	3	−6.833*	1.701	0.010	−11.207	−2.460
2	1	2.500	1.522	0.161	−1.413	6.413
	3	−4.333*	0.715	0.002	−6.171	−2.496
3	1	6.833*	1.701	0.010	2.460	11.207
	2	4.333*	0.715	0.002	2.496	6.171

Based on estimated marginal means

*. The mean difference is significant at the 0.05 level

b. Adjustment for multiple comparisons: least significant difference (equivalent to no adjustments)

Figure 17.54   Result of Pairwise Comparisons

17.9 SPSS for χ^2 Test

17.9.1 Group Design Four-Square Table χ^2 Test

Example 17.24 Bortezomib plus dexamethasone (BD) and bortezomib, epirubicin plus dexamethasone (PAD) are two chemotherapy regimens for multiple myeloma. The effects of treatments are shown in Table 17.14. Are the effects of the two chemotherapy regimens different?

Table 17.14 The Effects of Treatment for Multiple Myeloma by BD and PAD Chemotherapy Regimens

Treatment	Effective	Ineffective	Total	Effective rate/%
BD	23 (27.3)	15 (10.7)	38	60.5
PAD	33 (28.7)	7 (11.3)	40	82.5
Total	56	22	78	71.8

(1) Method one

Open Example 17.24.1.sav

Database 17.24.1.sav is the original database of this experiment.

The SPSS procedure

• Click "Analyze"→"Descriptive Statistics"→"Crosstabs"

• Move the "Treatment" variable into the "Row(s)" box and the "Effects" variable into the "Column(s)" box

• Click the "Statistics" button→"Chi-square"→"Continue"

• Click the "Cells" button →"Expected"

• Click "Continue"→"OK"

(2) Method two

Open Example 17.24.2.sav

Database 17.24.2.sav is the four-grid table made after the statistics of the experiment results, which is the most commonly used format of chi-square test.

(a) Weight cases by variable frequency

• Select "Data"→"Weight Cases"→ "Weight Case By"

• Move the "Frequency" variable into the edit frame "Frequency Variable"

(b) The SPSS procedure

The steps are the same as method one.

(c) Read and explain the results

The basic results of the chi-square test are given in the output results. Figure 17.55 shows the crosstabulation of the analysis data, while Figure 17.56 shows the chi-square values, degrees of freedom, and p-values of the chi-square test.

In this example, the result of Pearson chi-square produces the chi-square value of 4.647 and the p-value (two-sided) of 0.031, using $\alpha = 0.05$. The difference is statistically significant and we conclude that the two methods have different effects on the treatment of multiple myeloma.

Treatment × effects crosstabulation

			Effects		Total
			Ineffective	Effective	
Treatment	BD	Count	15	23	38
		Expected count	10.7	27.3	38.0
	PDD	Count	7	33	40
		Expected count	11.3	28.7	40.0
Total		Count	22	56	78
		Expected count	22.0	56.0	78.0

Figure 17.55　Output Window (Observed and Expected Count)

Chi-square tests

	Value	df	Asymptotic significance (two-sided)	Exact *sig.* (two-sided)	Exact *sig.* (one-sided)
Pearson chi-square	4.647[a]	1	0.031	—	—
Continuity correction[b]	3.625	1	0.057	—	—
Likelihood ratio	4.721	1	0.030	—	—
Fisher's exact test	—	—	—	0.044	0.028
Linear-by-linear association	4.587	1	0.032	—	—
N of valid cases	78	—	—	—	—

　　a. *0 cells (0.0%) have expected count less than 5; the minimum expected count is* 10.72

　　b. *Computed only for a* 2×2 *table*

Figure 17.56　Output Window (χ^2 test)

Example 17.25　Patients treated by PAD chemotherapy regimen from Example 17.24 can be divided into two groups: $\leqslant 4$ chemotherapy regimen cycles and > 4 chemotherapy regimen cycles. Are the effects of the PAD regimen different between the two groups?

Table 17.15　The Effects of Treatment by PAD Regimen for 2 Cycle Groups

Cycles	Effective	Ineffective	Total	Effective rate/%
$\leqslant 4$	14 (16.5)	6 (3.5)	20	70.0
> 4	19 (16.5)	1 (3.5)	20	90.0
Total	33	7	40	82.5

Open Example 17. 25. sav

(a) The SPSS procedure

Methods and steps are the same as Example 17. 24.

(b) Read and explain the results

The basic results of the chi-square test are given in the output results. Figure 17. 57 shows the crosstabulation of the analysis data. Figure 17. 58 shows the chi-square values, degrees of freedom, and p-values of the chi-square test.

According to Figure 17. 58, 2 cells (50. 0%) have expected count less than 5. The minimum expected count is 3. 50, and the sample size is equal to 40. As a result, we should choose the result of continuity correction.

Treatment × effects crosstabulation

			Effects		Total
			Ineffective	Effective	
Treatment	Cycle number smaller than 4	Count	6	14	20
		Expected count	3. 5	16. 5	20. 0
		Count	1	19	20
Total	Cycle number greater than 4	Expected count	3. 5	16. 5	20. 0
		Count	7	33	40
		Expected count	7. 0	33. 0	40. 0

Figure 17. 57   Output Window (Observed and Expected Count)

Chi-square tests

	Value	df	Asymptotic significance (two-sided)	Exact $sig.$ (two-sided)	Exact $sig.$ (one-sided)	Point probability
Pearson chi-square	4. 329[a]	1	0. 037	0. 091	0. 046	—
Continuity correction[b]	2. 771	1	0. 096	—	—	—
Likelihood ratio	4. 723	1	0. 030	0. 091	0. 046	—
Fisher's exact test	—	—	—	0. 091	0. 046	—
Linear-by-linear association	4. 221[c]	1	0. 040	0. 091	0. 046	0. 042
N of valid cases	40	—	—	—	—	—

a. *2 cells* (50. 0%) *have expected count less than* 5; *the minimum expected count is* 3. 50

b. *Computed only for a* 2×2 *table*

c. *The standardized statistic is* 2. 054

Figure 17. 58   Output Window (χ^2 Test)

17.9.2 χ^2 Test for Paired-Samples Four-Fold Table

Example 17.26   There were 100 systemic lupus erythematosus (SLE) serum samples, which were examined by chemiluminescent immunoassay (CLIA) and line immunoassay (LIA) to test the autoantibodies to ribonucleoprotein (RNP). The examination records are listed in Table 17.16. Can you evaluate whether two assays have the equal positive rate?

Table 17.16   The Comparison of the Testing Results by Two Assays

CLIA	LIA +	LIA −	Total
+	28 (a)	2 (b)	30
−	4 (c)	66 (d)	70
Total	32	68	100

Open Example 17.26. sav

(a) Weight cases by variable frequency

• Select "Data"→"Weight Cases"

• Click the radio button "Weight Case By" and move the "Frequency" variable into the edit frame "Frequency Variable"

(b) The SPSS procedure

• Select "Analyze"→"Descriptive Statistics"→ "Crosstabs"

• Move the "CLIA" variable into the edit frame "Row(s)" and the "LIA" variable into the edit frame "Column(s)"

• Click the "Statistics" button and tick the "McNemar" checkbox

• Click "Continue"→"OK"

(c) Read and explain the results

As shown in Figures 17.59 and 17.60, the p-value for χ^2 test for paired-samples four-fold table or so-called McNemar test is 0.687. Then H_0 (null hypothesis) should not be rejected and we concluded that we do not have enough evidence to prove that the positive testing rates of two tests are not equal.

CLIA×LIA crosstabulation

			LIA −	LIA +	Total
CLIA	−	Count	66	4	70
		Expected count	47.6	22.4	70.0

Continued

			LIA		Total
			−	+	
		Count	2	28	30
		Expected count	20. 4	9. 6	30. 0
Total	+	Count	68	32	100
		Expected count	68. 0	32. 0	100. 0

Figure 17. 59   Output 1 Window

Chi-square tests

	Value	Exact *sig.* (two-sided)
McNemar test	—	0. 687[a]
N of valid cases	100	—

a. Binomial distribution used

Figure 17. 60   Output 2 Window

17.9.3 χ^2 Test for the Comparison of Multiple Rates

Example 17. 27   Ninety-five acute pancreatitis patients were divided into three groups: mild acute pancreatitis (MAP), moderately severe acute pancreatitis (MSAP), and severe acute pancreatitis (SAP). The incidence rates of pleural effusion for these three acute pancreatitis groups are listed in Table 17. 17. Can you evaluate whether the incidence rates of the three groups are equal?

Table 17. 17   Comparison of Incidence Rates of Pleural Effusion among Acute Pancreatitis Groups

Groups	Pleural effusion		Total	Incidence rate/%
	Yes	No		
MAP	6	45	51	11. 8
MSAP	6	18	24	25. 0
SAP	10	10	20	50. 0
Total	22	73	95	23. 2

Open Example 17. 27. sav

(a) Weight cases by variable frequency

• Methods and steps are the same as Example 17. 24

(b) The SPSS procedure

• Methods and steps are the same as Example 17. 24

(c) Read and explain the results

As shown in Figures 17. 61 and 17. 62, only 1 cell (16. 7%) has expected count less than 5. The minimum expected count is 4.63. The result of Pearson chi-square should be chosen.

Acute_pancreatitis × pleural_effusion crosstabulation

			Pleural_effusion		Total
			No	Yes	
Acute_pancreatitis	MAP	Count	45	6	51
		Expected count	39.2	11.8	51.0
	MSAP	Count	18	6	24
		Expected count	18.4	5.6	24.0
	SAP	Count	10	10	20
		Expected count	15.4	4.6	20.0
Total		Count	73	22	95
		Expected count	73.0	22.0	95.0

Figure 17.61　Output Window (Observed and Expected Count)

Chi-square tests

	Value	df	Asymptotic significance (two-sided)	Exact *sig.* (two-sided)	Exact *sig.* (two-sided)	Point probability
Pearson chi-square	11.864[a]	2	0.003	0.002	—	—
Likelihood ratio	11.160	2	0.004	0.007	—	—
Fisher's exact test	11.089	—	—	0.004	—	—
Linear-by-linear association	11.413[b]	1	0.001	0.001	0.001	0.001
N of valid cases	95	—	—	—	—	—

a. 1 cell (16.7%) has expected count less than 5; the minimum expected count is 4.63

b. The standardized statistic is 3.378

Figure 17.62　Output Window (χ^2 Test)

17.9.4　χ^2 Test for the Comparison of Multiple Proportions

Example 17.28　There were 165 esophageal squamous cell carcinoma (ESCC) patients who were divided into two groups (early group and late group) according to the biochemical indices. Table 17.18 lists the proportions of the positions of carcinomas in the esophagus for two ESCC groups. Evaluate whether the proportions of the two groups are equal.

Table 17. 18　The Positions of Carcinomas in the Esophagus of ESCC Patients

Groups	Upper	Middle	Lower	Total
Early	20	34	7	61
Late	30	63	11	104
Total	50	97	18	165

Open Example 17. 28. sav

(a) Weight cases by variable frequency

• Methods and steps are the same as that in Example 17. 24

(b) The SPSS procedure

• Methods and steps are the same as that in Example 17. 24

(c) Read and explain the results

As shown in Figures 17. 63 and 17. 64, the result of chi-square tests—$\chi^2 = 0.379$ and $P = 0.828$, using $\alpha = 0.05$—shows we failed to reject the null hypothesis and we can conclude that we do not have sufficient evidence to prove the significant differences between the proportions of two groups.

ECSC_groups × position crosstabulation

			Position Upper	Position Middle	Position Lower	Total
ECSC_groups	Early	Count	20	34	7	61
		Expected count	18. 5	35. 9	6. 7	61. 0
	Late	Count	30	63	11	104
		Expected count	31. 5	61. 1	11. 3	104. 0
Total		Count	50	97	18	165
		Expected count	50. 0	97. 0	18. 0	165. 0

Figure 17. 63　Output Window (Observed and Expected Count)

Chi-square Tests

	Value	df	Asymptotic significance (two-sided)	Exact *sig.* (two-sided)	Exact *sig.* (one-sided)	Point probability
Pearson chi-square	0. 379[a]	2	0. 828	0. 839	—	—
Likelihood ratio	0. 378	2	0. 828	0. 839	—	—
Fisher's exact test	0. 446	—	—	0. 839	—	—
Linear-by-linear association	0. 094[b]	1	0. 759	0. 794	0. 431	0. 100
N of valid cases	165	—	—	—	—	—

a. 0 cell (0. 0%) has *expected count less than* 5; *the minimum expected count is* 6. 65

b. *The standardized statistic is* 0. 307

Figure 17. 64　Output Window (χ^2 test)

17.9.5 Fisher's Exact Test

Example 17.29 This is a randomized, double-blind, and placebo-controlled study. In total, 17 patients received new drug and 14 received placebo. After a course of treatment, the effect of treatment is assessed (Table 17.19). Evaluate whether the effects of treatment by the two treatments are different.

Table 17.19 Comparison of Effective Rates by Two Treatments

Group	Effective	Ineffective	Total	Effective rate/%
New drug	2	15	17	11.76
Placebo	4	10	14	28.57
Total	6	25	31	19.35

Open Example 17.29. sav

(a) Perform Fisher's exact test

We cannot use χ^2 test for the four-fold table because $n<40$. Instead, we need to use the 2×2 Fisher's exact test. Click the "Exact" button to open the Exact window, and select the option "Exact."

(b) Read and explain the results

The basic results of the chi-square test are given in the output results. Figure 17.65 shows the crosstabulation of the analysis data. The result of exact probability (Fisher's Exact Test) is displayed in Figure 17.66: P(two-sided)$=0.370$. Since the difference is not statistically significant, we cannot conclude that the two treatments have different effective rates.

Group✕effect crosstabulation

			Effect		Total
			Ineffective	Effective	
Group	Placebo	Count	10	4	14
		Expected count	11.3	2.7	14.0
Total	New drug	Count	15	2	17
		Expected count	13.7	3.3	17.0
		Count	25	6	31
		Expected count	25.0	6.0	31.0

Figure 17.65 Output Window (Observed and Expected Count)

Chi-square tests

	Value	df	Asymptotic significance (two-sided)	Exact *sig.* (two-sided)	Exact *sig.* (one-sided)	Point probability
Pearson chi-square	1.389[a]	1	0.239	0.370	0.235	—
Continuity correction[b]	0.521	1	0.470	—	—	—
Likelihood ratio	1.396	1	0.237	0.370	0.235	—
Fisher's exact test	—	—	—	0.370	0.235	—
Linear-by-linear Association	1.345[c]	1	0.246	0.370	0.235	0.185
N of valid cases	31	—	—	—	—	—

a. *2 cells (50.0%) have expected count less than 5; the minimum expected count is 2.71*

b. *Computed only for a 2×2 table*

c. *The standardized statistic is* −1.160

Figure 17.66   Output Window (Fisher's Exact Test)

17.9.6 χ^2 Test for Goodness-of-Fit Test

Example 17.30   A random sample of heights of 119 boys are recorded below.

119.3	121.2	116.6	126.4	120.0	115.5	119.9	116.5	121.6	116.9	122.1
123.4	119.2	117.3	114.4	119.9	118.7	123.2	119.8	122.3	122.6	127.6
110.4	115.9	129.4	115.2	115.9	113.0	126.3	125.3	114.6	122.4	125.7
124.0	130.4	118.9	122.1	118.6	117.2	116.7	121.3	115.6	120.5	125.2
122.2	112.8	117.3	125.3	116.7	132.2	119.3	116.4	118.2	121.7	118.6
115.2	118.0	109.7	120.5	110.3	117.2	113.7	120.0	117.0	121.3	112.9
110.2	116.1	118.5	120.0	120.7	121.4	119.6	114.2	121.7	123.6	120.6
112.7	119.8	123.4	122.3	113.2	120.1	124.3	120.5	127.8	123.7	125.9
108.9	119.7	114.3	127.8	120.3	114.5	130.6	120.8	120.5	114.6	119.1
114.5	121.9									

Question: Do the heights of the 119 boys follow the normal distribution?

Open Example 17.30.sav

(a) Normality test

• Methods and steps are the same as Example 17.14

(b) Read and explain the results

The histogram shows the distribution of height in the data set (Figure 17.67), and Figure 17.68 shows the descriptive statistics of height, with a mean of 119.54 cm and std. deviation of 4.77 cm.

The result of normality tests—$P=0.200$ (Kolmogorov-Smirnov test) and $P=0.674$ (Shapiro-Wilk test)—are both greater than 0.05, indicating that so we cannot reject the null hypothesis of a normal distribution. The data seem to fit the normal distribution reasonably well (Figure 17.69).

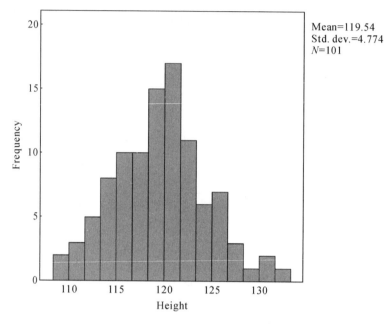

Figure 17.67 Histogram for Height

Descriptives

			Statistic	SE
Height	Mean		119.54	0.475
	95% CI for mean	Lower bound	118.60	—
		Upper bound	120.48	—
	5% Trimmed mean		119.49	—
	Median		119.80	—
	Variance		22.787	—
	Std. dev.		4.774	—
	Minimum		109	—
	Maximum		132	—
	Range		23	—
	IQR		6	—
	Skewness		0.182	0.240
	Kurtosis		0.031	0.476

Figure 17.68 Descriptive Output for Height

Normality tests

	Kolmogorov-Smirnov[a]			Shapiro-Wilk		
	Statistic	df	$sig.$	Statistic	df	$sig.$
Height	0.057	101	0.200*	0.990	101	0.674

a. *Lilliefors Significance Correction*

*. *A lower bound of the true significance*

Figure 17.69　Output Window

17.10　SPSS for Non-parametric Test

17.10.1　Non-parametric Test for Two Relate Samples

Example 17.31 An ophthalmologist wanted to assess the efficacy of a new operation on the visual acuity improvement. He randomly selected 12 of his inpatients and measured the visual acuity before and after the operation. Table 17.20 shows the data of 12 subjects' visual acuity in the study.

Table 17.20　Visual Acuity of 12 Subjects before and after Operation

Patients	1	2	3	4	5	6	7	8	9	10	11	12
Pre-operation	4.3	4.1	4.5	4.1	4.5	4.7	4.0	4.1	5.2	4.1	4.1	4.8
Post-operation	4.1	4.6	4.5	4.2	4.5	4.5	4.4	4.3	4.7	4.2	4.1	4.7

Open Example 17.31.sav

(a) Normal distribution test

Check the normality of D-value: methods and steps are the same as that in Example 17.14.

Since the p-value is less than 0.05, we should select the Wilcoxon signed rank test to perform the inference.

(b) Wilcoxon signed rank test

- "Analyze"→"Non-parametric Tests"→"Legacy Dialogs"→"2 Relate Samples"
- Move the "Pre-operation" and "Post-operation" variables to the "Test Pairs" box
- Highlight "Sign" and click "OK"

(c) Read and explain the results

Because the p-value = 1.000 > 0.05 (Figure 17.69), according to $\alpha = 0.05$ level, we cannot reject the null hypothesis and there is no statistically significant difference for visual acuity between pre- and post-operation. We conclude that the operation is not necessary for these patients.

Test statistics[a]

	Post-operation — pre-operation
Exact *sig.* (two-tailed)	1. 000[b]

a. Sign test

b. Binomial distribution used

Figure 17. 70   Result of Wilcoxon Signed Rank Test

17.10.2   Non-parametric Test for Two Independent Samples

Example 17. 32   A researcher wanted to know whether the protein level in the food will affect the weight. He randomly selected 19 rats from the university animal center and randomly assigned them into two groups. One group was given high-protein food and the other was fed with low-protein food. The weight of each rat at baseline and 3 months later was measured. The additive weight of rats is shown in Table 17. 21.

Table 17. 21   Additive Weight of Rats after Supplemented with Low- or High-Protein Food

Group	Rats number											
	1	2	3	4	5	6	7	8	9	10	11	12
Low-protein food	6	118	93	85	107	119	94	—	—	—	—	—
High-protein food	134	146	104	120	124	161	107	8	113	129	97	123

Open Example 17. 32. sav

(a) Normal distribution test

Methods and steps are the same as that in Example 17. 14

P-values of the two groups are less than 0. 05, and these two groups do not follow the normal distribution. So we should select independent samples non-parametric test to perform the inference.

(b) Independent samples non-parametric test

• Select "Analyze" → "Non-parametric Tests" → "Legacy Dialogs" → "2 Independent Samples"

• Highlight "Additive Weight" and move it into the "Test Variances List" box, and then move the "Group" variable to the "Grouping Variable" box

• Click the "Define Groups" button → input "1" and "2" in the blanks of Group 1 and Group 2, respectively

• Click "Continue" → "OK"

(c) Read and explain the results

The results of 2 independent samples non-parametric test are as follows: Figure 17. 71 shows the sample size, mean rank, and sum of ranks; and Figure 17. 72 shows a significant difference between the low-protein food group and high-protein food group ($Z = -2. 156$, $P = 0. 028$).

Ranks

	Group	N	Mean rank	Sum of ranks
Additive weight	Low-protein food	7	6.36	44.50
	High-protein food	12	12.13	145.50
	Total	19	—	—

Figure 17.71　Ranks of the Two Groups

Test statistics[a]

	Additive weight
Mann-Whitney U	16.500
Wilcoxon W	44.500
Z	-2.156
Asymp. *sig.* (two-tailed)	0.031
Exact *sig.* [2×(one-tailed *sig.*)]	0.028[b]

a. *Grouping Variable*: *group*

b. *Not corrected for ties*

Figure 17.72　Result of Mann-Whitney Test

Example 17.33　A physician wanted to know whether treatment A is different from a reference treatment for essential hypertension (EH) patients. He randomly selected 200 EH patients and assigned them into two groups in a random manner. Half of these 200 subjects were given treatment A (TRT group) and the other half were given the reference treatment (Control group) for 6 months (Table 17.22).

Table 17.22　Comparison of the Efficacy of Two Treatments in EH Patients

Group	Excellent	Valid	Invalid
TRT	50	30	20
Control	30	40	30

Open Example 17.33. sav

(a) Weighting the cases

• Select "Data"→"Weight Cases"→"Weight Cases By"

• Move the "Number" variable to the "Frequency Variable" box

• Click "OK"

(b) Two independent samples non-parametric test

• Select "Analyze"→"Non-parametric Tests"→"Legacy Dialogs"→"2 Independent Samples"

• Move the "Efficacy" variable to the "Test Variances List" box, and then move the "Group" variable to the "Grouping Variable" box

• Click the "Define Groups" button, and then input "1" and "2" in the blanks of Groups 1 and 2, respectively

　• Click "Continue"→"OK"

(c) Read and explain the results

Figure 17.73 shows the sample size, mean rank, and sum of ranks. Figure 17.74 shows that there is a significant difference between the TRT group and Control group ($Z = -2.739$, $P=0.006$). Since the value of efficacy is defined as Excellent$=1$, Valid$=2$, and Invalid$=3$, the mean rank of the TRT group is less than that of the Control group, suggesting the efficacy of the TRT group are better than the Control group.

Ranks

	Group	N	Mean rank	Sum of ranks
Efficacy	TRT	100	90.00	9,000.00
	Control	100	111.00	11,100.00
	Total	200	—	—

Figure 17.73　Ranks of the Two Groups

Test statistics[a]

	Efficacy
Mann-Whitney U	3,950.000
Wilcoxon W	9,000.000
Z	-2.739
Asymp. *sig.* (two-tailed)	0.006

a. Grouping Variable: group

Figure 17.74　Result of Mann-Whitney Test

17.10.3　Non-parametric Test for K-Independent Samples

Example 17.34　A physician wanted to know whether nutrient X is good for the growth of children. She randomly selected 120 primary school students from the childhood population in a city. These children were then randomly assigned into 4 groups and given either the placebo or different doses of the nutrient. Before the intervention, every kid's height was measured twice, strictly following the standard operating procedure (SOP). A year later, the height of each student was measured again. The average changes of height for each student between pre- and post-intervention were used to assess the efficacy of nutrient X on children's growth and development (Table 17.23).

Table 17. 23   Changes of Height（cm）among Different Groups

ID	Placebo	Low dose	Medium dose	High dose
1	8. 43	8. 79	9. 05	9. 40
2	8. 39	8. 99	8. 95	9. 43
3	8. 37	8. 89	8. 81	9. 22
4	8. 30	8. 90	8. 93	9. 36
5	8. 34	8. 86	8. 83	9. 30
6	8. 26	8. 65	8. 84	9. 32
⋮	⋮	⋮	⋮	⋮
22	8. 33	8. 79	8. 51	9. 03
23	8. 21	8. 66	9. 01	9. 31
24	8. 21	8. 90	8. 97	9. 41
25	8. 34	8. 84	8. 86	9. 31
26	8. 26	8. 89	8. 92	9. 44
27	8. 33	8. 79	8. 89	9. 41
28	8. 05	8. 77	9. 00	9. 41
29	8. 25	8. 89	8. 83	9. 41
30	8. 41	8. 74	9. 00	9. 26

Open Example 17. 34. sav

（a）K-independent samples non-parametric test

• "Analyze"→"Non-parametric Tests"→"Independent Samples"

• Click "Fields"

• Move the "Height_change" variable into the "Test Fields" blank，and the "Nutrient_X" variable into the "Groups" blank

• Click "Settings" → "Customize tests" → "Kruskal-Wallis One-Way ANOVA（K Samples）"

• Click "Run"

（b）Read and explain the results

The result of non-parametric test is as below：

Figure 17. 75 shows p-value（$P < 0.001$）and decision of the hypothesis test.

Hypothesis Test Summary

	Null Hypothesis	Test	Sig.	Decision
1	The distribution of Height_change is the same across categories of Nutrient_X.	Independent-Samples Kruskal-Wallis Test	.000	Reject the null hypothesis.

Asymptotic significances are displayed. The significance level is .05.

Figure 17. 75   Hypothesis Test Summary

Double-click the output window in Figure 17.75 to display the Model Viewer window. Figure 17.76 shows the boxplots and statistic of the test ($\chi^2 = 103.920$, $P < 0.001$).

Independent-Samples Kruskal-Wallis Test

Total N	120
Test Statistic	103.920
Degrees of Freedom	3
Asymptotic Sig. (2-sided test)	.000

Figure 17.76 Boxplots and the Result of Hypothesis Test

At the bottom of the Model Viewer window, expand the "View" menu and choose "Pairwise Comparisons" (Figure 17.77). The results of pairwise comparisons of groups are shown in Figure 17.78, suggesting that there are statistically significant differences among other groups, with the exception of the difference between Group Low and Group Medium (adjusted p-value $= 0.332$).

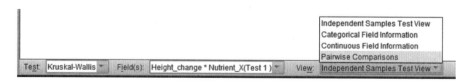

Figure 17.77 Boxplots and the Result of Hypothesis Test

Example 17.35 A physician wanted to know whether the efficacy of a special treatment significantly differs among doses. She randomly selected 240 participants from her outpatients and inpatients, who were randomly assigned into 4 groups, which received different doses of the treatment for 6 months. The outcome of the research is summarized in

Pairwise Comparisons of Nutrient_X

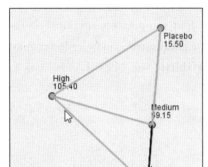

Each node shows the sample average rank of Nutrient_X.

Sample1-Sample2	Test Statistic	Std. Error	Std. Test Statistic	Sig.	Adj.Sig.
Placebo-Low	-36.450	8.979	-4.060	.000	.000
Placebo-Medium	-53.650	8.979	-5.975	.000	.000
Placebo-High	-89.900	8.979	-10.012	.000	.000
Low-Medium	-17.200	8.979	-1.916	.055	.332
Low-High	-53.450	8.979	-5.953	.000	.000
Medium-High	-36.250	8.979	-4.037	.000	.000

Each row tests the null hypothesis that the Sample 1 and Sample 2
distributions are the same.
Asymptotic significances (2-sided tests) are displayed. The significance level
is .05.

Figure 17. 78   Result of Pairwise Comparisons

Table 17. 24.

Table 17. 24   Efficacy of the Treatment at Different Doses

Dose	Excellent	Valid	Invalid
A	10	20	30
B	20	30	10
C	30	20	10
D	40	10	10

Open Example 17. 35. sav

(a) Weighting the cases

• Select "Data"→"Weight Cases"→"Weight Cases By"

- Move the "Number" variable to the "Frequency Variable" box
- Click "OK"

(b) Two or more independent samples non-parametric test
- Select "Analyze"→"Non-parametric Tests"→Independent Samples"→"Fields"
- Move the "Efficacy" variable to the "Test Fields" box and the "Group" variable to the "Groups" box
- Click "Settings"→"Customize Tests"→"Kruskal-Wallis One-Way ANOVA (K Samples)"
- Click "Run"

(c) Read and explain the results

Figure 17.79 shows the p-value ($P<0.001$) and the decision of the hypothesis test. Figure 17.80 shows the boxplots and statistic of the test ($\chi^2 = 36.751$, $P<0.001$). Double-click the Output window in Figure 17.80 to open the Model Viewer window. At the bottom of the Model Viewer window, expand the "View" menu and choose "Pairwise Comparisons" (Figure 17.81), with results shown in Figure 17.82, which suggests significant differences between Groups D and A, Groups C and A, and Groups B and A (adjusted p-value).

Hypothesis Test Summary

	Null Hypothesis	Test	Sig.	Decision
1	The distribution of efficacy is the same across categories of group.	Independent-Samples Kruskal-Wallis Test	.000	Reject the null hypothesis.

Asymptotic significances are displayed. The significance level is .05.

Figure 17.79   Hypothesis Test Summary

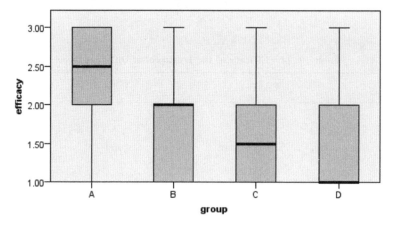

Independent-Samples Kruskal-Wallis Test

Total N	240
Test Statistic	36.751
Degrees of Freedom	3
Asymptotic Sig. (2-sided test)	.000

1. The test statistic is adjusted for ties.

Figure 17. 80　Boxplots and the Result of Hypothesis Test

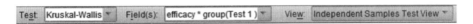

Figure 17. 81　Boxplots and the Result of Hypothesis Test

Pairwise Comparisons of group

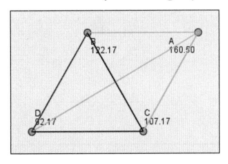

Each node shows the sample average rank of group.

Sample 1-Sam...	Test Statistic	Std. Error	Std. Test Statistic	Sig.	Adj.Sig.
D-C	15.000	11.857	1.265	.206	1.000
D-B	30.000	11.857	2.530	.011	.068
D-A	68.333	11.857	5.763	.000	.000
C-B	15.000	11.857	1.265	.206	1.000
C-A	53.333	11.857	4.498	.000	.000
B-A	38.333	11.857	3.233	.001	.007

Each row tests the null hypothesis that the Sample 1 and Sample 2 distributions are the same.
Asymptotic significances (2-sided tests) are displayed. The significance level is .05.

Figure 17. 82　Result of Pairwise Comparisons

17.11 SPSS for Linear Correlation and Regression

Example 17.36 Consider 15 adults whose BMI and waist circumference are measured and recorded in Table 17.25. Please determine if a correlation exists between the two measures.

Table 17.25 BMI (y, kg/m^2) and Waist Circumference (x, cm) of 15 Adults

No.	x (1)	y (2)
1	99.9	29.10
2	81.6	22.56
3	90.7	29.39
4	108.0	30.94
5	112.8	30.62
6	100.3	27.33
7	86.7	26.68
8	81.0	23.68
9	125.7	39.76
10	90.6	25.93
11	114.5	37.60
12	73.4	19.44
13	116.1	36.16
14	99.3	30.23
15	99.8	31.42
Total	1,480.4	440.84

Open Example 17.36. sav

(a) Draw the scatter plot

• Select "Graphs"→"Legacy Dialogs"→"Scatter/Dot"

• Select the "Simple Scatter" variable and click the "Define" button.

• Enter "y" into the "Y Axis", and "x" into the "X Axis" to find the scatter plot of variables "BMI" and "Waist Circumference"

The scatter plot is shown in Figure 17.83.

(b) Calculate the sample correlation coefficient r

• Select "Analyze"→"Correlate"→"Bivariate"

• Place "Waist Circumference (x)" and "BMI (y)" in the "Variables" field

• Tick the "Pearson" and "Two-Tailed" checkboxes

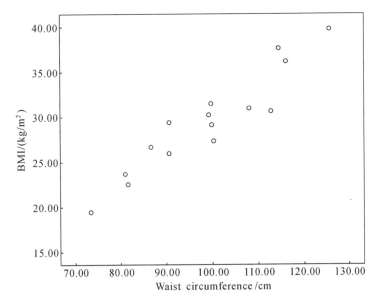

Figure 17. 83　The Output of Simple Scatterplot

• Click "OK"

As shown in Figure 17. 84, the sample correlation coefficient is $r=0.943$ ($P<0.001$). Therefore, there is a positive correlation between BMI and waist circumference of adults, and the correlation degree is 0. 943.

Correlations

		Waist circumference	BMI
Waist circumference	Pearson correlation	1	0. 943**
	sig. (two-tailed)		0. 000
	N	15	15
BMI	Pearson correlation	0. 943**	1
	sig. (two-tailed)	0. 000	—
	N	15	15

** . *Correlation is significant at the* 0. 01 *level* (*two-tailed*)

Figure 17. 84　The Output of Correlation

Example 17. 37

Derive the estimated regression line for the data in Example 17. 36.

Open Example 17. 36. sav

(a) The SPSS procedure

• Figure 17. 83 shows the linear tendency between waist circumference and BMI.

• Select "Analyze"→"Regression"→"Linear"

• Place "BMI" in the "Dependent" field, and "Waist Circumference" in the "Independent(s)" field. Then click the "Statistics" button

• Select "Estimate"→"Confidence Intervals"→"Model Fit"→"R-Squared Change"→"Descriptives"

• Click "Continue"→"OK"

(b) Read and explain the results

As shown in Figure 17.85, the F-value of ANOVA of the regression function is 103.399, and the p-value is 0.000 (Figures 17.85, 17.86, and 17.87), indicating that a significant linear relationship exists between the weight and body surface area. The model summary (Figure 17.84) shows that $R = 0.943$, $R^2 = 0.888$, and $R_{adj} = 0.880$, the proportion of the variance that is explained by the model. Since these numbers are quite high, the fitness of the function is appropriate.

In the coefficients figure (Figure 17.87), the constant term $b_0 = -5.358$ and covariate coefficient $b_1 = 0.352$. The linear equation is $\hat{y} = -5.358 + 0.352x$.

Model summary

Model	R	R-square	Adj. R-square	SE of the estimate	R-square change	F-change	df_1	df_2	sig. F-change
					Change statistics				
1	0.943[a]	0.888	0.880	1.92518	0.888	103.399	1	13	0.000

a. Predictors: (Constant), waist circumference

Figure 17.85   Output 1 Window of Linear Regression

ANOVA[a]

Model		Sum of squares	df	Mean square	F	sig.
1	Regression	383.232	1	383.232	103.399	0.000[b]
	Residual	48.182	13	3.706	—	—
	Total	431.415	14	—	—	—

a. Dependent Variable: BMI

b. Predictors: (Constant), waist circumference

Figure 17.86   Output 2 Window of Linear Regression

Coefficients[a]

Model		Unstandardized coefficients		Standardized coefficients	T	sig.	95% CI for B	
		B	SE	β			Lower bound	Upper bound
1	(Constant)	-5.358	3.453	—	-1.552	0.145	-12.818	2.102
	Waist circumference	0.352	0.035	0.943	10.169	0.000	0.277	0.427

a. Dependent Variable: BMI

Figure 17.87   Output 3 Window of Linear Regression

(c) Draw the regression line

• In the output window of the scatter plot, double-left-click the mouse to open the "Chart Editor" (Figure 17.88)

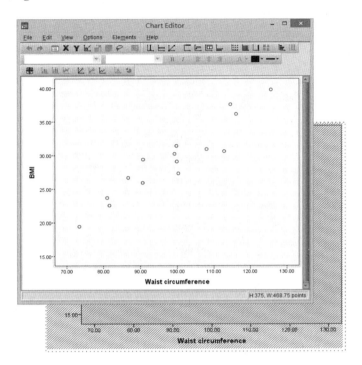

Figure 17.88　The Output of Scatter Plot

• Select "Elements"→"Fit Line"→"Linear"
• Click "Apply" to draw the regression line (Figure 17.89)

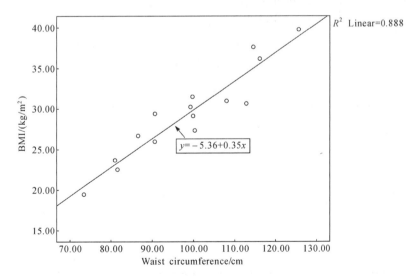

Figure 17.89　The Output of Linear Regression

Example 17.38 Please analyze if relationship exists between the burn area and length of stay of burn patients.

Open Example 17. 38. sav (Table 17. 26)

Table 17. 26   Burn Area and Length of Stay of 12 Burn Patients

Case No.	Burn area x_i(1)	Length of stay y_i(2)/d
1	Large	92
2	Large	83
3	Large	79
4	Severe	68
5	Severe	55
6	Small	11
7	Small	30
8	Small	35
9	Middle	9
10	Middle	10
11	Small	2
12	Small	3

(a) The SPSS procedure

• Select "Analyze"→"Correlate"→"Bivariate"

• Place "Burn Area (X)" and "Length of Stay (Days) (Y)" in the "Variables"

• Select "Spearman" and "Two-Tailed"

• Click "OK"

(b) Read and explain the results

The output window indicates the Spearman correlation coefficient r_s is 0. 689 and P is 0. 013, indicating statistical significance of the two variables and a relationship between the burn area and length of stay of burn patients (Figure 17. 90).

Correlations

			Burn area	Length of stay/d
Spearman's ρ	Burn area	Correlation coefficient	1. 000	0. 689*
		sig. (two-tailed)	—	0. 013
		N	12	12
	Length of stay/d	Correlation coefficient	0. 689*	1. 000
		sig. (two-tailed)	0. 013	—
		N	12	12

*. *Correlation is significant at the* 0. 05 *level* (*two-tailed*)

Figure 17. 90   The Output of Spearman Rand Correlations

17. 12   SPSS for Multiple Linear Regression

Example 17. 39   Suppose systolic blood pressure (SBP), age, BMI, and serum albumin (ALB) are measured for 8,366 subjects and the data are shown in Table 17. 27.

Table 17. 27   Sample Data for SBP, Age, BMI, and ALB for 8,366 Cases

ID	Age (X_1) /years	BMI (X_2) /(kg/m^2)	ALB (X_3) /(g/L)	SBP (y) /mmHg
5	49	29. 10	45	122
6	19	22. 56	51	114
7	59	29. 39	45	123
⋮	⋮	⋮	⋮	⋮
41,466	58	33. 65	44	151
41,468	66	26. 44	44	148
41,472	34	26. 23	50	127

Open Example 17. 39. sav

(a) The SPSS procedure

• Select "Analyze"→"Regression"→"Linear"

• Move the "SBP" variable to the "Dependent" box

• Move the "AGE," "BMI," and "ALB" variables into the "Independent(s)" box

• Click the "Statistics" button

• Tick "Estimates"→"Confidence Intervals"→"Model Fit"→"R-Square Change"→"Descriptives" checkboxes

• Click "Continue"→"OK"

(b) Read and explain the results

Figure 17.91 shows the model summary of the linear regression. With $R = 0.559$, $R^2 = 0.312$, $R^2_{adj} = 0.312$, the fitness of the function is acceptable.

Model Summary

Model	R	R-square	Adj. R-square	SE of the estimate	R-square change	F-change	df_1	df_2	$sig.$ F-change
					Change statistics				
1	0. 559[a]	0. 312	0. 312	14. 682	0. 312	1,264. 206	3	8,362	0. 000

a. Predictors: (Constant), ALB (g/L), age at screening adjudicated-recode, BMI (kg/m^2)

Figure 17.91   Model Summary of Linear Regression

Figure 17.92 shows the result of ANOVA of the regression function ($F = 1,264.206$, $P < 0.001$), suggesting that a significant linear relationship exists between the "SBP" variable and at least one independent variable.

ANOVA[a]

Model		Sum of squares	df	Mean square	F	$Sig.$
1	Regression	817,502.169	3	272,500.723	1,264.206	0.000[b]
	Residual	1,802,436.825	8,362	215.551	—	—
	Total	2,619,938.994	8,365	—	—	—

a. Dependent Variable: SBP average reported to examinee

b. Predictors: (Constant), ALB (g/L), age at screening adjudicated-recode, BMI (kg/m²)

Figure 17.92   The Result of ANOVA of Linear Regression

Figure 17.92 shows all the independent variables that influence the "SBP" variable (all the p-values of age, BMI, and ALB are less than 0.001). Among the three influencing factors, age has the strongest effect on SBP (Standardized Coefficients is 0.528), and ALB has the least effect on SBP (Standardized Coefficients is 0.090).

The regression equation is given by

$$\hat{y} = 67.621 + 0.488X_1 + 0.482X_2 + 0.441X_3$$

Coefficients[a]

Model		Unstandardized coefficients		Standardized coefficients	t	$sig.$	95% CI for B	
		B	SE	β			Lower bound	Upper bound
1	(Constant)	67.621	2.332	—	29.002	0.000	63.050	72.191
	Age at screening adjudicated-recode	0.488	0.008	0.528	57.630	0.000	0.471	0.504
	BMI/(kg/m²)	0.482	0.030	0.151	16.289	0.000	0.424	0.540
	ALB/(g/L)	0.441	0.046	0.090	9.662	0.000	0.352	0.530

a. Dependent Variable: SBP average reported to examinee

Figure 17.93   The Coefficients of Linear Regression

17.13   SPSS for Binary Logistic Regression

Example 17.40   In a case-control study of risk factors related to cancer of the esophagus, the data of two risk factors were listed in Table 17.28.

Table 17. 28   A Case-Control Study Data of Risk Factors Related to Cancer of the Esophagus

Smoking status (X_1)	Alcohol use (X_2)	Case ($Y=1$)	Control ($Y=0$)
Smoking	Drinking ($X_2=1$)	265	151
($X_1=1$)	Non-drinking ($X_2=0$)	44	57
Non-smoking	Drinking ($X_2=1$)	63	107
($X_1=0$)	Non-drinking ($X_2=0$)	63	136

Open Example 17. 40. sav

(a) Weight cases by variable frequency

• Select "Data"→"Weight Cases"

• Click the radio button "Weight Case By" and move the "Frequency" variable into the "Frequency Variable" box

(b) Perform binary logistic regression

• Select "Analyze"→"Regression"→"Binary Logistic"

• Move the "Disease (X_3)" variable into the "Dependent" box

• Move the "Smoking Status (X_1)" and "Alcohol Use (X_2)" variables into the "Covariates" box

• Click the "Options" Button

• Tick the "CI for exp(B)" checkbox (leave all other options to default) and click "Continue"

• Click "OK" to perform the binary logistic regression

(c) Read and explain the results

The binary logistic process defaults to building a model with a probability $P(Y=1)$ of a larger value of the dependent variable instead of $P(Y=0)$. Therefore, when observing the analysis results, it is necessary to check this part of the results to find out the assignment of the dependent variables and ensure that the interpretation of the analysis results is correct (Figures 17. 94, 17. 95, and 17. 96).

Dependent variable encoding

Original value	Internal value
Control	0
Case	1

Figure 17. 94   Table of Variable Assignments

Classification table[a]

Observed			Predicted		Percentage correct /%
			Disease		
			Control	Case	
Step 1	Disease	Control	300	151	66. 5
		Case	170	265	60. 9
	Overall percentage/%		—	—	63. 8

a. The cut value is 0. 500

Figure 17. 95　The Results of Classification Table

Variables in the equation

		B	SE	$Wald$	df	$sig.$	$\exp(B)$	95% CI for $\exp(B)$	
								Lower bound	Upper bound
Step 1[a]	X_1	0. 886	0. 150	34. 862	1	0. 000	2. 424	1. 807	3. 253
	X_2	0. 526	0. 157	11. 207	1	0. 001	1. 692	1. 244	2. 303
	Constant	−0. 910	0. 136	44. 870	1	0. 000	0. 403	—	—

a. Variable(s) entered on step 1: X_1, X_2

Figure 17. 96　The Results of Coefficients, Wald Test, OR, and 95% CI for OR

Figure 17. 96 is the most important part of the regression analysis, including the coefficient values of the variables and the constant term (B), standard error (SE), Wald chi-square values (Wald), degrees of freedom (df), p-values ($sig.$), and $\exp(B)$—the odds ratio (OR). The regression coefficient of the variable X_1 is 0. 886, with a p-value of 0. 000, showing X_1 is statistically significant. The coefficient of the variable X_2 is 0. 526, with a p-value of 0. 001, indicating X_2 is also statistically significant.

Example 17. 41　In order to find the risk factors related to the occurrence of coronary heart disease, a case-control study was conducted on 26 patients with coronary heart disease and 28 controls. The description and data on various risk factors are shown in Table 17. 29.

Table 17. 29　Eight Possible Risks Factors and Code for Coronary Heart Disease Study

Factors	Variable	Encoding
Age/years	X_1	<45=1, 45~54=2, 55~64=3, ≥65=4
Hypertension history	X_2	None=0, have=1
Hypertension family history	X_3	None=0, have=1
Smoking	X_4	Non-smoking=0, smoking=1
Hyperlipidemia history	X_5	None=0, have=1

Continued

Factors	Variable	Encoding
Animal fat intake	X_6	Low=0, high=1
BMI	X_7	<24=1, 24~25=2, ≥26=3
Type A personality	X_8	No=0, yes=1
Coronary heart disease	Y	Control=0, case=1

Open Example 17. 41. sav

(a) Perform binary logistic regression

- Select "Analyze"→"Regression"→"Binary Logistic"
- Move the "Coronary Heart Disease (Y)" variable into the "Dependent" box
- Move other variables into the "Covariates" box
- Change the "Method" from "Enter" to "Forward"
- Leave all other options with default values
- Click "OK" to perform the binary logistic regression

(b) Read and explain the results

Figure 17. 97 is the most important part of the regression analysis, including the coefficient values of the variables eventually introduced into the model and constant terms (B), standard error (SE), Wald chi-square values (Wald), degrees of freedom (df), p-values ($sig.$), and exp(B)—the odds ratio.

Four risk factors had been selected by the model: the age (X_1), hyperlipidemia history (X_5), animal fat intake amount (X_6), and type A personality (X_8). The coefficient of the variable X_1 is 0. 924 with a p-value of 0. 053, showing X_1 is statistically significant and the coefficient is positive ($OR = 2. 519$). The coefficient of the variable X_5 is 1. 496 with a p-value of 0. 044, showing X_5 was statistically significant and the coefficient is positive ($OR = 4. 464$). X_6 and X_8 can be explained in the same way.

Variables in the equation

		B	SE	$Wald$	df	$sig.$	exp(B)	95% CI for exp(B) Lower bound	95% CI for exp(B) Upper bound
Step 4[a]	X_1	0. 924	0. 477	3. 758	1	0. 053	2. 519	0. 990	6. 411
	X_5	1. 496	0. 744	4. 044	1	0. 044	4. 464	1. 039	19. 181
	X_6	3. 135	1. 249	6. 303	1	0. 012	23. 000	1. 989	265. 945
	X_8	1. 947	0. 847	5. 289	1	0. 021	7. 008	1. 333	36. 834
	Constant	−4. 705	1. 543	9. 295	1	0. 002	0. 009	—	—

a. Variable(s) entered on step 4: X_1

Figure 17. 97 The Results of Coefficients, Wald Test, OR, and 95% CI for OR

17. 14　SPSS for Survival Analysis

17. 14. 1　Life Table

Example 17. 42　A clinical trial was conducted to test the efficacy of different vitamin supplements in preventing visual loss in patients with retinitis pigmentosa (RP). Visual loss was measured by loss of retinal function as characterized by a 50% decline in the electroretinogram (ERG) 30 Hz amplitude, a measure of the electrical activity in the retina. In normal people, the normal range for ERG 30 Hz amplitude is $>50 \mu V$. In patients with RP, ERG 30 Hz amplitude is usually $<10 \mu V$ and is often $<1 \mu V$. Approximately 50% of patients with ERG 30 Hz amplitude near 0. 05 μV are legally blind compared with $<10\%$ of patients whose ERG 30 Hz amplitude is near 1. 3 μV (the average ERG amplitude for patients in this clinical trial). Patients in the study were randomized to one of the four treatment groups:

　　Group 1 received 15,000 IU of vitamin A and 3 IU (a trace amount) of vitamin E.

　　Group 2 received 75 IU (a trace amount) of vitamin A and 3 IU of vitamin E.

　　Group 3 received 15,000 IU of vitamin A and 400 IU of vitamin E.

　　Group 4 received 75 IU of vitamin A and 400 IU of vitamin E.

Let's call these four groups A group, trace group, AE group, and E group, respectively. We want to compare the proportion of patients who fails (i. e. loses 50% of initial ERG 30 Hz amplitude) in different treatment groups. Patients were enrolled from 1984 to 1987, and follow-up was terminated in September 1991. Because follow-up was terminated at the same point in chronological time, the period of follow-up differed for each patient. Patients who entered early in the study were followed for 6 years, whereas patients who enrolled later in the study were followed for 4 years. In addition, some patients dropped out of the study before September 1991 due to death, other diseases, side effects possibly due to the study medications or unwillingness to comply (take study medications). Estimate the survival probability at each of years $1 \sim 6$ for participants receiving 15,000 IU of vitamin A (i. e. groups A and AE combined) and participants receiving 75 IU of vitamin A (i. e. groups E and trace combined), respectively.

　　Open Example 17. 42. sav

　　(a) Perform Life Tables

　　• Select "Data"→"Transform"→"Weight Cases"→"Weight Cases By"→"Frequency Variable" column: number→"OK"

　　• Select "Analyze"→"Survival"→"Life Table"

　　• Move the "Time" variable into the "Time" box

　　• Change "Display Time Intervals" to "6" by "1"

　　• Move the "Result" variable into the "Status" box

- Define event: input "1" in "Single Value" box→"Continue"
- Move the "Group" variable into the "Factor" box
- Define Range: input "1" and "2" in "Minimum and Maximum" box →"Continue"
- Click the "Options" button
- Tick the "Life Table(s)" and "Survival" checkboxes
- Click "OK"

(b) The life table is listed as follows (Figure 17. 98)

The survival probability shows in "Proportion surviving" and "Cumulative proportion surviving at end of interval" columns. For the participants receiving 15,000 IU of vitamin A, the survival probability at year 1 is 0.98, and the survival probability is assumed to remain constant between year 1 and year 2. The probability of surviving to year 2 given that one survived to year 1 is 0.96. Thus, the survival probability at year 2 is 0.95 ("cumulative proportion surviving at end of interval" column).

17. 14. 2　Log-Rank Test

Example 17. 43　The researcher wanted to compare the efficacy of different vitamin supplements between the 15,000 IU daily group and 75 IU daily group.

Open Example 17. 43. sav

(a) Weight cases

Select "Data"→"Weight Cases"→"Weight Cases By"→"Frequency Variable" column: number→"OK"

(b) Perform Log-Rank Test

- Select "Analyze"→"Survival"→"Kaplan-Meier"
- Move the "Time" variable into the "Time" box
- Move the "Result" variable into the "Status" box
- Move the "Group" variable into the "Factor" box
- Click "Define Event," tick the "Single Value" checkbox, and input "1"
- Click the "Compare Factor" button
- Under the "Test Statistics" section, select "Log-Rank"→"Continue"
- Click the "Options" button→under the "Plots" section, select "Survival"
- Click "Continue"→"OK"

(c) Read and explain the results

Figure 17. 99 shows the total number of participants and the number of fails in each group. Figure 17. 100 shows the means and medians of survival time for each group. In this example, the median and 95% CI of survival time of 15,000 IU daily group and 75 IU daily group are 6.000 (5.080, 6.920) and 5.000 (4.356, 5.644).

The result of log-rank test in Figure 17. 101 shows that there is statistical difference of efficacy of different vitamin supplements between the 15,000 IU daily group and 75 IU daily

Life table

First-order controls	Interval start time	Number entering interval	Number withdrawing during interval	Number exposed to risk	Number of terminal events	Proportion terminating	Proportion surviving	Cumulative proportion surviving at end of interval	SE of cumulative proportion surviving at end of interval	Probability density	SE of probability density	Hazard rate	SE of hazard rate
15,000 IU daily group	0	172	0	172.000	0	0.00	1.00	1.00	0.00	0.000	0.000	0.00	0.00
	1	172	4	170.000	3	0.02	0.98	0.98	0.01	0.018	0.010	0.02	0.01
	2	165	0	165.000	6	0.04	0.96	0.95	0.02	0.036	0.014	0.04	0.02
	3	159	1	158.500	15	0.09	0.91	0.86	0.03	0.090	0.022	0.10	0.03
	4	143	26	130.000	21	0.16	0.84	0.72	0.04	0.138	0.028	0.18	0.04
	5	96	35	78.500	15	0.19	0.81	0.58	0.04	0.137	0.033	0.21	0.05
	6	46	41	25.500	5	0.20	0.80	0.47	0.06	0.000	0.000	0.00	0.00
75 IU daily group	0	182	0	182.000	0	0.00	1.00	1.00	0.00	0.000	0.000	0.00	0.00
	1	182	0	182.000	8	0.04	0.96	0.96	0.02	0.044	0.015	0.04	0.02
	2	174	3	172.500	13	0.08	0.92	0.88	0.02	0.072	0.019	0.08	0.02
	3	158	2	157.000	21	0.13	0.87	0.77	0.03	0.118	0.024	0.14	0.03
	4	135	28	121.000	21	0.17	0.83	0.63	0.04	0.133	0.027	0.19	0.04
	5	86	31	70.500	13	0.18	0.82	0.52	0.04	0.117	0.030	0.20	0.06
	6	42	29	27.500	13	0.47	0.53	0.27	0.05	0.000	0.000	0.00	0.00

Figure 17.98 Life Table

group ($\chi^2 = 4.348$, $P = 0.037$), according to the median and 95% CI of survival time in Figure 17.99. The efficacy of 15,000 IU daily vitamin supplements is better.

Figure 17.102 shows the cumulative survival curve of two groups, with the cumulative survival curve of 15,000 IU daily group higher than that of 75 IU daily group, which means the efficacy of 15,000 IU daily vitamin supplements is better.

Case processing summary

Group	Total N	N of Events	Censored	
			N	Percent/%
15,000 IU daily	134	65	69	51.5
75 IU daily	149	82	67	45.0
Overall	283	147	136	48.1

Figure 17.99   Means and Medians for Survival Time

Means and medians for survival time

Group	Mean[a]				Median			
			95% CI				95% CI	
	Estimate	SE	Lower bound	Upper bound	Estimate	SE	Lower bound	Upper bound
15,000 IU daily	4.893	0.122	4.653	5.133	6.000	0.469	5.080	6.920
75 IU daily	4.516	0.134	4.253	4.779	5.000	0.328	4.356	5.644
Overall	4.694	0.092	4.514	4.875	5.000	0.275	4.461	5.539

a. *Estimation is limited to the largest survival time if it is censored*

Figure 17.100   Means and Medians for Survival Time

Overall Comparisons

	Chi-square	df	sig.
Log-rank (Mantel-Cox)	4.348	1	0.037

Test of equality of survival distributions for the different levels of group

Figure 17.101   The Result of Log-Rank Test

17.14.3 Cox Regression

Example 17.44   If the researcher wanted to compare the efficacy of different vitamin supplements between 15,000 IU daily group and 75 IU daily group, he might use the Cox regression besides log-rank test.

$$x = \begin{cases} 1, & 15,000 \text{ IU group} \\ 0, & 75 \text{ IU group} \end{cases} \qquad y = \begin{cases} 1, & \text{Fail} \\ 0, & \text{Censored} \end{cases}$$

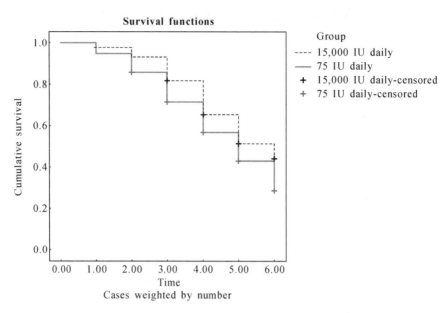

Figure 17. 101　Cumulative Survival Curve of Two Groups

Open Example 17. 44. sav

(a) Weight cases

● "Data"→"Weight Cases"→"Weight Cases By"→"Frequency Variable" column:
number→"OK"

(b) Perforem Cox Regression

● Select "Analyze"→"Survival"→" Cox Regression"

● Move the "Time" variable into the "Time" box

● Move the "Result" variable into the "Status" box

● Move the "Group" variable into the "Covariates" box

● Click the "Define Event" button, tick the "Single Value" checkbox, and input "1"

● Click the "Plots" button, tick the "Survival" checkbox, and click "Continue"

● Click the "Options" button→Under the "Model Statistics" section, select "CI for exp(B)
95%"

● Click "Continue"→"OK"

(c) Read and explain the results

Figure 17. 103 shows the number of fails, censored and total participants. Figures
17. 104 and 17. 105 show that the value of -2 log-likelihood of the Cox regression model
was decreased from 1,690. 482 to 1,684. 830 after the independent variables enter the model
(p-value equals 0. 060).

The coefficients of the Cox regression (shown in Figure 17. 106), for vitamin
supplements, are HR (95% CI): 0. 694(0. 504, 0. 957) with $P=0. 026$, indicating that the
participants of 15,000 IU daily group have lower hazard to fail compared with 75 IU daily
group. For the "Sex" variable, the coefficients are HR (95% CI): 0. 844(0. 597,0. 193)

with $P=0.336$, meaning that females have a lower hazard to fail compared with males, but there is no statistically significant difference between them since the p-value is quite high.

Figure 17.107 shows that the median of survival time for all participants is 6 years.

Case processing summary

		Unweighted		Weighted[b]	
		N	Percent/%	N	Percent/%
Cases available in analysis	Event[a]	24	55.8	154	43.5
	Censored	19	44.2	200	56.5
	Total	43	100.0	354	100.0
Cases dropped	Cases with missing values	0	0.0		
	Cases with negative time	0	0.0		
	Censored cases before the earliest event in a stratum	0	0.0		
	Total	0	0.0		
Total		43	100.0		

a. Dependent Variable: time

b. Weighted by: number

Figure 17.103　Summary of the Case Processing

Omnibus tests of model coefficients

-2 Log-likelihood
1,690.482

Figure 17.104　Omnibus Tests of Model Coefficients

Omnibus tests of model coefficients[a]

-2 Log-likelihood	Overall (score)			Change from previous step			Change from previous block		
	Chi-square	df	*sig.*	Chi-square	df	*sig.*	Chi-square	df	*sig.*
1,684.830	5.630	2	0.060	5.652	2	0.059	5.652	2	0.059

a. Beginning block number 1; Method=Enter

Figure 17.105　Model Coefficients after the Independent Variables Enter

Variables in the equation

	B	SE	$Wald$	df	*sig.*	$\exp(B)$	95% CI for $\exp(B)$	
							Lower bound	Upper bound
x_1	-0.365	0.164	4.970	1	0.026	0.694	0.504	0.957
x_2	-0.170	0.177	0.927	1	0.336	0.844	0.597	1.193

Figure 17.106　Coefficients of Cox Regression

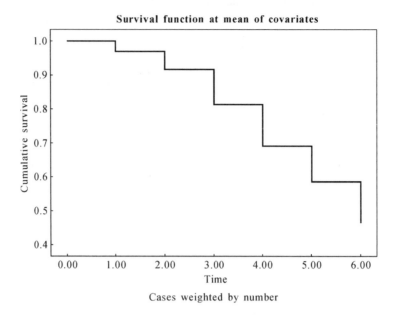

Figure 17. 107   Survival Function

（Leng Ruixue，Fan Yinguang，Shi Hongying）

Appendixes

Appendix 1

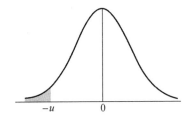

Table of Standard Normal Curve Areas

u	0.00	0.01	0.02	0.03	0.04	0.05	0.06	0.07	0.08	0.09
-3.0	0.0013	0.0013	0.0013	0.0012	0.0012	0.0011	0.0011	0.0011	0.0010	0.0010
-2.9	0.0019	0.0018	0.0018	0.0017	0.0016	0.0016	0.0015	0.0015	0.0014	0.0014
-2.8	0.0026	0.0025	0.0024	0.0023	0.0023	0.0022	0.0021	0.0021	0.0020	0.0019
-2.7	0.0035	0.0034	0.0033	0.0032	0.0031	0.0030	0.0029	0.0028	0.0027	0.0026
-2.6	0.0047	0.0045	0.0044	0.0043	0.0041	0.0040	0.0039	0.0038	0.0037	0.0036
-2.5	0.0062	0.0060	0.0059	0.0057	0.0055	0.0054	0.0052	0.0051	0.0049	0.0048
-2.4	0.0082	0.0080	0.0078	0.0075	0.0073	0.0071	0.0069	0.0068	0.0066	0.0064
-2.3	0.0107	0.0104	0.0102	0.0099	0.0096	0.0094	0.0091	0.0089	0.0087	0.0084
-2.2	0.0139	0.0136	0.0132	0.0129	0.0125	0.0122	0.0119	0.0116	0.0113	0.0110
-2.1	0.0179	0.0174	0.0170	0.0166	0.0162	0.0158	0.0154	0.0150	0.0146	0.0143
-2.0	0.0228	0.0222	0.0217	0.0212	0.0207	0.0202	0.0197	0.0192	0.0188	0.0183

Continued

u	0.00	0.01	0.02	0.03	0.04	0.05	0.06	0.07	0.08	0.09
−1.9	0.0287	0.0281	0.0274	0.0268	0.0262	0.0256	0.0250	0.0244	0.0239	0.0233
−1.8	0.0359	0.0351	0.0344	0.0336	0.0329	0.0322	0.0314	0.0307	0.0301	0.0294
−1.7	0.0446	0.0436	0.0427	0.0418	0.0409	0.0401	0.0392	0.0384	0.0375	0.0367
−1.6	0.0548	0.0537	0.0526	0.0516	0.0505	0.0495	0.0485	0.0475	0.0465	0.0455
−1.5	0.0668	0.0655	0.0643	0.0630	0.0618	0.0606	0.0594	0.0582	0.0571	0.0559
−1.4	0.0808	0.0793	0.0778	0.0764	0.0749	0.0735	0.0721	0.0708	0.0694	0.0681
−1.3	0.0968	0.0951	0.0934	0.0918	0.0901	0.0885	0.0869	0.0853	0.0838	0.0823
−1.2	0.1151	0.1131	0.1112	0.1093	0.1075	0.1056	0.1038	0.1020	0.1003	0.0985
−1.1	0.1357	0.1335	0.1314	0.1292	0.1271	0.1251	0.1230	0.1210	0.1190	0.1170
−1.0	0.1587	0.1562	0.1539	0.1515	0.1492	0.1469	0.1446	0.1423	0.1401	0.1379
−0.9	0.1841	0.1814	0.1788	0.1762	0.1736	0.1711	0.1685	0.1660	0.1635	0.1611
−0.8	0.2119	0.2090	0.2061	0.2033	0.2005	0.1977	0.1949	0.1922	0.1894	0.1867
−0.7	0.2420	0.2389	0.2358	0.2327	0.2296	0.2266	0.2236	0.2206	0.2177	0.2148
−0.6	0.2743	0.2709	0.2676	0.2643	0.2611	0.2578	0.2546	0.2514	0.2483	0.2451
−0.5	0.3085	0.3050	0.3015	0.2981	0.2946	0.2912	0.2877	0.2843	0.2810	0.2776
−0.4	0.3446	0.3409	0.3372	0.3336	0.3300	0.3264	0.3228	0.3192	0.3156	0.3121
−0.3	0.3821	0.3783	0.3745	0.3707	0.3669	0.3632	0.3594	0.3557	0.3520	0.3483
−0.2	0.4207	0.4168	0.4129	0.4090	0.4052	0.4013	0.3974	0.3936	0.3897	0.3859
−0.1	0.4602	0.4562	0.4522	0.4483	0.4443	0.4404	0.4364	0.4325	0.4286	0.4247
−0.0	0.5000	0.4960	0.4920	0.4880	0.4840	0.4801	0.4761	0.4721	0.4681	0.4641

Appendix 2

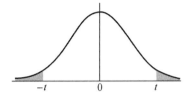

Table of Student's *t*-Distribution Critical Value

Degree of freedom, υ		Probability, P									
	One-tailed	0.25	0.20	0.10	0.05	0.025	0.01	0.005	0.0025	0.001	0.0005
	Two-tailed	0.50	0.40	0.20	0.10	0.05	0.02	0.01	0.005	0.002	0.001
1		1.000	1.376	3.078	6.314	12.706	31.821	63.657	127.321	318.309	636.619
2		0.816	1.061	1.886	2.920	4.303	6.965	9.925	14.089	22.327	31.599
3		0.765	0.978	1.638	2.353	3.182	4.541	5.841	7.453	10.215	12.924
4		0.741	0.941	1.533	2.132	2.776	3.747	4.604	5.598	7.173	8.610
5		0.727	0.920	1.476	2.015	2.571	3.365	4.032	4.773	5.893	6.869
6		0.718	0.906	1.440	1.943	2.447	3.143	3.707	4.317	5.208	5.959
7		0.711	0.896	1.415	1.895	2.365	2.998	3.499	4.029	4.785	5.408
8		0.706	0.889	1.397	1.860	2.306	2.896	3.355	3.833	4.501	5.041
9		0.703	0.883	1.383	1.833	2.262	2.821	3.250	3.690	4.297	4.781
10		0.700	0.879	1.372	1.812	2.228	2.764	3.169	3.581	4.144	4.587
11		0.697	0.876	1.363	1.796	2.201	2.718	3.106	3.497	4.025	4.437
12		0.695	0.873	1.356	1.782	2.179	2.681	3.055	3.428	3.930	4.318
13		0.694	0.870	1.350	1.771	2.160	2.650	3.012	3.372	3.852	4.221
14		0.692	0.868	1.345	1.761	2.145	2.624	2.977	3.326	3.787	4.140
15		0.691	0.866	1.341	1.753	2.131	2.602	2.947	3.286	3.733	4.073
16		0.690	0.865	1.337	1.746	2.120	2.583	2.921	3.252	3.686	4.015
17		0.689	0.863	1.333	1.740	2.110	2.567	2.898	3.222	3.646	3.965
18		0.688	0.862	1.330	1.734	2.101	2.552	2.878	3.197	3.610	3.922
19		0.688	0.861	1.328	1.729	2.093	2.539	2.861	3.174	3.579	3.883
20		0.687	0.860	1.325	1.725	2.086	2.528	2.845	3.153	3.552	3.850

Continued

Degree of freedom, υ		0.25	0.20	0.10	0.05	0.025	0.01	0.005	0.0025	0.001	0.0005
	One-tailed										
	Two-tailed	0.50	0.40	0.20	0.10	0.05	0.02	0.01	0.005	0.002	0.001
21		0.686	0.859	1.323	1.721	2.080	2.518	2.831	3.135	3.527	3.819
22		0.686	0.858	1.321	1.717	2.074	2.508	2.819	3.119	3.505	3.792
23		0.685	0.858	1.319	1.714	2.069	2.500	2.807	3.104	3.485	3.768
24		0.685	0.857	1.318	1.711	2.064	2.492	2.797	3.091	3.467	3.745
25		0.684	0.856	1.316	1.708	2.060	2.485	2.787	3.078	3.450	3.725
26		0.684	0.856	1.315	1.706	2.056	2.479	2.779	3.067	3.435	3.707
27		0.684	0.855	1.314	1.703	2.052	2.473	2.771	3.057	3.421	3.690
28		0.683	0.855	1.313	1.701	2.048	2.467	2.763	3.047	3.408	3.674
29		0.683	0.854	1.311	1.699	2.045	2.462	2.756	3.038	3.396	3.659
30		0.683	0.854	1.310	1.697	2.042	2.457	2.750	3.030	3.385	3.646
31		0.682	0.853	1.309	1.696	2.040	2.453	2.744	3.022	3.375	3.633
32		0.682	0.853	1.309	1.694	2.037	2.449	2.738	3.015	3.365	3.622
33		0.682	0.853	1.308	1.692	2.035	2.445	2.733	3.008	3.356	3.611
34		0.682	0.852	1.307	1.691	2.032	2.441	2.728	3.002	3.348	3.601
35		0.682	0.852	1.306	1.690	2.030	2.438	2.724	2.996	3.340	3.591
36		0.681	0.852	1.306	1.688	2.028	2.434	2.719	2.990	3.333	3.582
37		0.681	0.851	1.305	1.687	2.026	2.431	2.715	2.985	3.326	3.574
38		0.681	0.851	1.304	1.686	2.024	2.429	2.712	2.980	3.319	3.566
39		0.681	0.851	1.304	1.685	2.023	2.426	2.708	2.976	3.313	3.558
40		0.681	0.851	1.303	1.684	2.021	2.423	2.704	2.971	3.307	3.551
50		0.679	0.849	1.299	1.676	2.009	2.403	2.678	2.937	3.261	3.496
60		0.679	0.848	1.296	1.671	2.000	2.390	2.660	2.915	3.232	3.460
70		0.678	0.847	1.294	1.667	1.994	2.381	2.648	2.899	3.211	3.435
80		0.678	0.846	1.292	1.664	1.990	2.374	2.639	2.887	3.195	3.416
90		0.677	0.846	1.291	1.662	1.987	2.368	2.632	2.878	3.183	3.402
100		0.677	0.845	1.290	1.660	1.984	2.364	2.626	2.871	3.174	3.390
200		0.676	0.843	1.286	1.653	1.972	2.345	2.601	2.839	3.131	3.340
500		0.675	0.842	1.283	1.648	1.965	2.334	2.586	2.820	3.107	3.310
1000		0.675	0.842	1.282	1.646	1.962	2.330	2.581	2.813	3.098	3.300
∞		0.6745	0.8416	1.2816	1.6449	1.9600	2.3264	2.5758	2.8070	3.0902	3.2905

Probability, P

Appendix 3-1

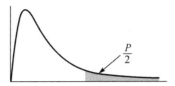

Table of F-Critical Value (Homogeneity Test of Variances)

$P=0.20$

Degree of freedom in denominator (v_2)	Degree of freedom in numerator (v_1)															
	1	2	3	4	5	6	7	8	9	10	12	15	20	30	60	∞
1	39.86	49.50	53.59	55.83	57.24	58.20	58.91	59.44	59.86	60.19	60.71	61.22	61.74	62.26	62.79	63.33
2	8.53	9.00	9.16	9.24	9.29	9.33	9.35	9.37	9.38	9.39	9.41	9.42	9.44	9.46	9.47	9.49
3	5.54	5.46	5.39	5.34	5.31	5.28	5.27	5.25	5.24	5.23	5.22	5.20	5.18	5.17	5.15	5.13
4	4.54	4.32	4.19	4.11	4.05	4.01	3.98	3.95	3.94	3.92	3.90	3.87	3.84	3.82	3.79	3.76
5	4.06	3.78	3.62	3.52	3.45	3.40	3.37	3.34	3.32	3.30	3.27	3.24	3.21	3.17	3.14	3.10
6	3.78	3.46	3.29	3.18	3.11	3.05	3.01	2.98	2.96	2.94	2.90	2.87	2.84	2.80	2.76	2.72
7	3.59	3.26	3.07	2.96	2.88	2.83	2.78	2.75	2.72	2.70	2.67	2.63	2.59	2.56	2.51	2.47
8	3.46	3.11	2.92	2.81	2.73	2.67	2.62	2.59	2.56	2.54	2.50	2.46	2.42	2.38	2.34	2.29
9	3.36	3.01	2.81	2.69	2.61	2.55	2.51	2.47	2.44	2.42	2.38	2.34	2.30	2.25	2.21	2.16
10	3.29	2.92	2.73	2.61	2.52	2.46	2.41	2.38	2.35	2.32	2.28	2.24	2.20	2.16	2.11	2.06
11	3.23	2.86	2.66	2.54	2.45	2.39	2.34	2.30	2.27	2.25	2.21	2.17	2.12	2.08	2.03	1.97
12	3.18	2.81	2.61	2.48	2.39	2.33	2.28	2.24	2.21	2.19	2.15	2.10	2.06	2.01	1.96	1.90
13	3.14	2.76	2.56	2.43	2.35	2.28	2.23	2.20	2.16	2.14	2.10	2.05	2.01	1.96	1.90	1.85
14	3.10	2.73	2.52	2.39	2.31	2.24	2.19	2.15	2.12	2.10	2.05	2.01	1.96	1.91	1.86	1.80
15	3.07	2.70	2.49	2.36	2.27	2.21	2.16	2.12	2.09	2.06	2.02	1.97	1.92	1.87	1.82	1.76
16	3.05	2.67	2.46	2.33	2.24	2.18	2.13	2.09	2.06	2.03	1.99	1.94	1.89	1.84	1.78	1.72
17	3.03	2.64	2.44	2.31	2.22	2.15	2.10	2.06	2.03	2.00	1.96	1.91	1.86	1.81	1.75	1.69
18	3.01	2.62	2.42	2.29	2.20	2.13	2.08	2.04	2.00	1.98	1.93	1.89	1.84	1.78	1.72	1.66
19	2.99	2.61	2.40	2.27	2.18	2.11	2.06	2.02	1.98	1.96	1.91	1.86	1.81	1.76	1.70	1.63
20	2.97	2.59	2.38	2.25	2.16	2.09	2.04	2.00	1.96	1.94	1.89	1.84	1.79	1.74	1.68	1.61

Continued

Degree of freedom in denominator (v_2)	Degree of freedom in numerator (v_1)															
	1	2	3	4	5	6	7	8	9	10	12	15	20	30	60	∞
21	2.96	2.57	2.36	2.23	2.14	2.08	2.02	1.98	1.95	1.92	1.87	1.83	1.78	1.72	1.66	1.59
22	2.95	2.56	2.35	2.22	2.13	2.06	2.01	1.97	1.93	1.90	1.86	1.81	1.76	1.70	1.64	1.57
23	2.94	2.55	2.34	2.21	2.11	2.05	1.99	1.95	1.92	1.89	1.84	1.80	1.74	1.69	1.62	1.55
24	2.93	2.54	2.33	2.19	2.10	2.04	1.98	1.94	1.91	1.88	1.83	1.78	1.73	1.67	1.61	1.53
25	2.92	2.53	2.32	2.18	2.09	2.02	1.97	1.93	1.89	1.87	1.82	1.77	1.72	1.66	1.59	1.52
26	2.91	2.52	2.31	2.17	2.08	2.01	1.96	1.92	1.88	1.86	1.81	1.76	1.71	1.65	1.58	1.50
27	2.90	2.51	2.30	2.17	2.07	2.00	1.95	1.91	1.87	1.85	1.80	1.75	1.70	1.64	1.57	1.49
28	2.89	2.50	2.29	2.16	2.06	2.00	1.94	1.90	1.87	1.84	1.79	1.74	1.69	1.63	1.56	1.48
29	2.89	2.50	2.28	2.15	2.06	1.99	1.93	1.89	1.86	1.83	1.78	1.73	1.68	1.62	1.55	1.47
30	2.88	2.49	2.28	2.14	2.05	1.98	1.93	1.88	1.85	1.82	1.77	1.72	1.67	1.61	1.54	1.46
40	2.84	2.44	2.23	2.09	2.00	1.93	1.87	1.83	1.79	1.76	1.71	1.66	1.61	1.54	1.47	1.38
60	2.79	2.39	2.18	2.04	1.95	1.87	1.82	1.77	1.74	1.71	1.66	1.60	1.54	1.48	1.40	1.29
120	2.75	2.35	2.13	1.99	1.90	1.82	1.77	1.72	1.68	1.65	1.60	1.55	1.48	1.41	1.32	1.19
∞	2.71	2.30	2.08	1.94	1.85	1.77	1.72	1.67	1.63	1.60	1.55	1.49	1.42	1.34	1.24	1.00

Appendix 3-2

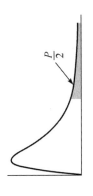

Table of F-Critical Value (Homogeneity Test of Variances)

$P=0.05$

Degree of freedom in denominator (v_2)	Degree of freedom in numerator (v_1)															
	1	2	3	4	5	6	7	8	9	10	12	15	20	30	60	∞
1	647.79	799.50	864.16	899.58	921.85	937.11	948.22	956.66	963.28	968.63	976.71	984.87	993.10	1,001.41	1,009.80	1,018.26
2	38.51	39.00	39.17	39.25	39.30	39.33	39.36	39.37	39.39	39.40	39.41	39.43	39.45	39.46	39.48	39.50
3	17.44	16.04	15.44	15.10	14.88	14.73	14.62	14.54	14.47	14.42	14.34	14.25	14.17	14.08	13.99	13.90
4	12.22	10.65	9.98	9.60	9.36	9.20	9.07	8.98	8.90	8.84	8.75	8.66	8.56	8.46	8.36	8.26
5	10.01	8.43	7.76	7.39	7.15	6.98	6.85	6.76	6.68	6.62	6.52	6.43	6.33	6.23	6.12	6.02
6	8.81	7.26	6.60	6.23	5.99	5.82	5.70	5.60	5.52	5.46	5.37	5.27	5.17	5.07	4.96	4.85
7	8.07	6.54	5.89	5.52	5.29	5.12	4.99	4.90	4.82	4.76	4.67	4.57	4.47	4.36	4.25	4.14
8	7.57	6.06	5.42	5.05	4.82	4.65	4.53	4.43	4.36	4.30	4.20	4.10	4.00	3.89	3.78	3.67
9	7.21	5.71	5.08	4.72	4.48	4.32	4.20	4.10	4.03	3.96	3.87	3.77	3.67	3.56	3.45	3.33
10	6.94	5.46	4.83	4.47	4.24	4.07	3.95	3.85	3.78	3.72	3.62	3.52	3.42	3.31	3.20	3.08

Continued

Degree of freedom in numerator (v_1)

Degree of freedom in denominator (v_2)	1	2	3	4	5	6	7	8	9	10	12	15	20	30	60	∞
11	6.72	5.26	4.63	4.28	4.04	3.88	3.76	3.66	3.59	3.53	3.43	3.33	3.23	3.12	3.00	2.88
12	6.55	5.10	4.47	4.12	3.89	3.73	3.61	3.51	3.44	3.37	3.28	3.18	3.07	2.96	2.85	2.72
13	6.41	4.97	4.35	4.00	3.77	3.60	3.48	3.39	3.31	3.25	3.15	3.05	2.95	2.84	2.72	2.60
14	6.30	4.86	4.24	3.89	3.66	3.50	3.38	3.29	3.21	3.15	3.05	2.95	2.84	2.73	2.61	2.49
15	6.20	4.77	4.15	3.80	3.58	3.41	3.29	3.20	3.12	3.06	2.96	2.86	2.76	2.64	2.52	2.40
16	6.12	4.69	4.08	3.73	3.50	3.34	3.22	3.12	3.05	2.99	2.89	2.79	2.68	2.57	2.45	2.32
17	6.04	4.62	4.01	3.66	3.44	3.28	3.16	3.06	2.98	2.92	2.82	2.72	2.62	2.50	2.38	2.25
18	5.98	4.56	3.95	3.61	3.38	3.22	3.10	3.01	2.93	2.87	2.77	2.67	2.56	2.44	2.32	2.19
19	5.92	4.51	3.90	3.56	3.33	3.17	3.05	2.96	2.88	2.82	2.72	2.62	2.51	2.39	2.27	2.13
20	5.87	4.46	3.86	3.51	3.29	3.13	3.01	2.91	2.84	2.77	2.68	2.57	2.46	2.35	2.22	2.09
21	5.83	4.42	3.82	3.48	3.25	3.09	2.97	2.87	2.80	2.73	2.64	2.53	2.42	2.31	2.18	2.04
22	5.79	4.38	3.78	3.44	3.22	3.05	2.93	2.84	2.76	2.70	2.60	2.50	2.39	2.27	2.14	2.00
23	5.75	4.35	3.75	3.41	3.18	3.02	2.90	2.81	2.73	2.67	2.57	2.47	2.36	2.24	2.11	1.97
24	5.72	4.32	3.72	3.38	3.15	2.99	2.87	2.78	2.70	2.64	2.54	2.44	2.33	2.21	2.08	1.94
25	5.69	4.29	3.69	3.35	3.13	2.97	2.85	2.75	2.68	2.61	2.51	2.41	2.30	2.18	2.05	1.91
26	5.66	4.27	3.67	3.33	3.10	2.94	2.82	2.73	2.65	2.59	2.49	2.39	2.28	2.16	2.03	1.88
27	5.63	4.24	3.65	3.31	3.08	2.92	2.80	2.71	2.63	2.57	2.47	2.36	2.25	2.13	2.00	1.85
28	5.61	4.22	3.63	3.29	3.06	2.90	2.78	2.69	2.61	2.55	2.45	2.34	2.23	2.11	1.98	1.83
29	5.59	4.20	3.61	3.27	3.04	2.88	2.76	2.67	2.59	2.53	2.43	2.32	2.21	2.09	1.96	1.81
30	5.57	4.18	3.59	3.25	3.03	2.87	2.75	2.65	2.57	2.51	2.41	2.31	2.20	2.07	1.94	1.79
40	5.42	4.05	3.46	3.13	2.90	2.74	2.62	2.53	2.45	2.39	2.29	2.18	2.07	1.94	1.80	1.64
60	5.29	3.93	3.34	3.01	2.79	2.63	2.51	2.41	2.33	2.27	2.17	2.06	1.94	1.82	1.67	1.48
120	5.15	3.80	3.23	2.89	2.67	2.52	2.39	2.30	2.22	2.16	2.05	1.94	1.82	1.69	1.53	1.31
∞	5.02	3.69	3.12	2.79	2.57	2.41	2.29	2.19	2.11	2.05	1.94	1.83	1.71	1.57	1.39	1.00

Appendix 4

F-Critical Value (ANOVA Analysis)

First Line: $P=0.05$　　Second Line: $P=0.01$

Degree of freedom in denominator (v_2)	Degree of freedom in numerator (v_1)											
	1	2	3	4	5	6	7	8	9	10	11	12
1	161.45	199.50	215.71	224.58	230.16	233.99	236.77	238.88	240.54	241.88	242.98	243.91
	4,052.18	4,999.50	5,403.35	5,624.58	5,763.65	5,858.99	5,928.36	5,981.07	6,022.47	6,055.85	6,083.32	6,106.32
2	18.51	19.00	19.16	19.25	19.30	19.33	19.35	19.37	19.38	19.40	19.40	19.41
	98.50	99.00	99.17	99.25	99.30	99.33	99.36	99.37	99.39	99.40	99.41	99.42
3	10.13	9.55	9.28	9.12	9.01	8.94	8.89	8.85	8.81	8.79	8.76	8.74
	34.12	30.82	29.46	28.71	28.24	27.91	27.67	27.49	27.35	27.23	27.13	27.05
4	7.71	6.94	6.59	6.39	6.26	6.16	6.09	6.04	6.00	5.96	5.94	5.91
	21.20	18.00	16.69	15.98	15.52	15.21	14.98	14.80	14.66	14.55	14.45	14.37
5	6.61	5.79	5.41	5.19	5.05	4.95	4.88	4.82	4.77	4.74	4.70	4.68
	16.26	13.27	12.06	11.39	10.97	10.67	10.46	10.29	10.16	10.05	9.96	9.89
6	5.99	5.14	4.76	4.53	4.39	4.28	4.21	4.15	4.10	4.06	4.03	4.00
	13.75	10.92	9.78	9.15	8.75	8.47	8.26	8.10	7.98	7.87	7.79	7.72
7	5.59	4.74	4.35	4.12	3.97	3.87	3.79	3.73	3.68	3.64	3.60	3.57
	12.25	9.55	8.45	7.85	7.46	7.19	6.99	6.84	6.72	6.62	6.54	6.47
8	5.32	4.46	4.07	3.84	3.69	3.58	3.50	3.44	3.39	3.35	3.31	3.28
	11.26	8.65	7.59	7.01	6.63	6.37	6.18	6.03	5.91	5.81	5.73	5.67

Continued

Degree of freedom in numerator (v_1)

Degree of freedom in denominator (v_2)	1	2	3	4	5	6	7	8	9	10	11	12
9	5.12	4.26	3.86	3.63	3.48	3.37	3.29	3.23	3.18	3.14	3.10	3.07
	10.56	8.02	6.99	6.42	6.06	5.80	5.61	5.47	5.35	5.26	5.18	5.11
10	4.96	4.10	3.71	3.48	3.33	3.22	3.14	3.07	3.02	2.98	2.94	2.91
	10.04	7.56	6.55	5.99	5.64	5.39	5.20	5.06	4.94	4.85	4.77	4.71
11	4.84	3.98	3.59	3.36	3.20	3.09	3.01	2.95	2.90	2.85	2.82	2.79
	9.65	7.21	6.22	5.67	5.32	5.07	4.89	4.74	4.63	4.54	4.46	4.40
12	4.75	3.89	3.49	3.26	3.11	3.00	2.91	2.85	2.80	2.75	2.72	2.69
	9.33	6.93	5.95	5.41	5.06	4.82	4.64	4.50	4.39	4.30	4.22	4.16
13	4.67	3.81	3.41	3.18	3.03	2.92	2.83	2.77	2.71	2.67	2.63	2.60
	9.07	6.70	5.74	5.21	4.86	4.62	4.44	4.30	4.19	4.10	4.02	3.96
14	4.60	3.74	3.34	3.11	2.96	2.85	2.76	2.70	2.65	2.60	2.57	2.53
	8.86	6.51	5.56	5.04	4.69	4.46	4.28	4.14	4.03	3.94	3.86	3.80
15	4.54	3.68	3.29	3.06	2.90	2.79	2.71	2.64	2.59	2.54	2.51	2.48
	8.68	6.36	5.42	4.89	4.56	4.32	4.14	4.00	3.89	3.80	3.73	3.67
16	4.49	3.63	3.24	3.01	2.85	2.74	2.66	2.59	2.54	2.49	2.46	2.42
	8.53	6.23	5.29	4.77	4.44	4.20	4.03	3.89	3.78	3.69	3.62	3.55
17	4.45	3.59	3.20	2.96	2.81	2.70	2.61	2.55	2.49	2.45	2.41	2.38
	8.40	6.11	5.18	4.67	4.34	4.10	3.93	3.79	3.68	3.59	3.52	3.46

Continued

Degree of freedom in numerator (v_1)

Degree of freedom in denominator (v_2)	1	2	3	4	5	6	7	8	9	10	11	12
18	4.41	3.55	3.16	2.93	2.77	2.66	2.58	2.51	2.46	2.41	2.37	2.34
	8.29	6.01	5.09	4.58	4.25	4.01	3.84	3.71	3.60	3.51	3.43	3.37
19	4.38	3.52	3.13	2.90	2.74	2.63	2.54	2.48	2.42	2.38	2.34	2.31
	8.18	5.93	5.01	4.50	4.17	3.94	3.77	3.63	3.52	3.43	3.36	3.30
20	4.35	3.49	3.10	2.87	2.71	2.60	2.51	2.45	2.39	2.35	2.31	2.28
	8.10	5.85	4.94	4.43	4.10	3.87	3.70	3.56	3.46	3.37	3.29	3.23
21	4.32	3.47	3.07	2.84	2.68	2.57	2.49	2.42	2.37	2.32	2.28	2.25
	8.02	5.78	4.87	4.37	4.04	3.81	3.64	3.51	3.40	3.31	3.24	3.17
22	4.30	3.44	3.05	2.82	2.66	2.55	2.46	2.40	2.34	2.30	2.26	2.23
	7.95	5.72	4.82	4.31	3.99	3.76	3.59	3.45	3.35	3.26	3.18	3.12
23	4.28	3.42	3.03	2.80	2.64	2.53	2.44	2.37	2.32	2.27	2.24	2.20
	7.88	5.66	4.76	4.26	3.94	3.71	3.54	3.41	3.30	3.21	3.14	3.07
24	4.26	3.40	3.01	2.78	2.62	2.51	2.42	2.36	2.30	2.25	2.22	2.18
	7.82	5.61	4.72	4.22	3.90	3.67	3.50	3.36	3.26	3.17	3.09	3.03
25	4.24	3.39	2.99	2.76	2.60	2.49	2.40	2.34	2.28	2.24	2.20	2.16
	7.77	5.57	4.68	4.18	3.85	3.63	3.46	3.32	3.22	3.13	3.06	2.99

Appendix 4 (Continued)

F-Critical Value (ANOVA Analysis)

First Line: $P=0.05$ Second Line: $P=0.01$

Degree of freedom in denominator (v_2)	Degree of freedom in numerator (v_1)											
	14	16	20	24	30	40	50	75	100	200	500	∞
1	245.36	246.46	248.01	249.05	250.10	251.14	251.77	252.62	253.04	253.68	254.06	254.31
	6,142.67	6,170.10	6,208.73	6,234.63	6,260.65	6,286.78	6,302.52	6,323.56	6,334.11	6,349.97	6,359.50	6,365.86
2	19.42	19.43	19.45	19.45	19.46	19.47	19.48	19.48	19.49	19.49	19.49	19.50
	99.43	99.44	99.45	99.46	99.47	99.47	99.48	99.49	99.49	99.49	99.50	99.50
3	8.71	8.69	8.66	8.64	8.62	8.59	8.58	8.56	8.55	8.54	8.53	8.53
	26.92	26.83	26.69	26.60	26.50	26.41	26.35	26.28	26.24	26.18	26.15	26.13
4	5.87	5.84	5.80	5.77	5.75	5.72	5.70	5.68	5.66	5.65	5.64	5.63
	14.25	14.15	14.02	13.93	13.84	13.75	13.69	13.61	13.58	13.52	13.49	13.46
5	4.64	4.60	4.56	4.53	4.50	4.46	4.44	4.42	4.41	4.39	4.37	4.37
	9.77	9.68	9.55	9.47	9.38	9.29	9.24	9.17	9.13	9.08	9.04	9.02
6	3.96	3.92	3.87	3.84	3.81	3.77	3.75	3.73	3.71	3.69	3.68	3.67
	7.60	7.52	7.40	7.31	7.23	7.14	7.09	7.02	6.99	6.93	6.90	6.88
7	3.53	3.49	3.44	3.41	3.38	3.34	3.32	3.29	3.27	3.25	3.24	3.23
	6.36	6.28	6.16	6.07	5.99	5.91	5.86	5.79	5.75	5.70	5.67	5.65
8	3.24	3.20	3.15	3.12	3.08	3.04	3.02	2.99	2.97	2.95	2.94	2.93
	5.56	5.48	5.36	5.28	5.20	5.12	5.07	5.00	4.96	4.91	4.88	4.86

Continued

Degree of freedom in denominator (v_2)	Degree of freedom in numerator (v_1)											
	14	16	20	24	30	40	50	75	100	200	500	∞
9	3.03	2.99	2.94	2.90	2.86	2.83	2.80	2.77	2.76	2.73	2.72	2.71
	5.01	4.92	4.81	4.73	4.65	4.57	4.52	4.45	4.41	4.36	4.33	4.31
10	2.86	2.83	2.77	2.74	2.70	2.66	2.64	2.60	2.59	2.56	2.55	2.54
	4.60	4.52	4.41	4.33	4.25	4.17	4.12	4.05	4.01	3.96	3.93	3.91
11	2.74	2.70	2.65	2.61	2.57	2.53	2.51	2.47	2.46	2.43	2.42	2.40
	4.29	4.21	4.10	4.02	3.94	3.86	3.81	3.74	3.71	3.66	3.62	3.60
12	2.64	2.60	2.54	2.51	2.47	2.43	2.40	2.37	2.35	2.32	2.31	2.30
	4.05	3.97	3.86	3.78	3.70	3.62	3.57	3.50	3.47	3.41	3.38	3.36
13	2.55	2.51	2.46	2.42	2.38	2.34	2.31	2.28	2.26	2.23	2.22	2.21
	3.86	3.78	3.66	3.59	3.51	3.43	3.38	3.31	3.27	3.22	3.19	3.17
14	2.48	2.44	2.39	2.35	2.31	2.27	2.24	2.21	2.19	2.16	2.14	2.13
	3.70	3.62	3.51	3.43	3.35	3.27	3.22	3.15	3.11	3.06	3.03	3.00
15	2.42	2.38	2.33	2.29	2.25	2.20	2.18	2.14	2.12	2.10	2.08	2.07
	3.56	3.49	3.37	3.29	3.21	3.13	3.08	3.01	2.98	2.92	2.89	2.87
16	2.37	2.33	2.28	2.24	2.19	2.15	2.12	2.09	2.07	2.04	2.02	2.01
	3.45	3.37	3.26	3.18	3.10	3.02	2.97	2.90	2.86	2.81	2.78	2.75
17	2.33	2.29	2.23	2.19	2.15	2.10	2.08	2.04	2.02	1.99	1.97	1.96
	3.35	3.27	3.16	3.08	3.00	2.92	2.87	2.80	2.76	2.71	2.68	2.65

Continued

Degree of freedom in denominator (v_2)	Degree of freedom in numerator (v_1)											
	14	16	20	24	30	40	50	75	100	200	500	∞
18	2.29	2.25	2.19	2.15	2.11	2.06	2.04	2.00	1.98	1.95	1.93	1.92
	3.27	3.19	3.08	3.00	2.92	2.84	2.78	2.71	2.68	2.62	2.59	2.57
19	2.26	2.21	2.16	2.11	2.07	2.03	2.00	1.96	1.94	1.91	1.89	1.88
	3.19	3.12	3.00	2.92	2.84	2.76	2.71	2.64	2.60	2.55	2.51	2.49
20	2.22	2.18	2.12	2.08	2.04	1.99	1.97	1.93	1.91	1.88	1.86	1.84
	3.13	3.05	2.94	2.86	2.78	2.69	2.64	2.57	2.54	2.48	2.44	2.42
21	2.20	2.16	2.10	2.05	2.01	1.96	1.94	1.90	1.88	1.84	1.83	1.81
	3.07	2.99	2.88	2.80	2.72	2.64	2.58	2.51	2.48	2.42	2.38	2.36
22	2.17	2.13	2.07	2.03	1.98	1.94	1.91	1.87	1.85	1.82	1.80	1.78
	3.02	2.94	2.83	2.75	2.67	2.58	2.53	2.46	2.42	2.36	2.33	2.31
23	2.15	2.11	2.05	2.01	1.96	1.91	1.88	1.84	1.82	1.79	1.77	1.76
	2.97	2.89	2.78	2.70	2.62	2.54	2.48	2.41	2.37	2.32	2.28	2.26
24	2.13	2.09	2.03	1.98	1.94	1.89	1.86	1.82	1.80	1.77	1.75	1.73
	2.93	2.85	2.74	2.66	2.58	2.49	2.44	2.37	2.33	2.27	2.24	2.21
25	2.11	2.07	2.01	1.96	1.92	1.87	1.84	1.80	1.78	1.75	1.73	1.71
	2.89	2.81	2.70	2.62	2.54	2.45	2.40	2.33	2.29	2.23	2.19	2.17

Appendix 4 (Continued)

F-Critical Value (ANOVA Analysis)

First Line: $P=0.05$ Second Line: $P=0.01$

Degree of freedom in denominator (v_2)	\multicolumn{12}{c}{Degree of freedom in numerator (v_1)}

(v_2)	1	2	3	4	5	6	7	8	9	10	11	12
26	4.23	3.37	2.98	2.74	2.59	2.47	2.39	2.32	2.27	2.22	2.18	2.15
	7.72	5.53	4.64	4.14	3.82	3.59	3.42	3.29	3.18	3.09	3.02	2.96
27	4.21	3.35	2.96	2.73	2.57	2.46	2.37	2.31	2.25	2.20	2.17	2.13
	7.68	5.49	4.60	4.11	3.78	3.56	3.39	3.26	3.15	3.06	2.99	2.93
28	4.20	3.34	2.95	2.71	2.56	2.45	2.36	2.29	2.24	2.19	2.15	2.12
	7.64	5.45	4.57	4.07	3.75	3.53	3.36	3.23	3.12	3.03	2.96	2.90
29	4.18	3.33	2.93	2.70	2.55	2.43	2.35	2.28	2.22	2.18	2.14	2.10
	7.60	5.42	4.54	4.04	3.73	3.50	3.33	3.20	3.09	3.00	2.93	2.87
30	4.17	3.32	2.92	2.69	2.53	2.42	2.33	2.27	2.21	2.16	2.13	2.09
	7.56	5.39	4.51	4.02	3.70	3.47	3.30	3.17	3.07	2.98	2.91	2.84
32	4.15	3.29	2.90	2.67	2.51	2.40	2.31	2.24	2.19	2.14	2.10	2.07
	7.50	5.34	4.46	3.97	3.65	3.43	3.26	3.13	3.02	2.93	2.86	2.80
34	4.13	3.28	2.88	2.65	2.49	2.38	2.29	2.23	2.17	2.12	2.08	2.05
	7.44	5.29	4.42	3.93	3.61	3.39	3.22	3.09	2.98	2.89	2.82	2.76
36	4.11	3.26	2.87	2.63	2.48	2.36	2.28	2.21	2.15	2.11	2.07	2.03
	7.40	5.25	4.38	3.89	3.57	3.35	3.18	3.05	2.95	2.86	2.79	2.72

Medical Statistics

Continued

Degree of freedom in denominator (v_2)	Degree of freedom in numerator (v_1)											
	1	2	3	4	5	6	7	8	9	10	11	12
38	4.10	3.24	2.85	2.62	2.46	2.35	2.26	2.19	2.14	2.09	2.05	2.02
	7.35	5.21	4.34	3.86	3.54	3.32	3.15	3.02	2.92	2.83	2.75	2.69
40	4.08	3.23	2.84	2.61	2.45	2.34	2.25	2.18	2.12	2.08	2.04	2.00
	7.31	5.18	4.31	3.83	3.51	3.29	3.12	2.99	2.89	2.80	2.73	2.66
42	4.07	3.22	2.83	2.59	2.44	2.32	2.24	2.17	2.11	2.06	2.03	1.99
	7.28	5.15	4.29	3.80	3.49	3.27	3.10	2.97	2.86	2.78	2.70	2.64
44	4.06	3.21	2.82	2.58	2.43	2.31	2.23	2.16	2.10	2.05	2.01	1.98
	7.25	5.12	4.26	3.78	3.47	3.24	3.08	2.95	2.84	2.75	2.68	2.62
46	4.05	3.20	2.81	2.57	2.42	2.30	2.22	2.15	2.09	2.04	2.00	1.97
	7.22	5.10	4.24	3.76	3.44	3.22	3.06	2.93	2.82	2.73	2.66	2.60
48	4.04	3.19	2.80	2.57	2.41	2.29	2.21	2.14	2.08	2.03	1.99	1.96
	7.19	5.08	4.22	3.74	3.43	3.20	3.04	2.91	2.80	2.71	2.64	2.58
50	4.03	3.18	2.79	2.56	2.40	2.29	2.20	2.13	2.07	2.03	1.99	1.95
	7.17	5.06	4.20	3.72	3.41	3.19	3.02	2.89	2.78	2.70	2.63	2.56
60	4.00	3.15	2.76	2.53	2.37	2.25	2.17	2.10	2.04	1.99	1.95	1.92
	7.08	4.98	4.13	3.65	3.34	3.12	2.95	2.82	2.72	2.63	2.56	2.50
70	3.98	3.13	2.74	2.50	2.35	2.23	2.14	2.07	2.02	1.97	1.93	1.89
	7.01	4.92	4.07	3.60	3.29	3.07	2.91	2.78	2.67	2.59	2.51	2.45

Continued

Degree of freedom in denominator $(v)_2$	Degree of freedom in numerator (v_1)											
	1	2	3	4	5	6	7	8	9	10	11	12
80	3.96	3.11	2.72	2.49	2.33	2.21	2.13	2.06	2.00	1.95	1.91	1.88
	6.96	4.88	4.04	3.56	3.26	3.04	2.87	2.74	2.64	2.55	2.48	2.42
100	3.94	3.09	2.70	2.46	2.31	2.19	2.10	2.03	1.97	1.93	1.89	1.85
	6.90	4.82	3.98	3.51	3.21	2.99	2.82	2.69	2.59	2.50	2.43	2.37
125	3.92	3.07	2.68	2.44	2.29	2.17	2.08	2.01	1.96	1.91	1.87	1.83
	6.84	4.78	3.94	3.47	3.17	2.95	2.79	2.66	2.55	2.47	2.39	2.33
150	3.90	3.06	2.66	2.43	2.27	2.16	2.07	2.00	1.94	1.89	1.85	1.82
	6.81	4.75	3.91	3.45	3.14	2.92	2.76	2.63	2.53	2.44	2.37	2.31
200	3.89	3.04	2.65	2.42	2.26	2.14	2.06	1.98	1.93	1.88	1.84	1.80
	6.76	4.71	3.88	3.41	3.11	2.89	2.73	2.60	2.50	2.41	2.34	2.27
400	3.86	3.02	2.63	2.39	2.24	2.12	2.03	1.96	1.90	1.85	1.81	1.78
	6.70	4.66	3.83	3.37	3.06	2.85	2.68	2.56	2.45	2.37	2.29	2.23
1000	3.85	3.00	2.61	2.38	2.22	2.11	2.02	1.95	1.89	1.84	1.80	1.76
	6.66	4.63	3.80	3.34	3.04	2.82	2.66	2.53	2.43	2.34	2.27	2.20
∞	3.84	3.00	2.60	2.37	2.21	2.10	2.01	1.94	1.88	1.83	1.79	1.75
	6.64	4.60	3.78	3.32	3.02	2.80	2.64	2.51	2.41	2.32	2.24	2.18

Appendix 4 (Continued)

F-Critical Value (ANOVA Analysis)

First Line: $P=0.05$　Second Line: $P=0.01$

Degree of freedom in denominator (v_2)	Degree of freedom in numerator (v_1)											
	14	16	20	24	30	40	50	75	100	200	500	∞
26	2.09	2.05	1.99	1.95	1.90	1.85	1.82	1.78	1.76	1.73	1.71	1.69
	2.86	2.78	2.66	2.58	2.50	2.42	2.36	2.29	2.25	2.19	2.16	2.13
27	2.08	2.04	1.97	1.93	1.88	1.84	1.81	1.76	1.74	1.71	1.69	1.67
	2.82	2.75	2.63	2.55	2.47	2.38	2.33	2.26	2.22	2.16	2.12	2.10
28	2.06	2.02	1.96	1.91	1.87	1.82	1.79	1.75	1.73	1.69	1.67	1.65
	2.79	2.72	2.60	2.52	2.44	2.35	2.30	2.23	2.19	2.13	2.09	2.06
29	2.05	2.01	1.94	1.90	1.85	1.81	1.77	1.73	1.71	1.67	1.65	1.64
	2.77	2.69	2.57	2.49	2.41	2.33	2.27	2.20	2.16	2.10	2.06	2.03
30	2.04	1.99	1.93	1.89	1.84	1.79	1.76	1.72	1.70	1.66	1.64	1.62
	2.74	2.66	2.55	2.47	2.39	2.30	2.25	2.17	2.13	2.07	2.03	2.01
32	2.01	1.97	1.91	1.86	1.82	1.77	1.74	1.69	1.67	1.63	1.61	1.59
	2.70	2.62	2.50	2.42	2.34	2.25	2.20	2.12	2.08	2.02	1.98	1.96
34	1.99	1.95	1.89	1.84	1.80	1.75	1.71	1.67	1.65	1.61	1.59	1.57
	2.66	2.58	2.46	2.38	2.30	2.21	2.16	2.08	2.04	1.98	1.94	1.91
36	1.98	1.93	1.87	1.82	1.78	1.73	1.69	1.65	1.62	1.59	1.56	1.55
	2.62	2.54	2.43	2.35	2.26	2.18	2.12	2.04	2.00	1.94	1.90	1.87

Continued

Degree of freedom in denominator (v_2)	Degree of freedom in numerator (v_1)											
	14	16	20	24	30	40	50	75	100	200	500	∞
38	1.96	1.92	1.85	1.81	1.76	1.71	1.68	1.63	1.61	1.57	1.54	1.53
	2.59	2.51	2.40	2.32	2.23	2.14	2.09	2.01	1.97	1.90	1.86	1.84
40	1.95	1.90	1.84	1.79	1.74	1.69	1.66	1.61	1.59	1.55	1.53	1.51
	2.56	2.48	2.37	2.29	2.20	2.11	2.06	1.98	1.94	1.87	1.83	1.80
42	1.94	1.89	1.83	1.78	1.73	1.68	1.65	1.60	1.57	1.53	1.51	1.49
	2.54	2.46	2.34	2.26	2.18	2.09	2.03	1.95	1.91	1.85	1.80	1.78
44	1.92	1.88	1.81	1.77	1.72	1.67	1.63	1.59	1.56	1.52	1.49	1.48
	2.52	2.44	2.32	2.24	2.15	2.07	2.01	1.93	1.89	1.82	1.78	1.75
46	1.91	1.87	1.80	1.76	1.71	1.65	1.62	1.57	1.55	1.51	1.48	1.46
	2.50	2.42	2.30	2.22	2.13	2.04	1.99	1.91	1.86	1.80	1.76	1.73
48	1.90	1.86	1.79	1.75	1.70	1.64	1.61	1.56	1.54	1.49	1.47	1.45
	2.48	2.40	2.28	2.20	2.12	2.02	1.97	1.89	1.84	1.78	1.73	1.70
50	1.89	1.85	1.78	1.74	1.69	1.63	1.60	1.55	1.52	1.48	1.46	1.44
	2.46	2.38	2.27	2.18	2.10	2.01	1.95	1.87	1.82	1.76	1.71	1.68
60	1.86	1.82	1.75	1.70	1.65	1.59	1.56	1.51	1.48	1.44	1.41	1.39
	2.39	2.31	2.20	2.12	2.03	1.94	1.88	1.79	1.75	1.68	1.63	1.60
70	1.84	1.79	1.72	1.67	1.62	1.57	1.53	1.48	1.45	1.40	1.37	1.35
	2.35	2.27	2.15	2.07	1.98	1.89	1.83	1.74	1.70	1.62	1.57	1.54

Continued

Degree of freedom in denominator (ν_2)	Degree of freedom in numerator (ν_1)											
	14	16	20	24	30	40	50	75	100	200	500	∞
80	1.82	1.77	1.70	1.65	1.60	1.54	1.51	1.45	1.43	1.38	1.35	1.32
	2.31	2.23	2.12	2.03	1.94	1.85	1.79	1.70	1.65	1.58	1.53	1.49
100	1.79	1.75	1.68	1.63	1.57	1.52	1.48	1.42	1.39	1.34	1.31	1.28
	2.27	2.19	2.07	1.98	1.89	1.80	1.74	1.65	1.60	1.52	1.47	1.43
125	1.77	1.73	1.66	1.60	1.55	1.49	1.45	1.40	1.36	1.31	1.27	1.25
	2.23	2.15	2.03	1.94	1.85	1.76	1.69	1.60	1.55	1.47	1.41	1.37
150	1.76	1.71	1.64	1.59	1.54	1.48	1.44	1.38	1.34	1.29	1.25	1.22
	2.20	2.12	2.00	1.92	1.83	1.73	1.66	1.57	1.52	1.43	1.38	1.33
200	1.74	1.69	1.62	1.57	1.52	1.46	1.41	1.35	1.32	1.26	1.22	1.19
	2.17	2.09	1.97	1.89	1.79	1.69	1.63	1.53	1.48	1.39	1.33	1.28
400	1.72	1.67	1.60	1.54	1.49	1.42	1.38	1.32	1.28	1.22	1.17	1.13
	2.13	2.05	1.92	1.84	1.75	1.64	1.58	1.48	1.42	1.32	1.25	1.19
1000	1.70	1.65	1.58	1.53	1.47	1.41	1.36	1.30	1.26	1.19	1.13	1.08
	2.10	2.02	1.90	1.81	1.72	1.61	1.54	1.44	1.38	1.28	1.19	1.11
∞	1.69	1.64	1.57	1.52	1.46	1.39	1.35	1.28	1.24	1.17	1.11	1.00
	2.08	2.00	1.88	1.79	1.70	1.59	1.52	1.42	1.36	1.25	1.15	1.00

Appendix 5

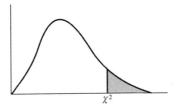

χ^2 Distribution Critical Value

Degree of freedom (υ)	Probability (P)												
	0.995	0.990	0.975	0.950	0.900	0.750	0.500	0.250	0.100	0.050	0.025	0.010	0.005
1	—	—	—	—	0.02	0.10	0.45	1.32	2.71	3.84	5.02	6.63	7.88
2	0.01	0.02	0.05	0.10	0.21	0.58	1.39	2.77	4.61	5.99	7.38	9.21	10.60
3	0.07	0.11	0.22	0.35	0.58	1.21	2.37	4.11	6.25	7.81	9.35	11.34	12.84
4	0.21	0.30	0.48	0.71	1.06	1.92	3.36	5.39	7.78	9.49	11.14	13.28	14.86
5	0.41	0.55	0.83	1.15	1.61	2.67	4.35	6.63	9.24	11.07	12.83	15.09	16.75
6	0.68	0.87	1.24	1.64	2.20	3.45	5.35	7.84	10.64	12.59	14.45	16.81	18.55
7	0.99	1.24	1.69	2.17	2.83	4.25	6.35	9.04	12.02	14.07	16.01	18.48	20.28
8	1.34	1.65	2.18	2.73	3.49	5.07	7.34	10.22	13.36	15.51	17.53	20.09	21.95
9	1.73	2.09	2.70	3.33	4.17	5.90	8.34	11.39	14.68	16.92	19.02	21.67	23.59
10	2.16	2.56	3.25	3.94	4.87	6.74	9.34	12.55	15.99	18.31	20.48	23.21	25.19
11	2.60	3.05	3.82	4.57	5.58	7.58	10.34	13.70	17.28	19.68	21.92	24.72	26.76
12	3.07	3.57	4.40	5.23	6.30	8.44	11.34	14.85	18.55	21.03	23.34	26.22	28.30
13	3.57	4.11	5.01	5.89	7.04	9.30	12.34	15.98	19.81	22.36	24.74	27.69	29.82
14	4.07	4.66	5.63	6.57	7.79	10.17	13.34	17.12	21.06	23.68	26.12	29.14	31.32
15	4.60	5.23	6.26	7.26	8.55	11.04	14.34	18.25	22.31	25.00	27.49	30.58	32.80
16	5.14	5.81	6.91	7.96	9.31	11.91	15.34	19.37	23.54	26.30	28.85	32.00	34.27
17	5.70	6.41	7.56	8.67	10.09	12.79	16.34	20.49	24.77	27.59	30.19	33.41	35.72
18	6.26	7.01	8.23	9.39	10.86	13.68	17.34	21.60	25.99	28.87	31.53	34.81	37.16
19	6.84	7.63	8.91	10.12	11.65	14.56	18.34	22.72	27.20	30.14	32.85	36.19	38.58
20	7.43	8.26	9.59	10.85	12.44	15.45	19.34	23.83	28.41	31.41	34.17	37.57	40.00

Continued

Degree of freedom (v)	Probability (P)												
	0.995	0.990	0.975	0.950	0.900	0.750	0.500	0.250	0.100	0.050	0.025	0.010	0.005
21	8.03	8.90	10.28	11.59	13.24	16.34	20.34	24.93	29.62	32.67	35.48	38.93	41.40
22	8.64	9.54	10.98	12.34	14.04	17.24	21.34	26.04	30.81	33.92	36.78	40.29	42.80
23	9.26	10.20	11.69	13.09	14.85	18.14	22.34	27.14	32.01	35.17	38.08	41.64	44.18
24	9.89	10.86	12.40	13.85	15.66	19.04	23.34	28.24	33.20	36.42	39.36	42.98	45.56
25	10.52	11.52	13.12	14.61	16.47	19.94	24.34	29.34	34.38	37.65	40.65	44.31	46.93
26	11.16	12.20	13.84	15.38	17.29	20.84	25.34	30.43	35.56	38.89	41.92	45.64	48.29
27	11.81	12.88	14.57	16.15	18.11	21.75	26.34	31.53	36.74	40.11	43.19	46.96	49.64
28	12.46	13.56	15.31	16.93	18.94	22.66	27.34	32.62	37.92	41.34	44.46	48.28	50.99
29	13.12	14.26	16.05	17.71	19.77	23.57	28.34	33.71	39.09	42.56	45.72	49.59	52.34
30	13.79	14.95	16.79	18.49	20.60	24.48	29.34	34.80	40.26	43.77	46.98	50.89	53.67
40	20.71	22.16	24.43	26.51	29.05	33.66	39.34	45.62	51.81	55.76	59.34	63.69	66.77
50	27.99	29.71	32.36	34.76	37.69	42.94	49.33	56.33	63.17	67.50	71.42	76.15	79.49
60	35.53	37.48	40.48	43.19	46.46	52.29	59.33	66.98	74.40	79.08	83.30	88.38	91.95
70	43.28	45.44	48.76	51.74	55.33	61.70	69.33	77.58	85.53	90.53	95.02	100.42	104.22
80	51.17	53.54	57.15	60.39	64.28	71.14	79.33	88.13	96.58	101.88	106.63	112.33	116.32
90	59.20	61.75	65.65	69.13	73.29	80.62	89.33	98.64	107.56	113.14	118.14	124.12	128.30
100	67.33	70.06	74.22	77.93	82.36	90.13	99.33	109.14	118.50	124.34	129.56	135.81	140.17

Appendix 6

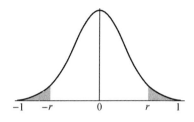

r-Critical Value

Degree of freedom (υ)		Probability (P)								
	One-tailed	0.25	0.10	0.05	0.025	0.01	0.005	0.0025	0.001	0.0005
	Two-tailed	0.50	0.20	0.10	0.05	0.02	0.01	0.005	0.002	0.001
1		0.707	0.951	0.988	0.997	1.000	1.000	1.000	1.000	1.000
2		0.500	0.800	0.900	0.950	0.980	0.990	0.995	0.998	0.999
3		0.404	0.687	0.805	0.878	0.934	0.959	0.974	0.986	0.991
4		0.347	0.608	0.729	0.811	0.882	0.917	0.942	0.963	0.974
5		0.309	0.551	0.669	0.755	0.833	0.875	0.906	0.935	0.951
6		0.281	0.507	0.621	0.707	0.789	0.834	0.870	0.905	0.925
7		0.260	0.472	0.582	0.666	0.750	0.798	0.836	0.875	0.898
8		0.242	0.443	0.549	0.632	0.715	0.765	0.805	0.847	0.872
9		0.228	0.419	0.521	0.602	0.685	0.735	0.776	0.820	0.847
10		0.216	0.398	0.497	0.576	0.658	0.708	0.750	0.795	0.823
11		0.206	0.380	0.476	0.553	0.634	0.684	0.726	0.772	0.801
12		0.197	0.365	0.457	0.532	0.612	0.661	0.703	0.750	0.780
13		0.189	0.351	0.441	0.514	0.592	0.641	0.683	0.730	0.760
14		0.182	0.338	0.426	0.497	0.574	0.623	0.664	0.711	0.742
15		0.176	0.327	0.412	0.482	0.558	0.606	0.647	0.694	0.725
16		0.170	0.317	0.400	0.468	0.542	0.590	0.631	0.678	0.708
17		0.165	0.308	0.389	0.456	0.529	0.575	0.616	0.662	0.693
18		0.160	0.299	0.378	0.444	0.515	0.561	0.602	0.648	0.679
19		0.156	0.291	0.369	0.433	0.503	0.549	0.589	0.635	0.665
20		0.152	0.284	0.360	0.423	0.492	0.537	0.576	0.622	0.652
21		0.148	0.277	0.352	0.413	0.482	0.526	0.565	0.610	0.640

Continued

Degree of freedom (υ)		0.25	0.10	0.05	0.025	0.01	0.005	0.0025	0.001	0.0005
	One-tailed									
	Two-tailed	0.50	0.20	0.10	0.05	0.02	0.01	0.005	0.002	0.001
22		0.145	0.271	0.344	0.404	0.472	0.515	0.554	0.599	0.629
23		0.141	0.265	0.337	0.396	0.462	0.505	0.543	0.588	0.618
24		0.138	0.260	0.330	0.388	0.453	0.496	0.534	0.578	0.607
25		0.136	0.255	0.323	0.381	0.445	0.487	0.524	0.568	0.597
26		0.133	0.250	0.317	0.374	0.437	0.479	0.515	0.559	0.588
27		0.131	0.245	0.311	0.367	0.430	0.471	0.507	0.550	0.579
28		0.128	0.241	0.306	0.361	0.423	0.463	0.499	0.541	0.570
29		0.126	0.237	0.301	0.355	0.416	0.456	0.491	0.533	0.562
30		0.124	0.233	0.296	0.349	0.409	0.449	0.484	0.526	0.554
31		0.122	0.229	0.291	0.344	0.403	0.442	0.477	0.518	0.546
32		0.120	0.225	0.287	0.339	0.397	0.436	0.470	0.511	0.539
33		0.118	0.222	0.283	0.334	0.392	0.430	0.464	0.504	0.532
34		0.116	0.219	0.279	0.329	0.386	0.424	0.458	0.498	0.525
35		0.115	0.216	0.275	0.325	0.381	0.418	0.452	0.492	0.519
36		0.113	0.213	0.271	0.320	0.376	0.413	0.446	0.486	0.513
37		0.111	0.210	0.267	0.316	0.371	0.408	0.441	0.480	0.507
38		0.110	0.207	0.264	0.312	0.367	0.403	0.435	0.474	0.501
39		0.108	0.204	0.261	0.308	0.362	0.398	0.430	0.469	0.495
40		0.107	0.202	0.257	0.304	0.358	0.393	0.425	0.463	0.490
41		0.106	0.199	0.254	0.301	0.354	0.389	0.420	0.458	0.484
42		0.104	0.197	0.251	0.297	0.350	0.384	0.416	0.453	0.479
43		0.103	0.195	0.248	0.294	0.346	0.380	0.411	0.449	0.474
44		0.102	0.192	0.246	0.291	0.342	0.376	0.407	0.444	0.469
45		0.101	0.190	0.243	0.288	0.338	0.372	0.403	0.439	0.465
46		0.100	0.188	0.240	0.285	0.335	0.368	0.399	0.435	0.460
47		0.099	0.186	0.238	0.282	0.331	0.365	0.395	0.431	0.456
48		0.098	0.184	0.235	0.279	0.328	0.361	0.391	0.427	0.451
49		0.097	0.182	0.233	0.276	0.325	0.358	0.387	0.423	0.447
50		0.096	0.181	0.231	0.273	0.322	0.354	0.384	0.419	0.443

Appendix 7

r_s-Critical Value

n		Probability (P)								
	One-tailed	0.25	0.10	0.05	0.025	0.01	0.005	0.0025	0.001	0.0005
	Two-tailed	0.50	0.20	0.10	0.05	0.02	0.01	0.005	0.002	0.001
4		0.600	1.000	1.000	—	—	—	—	—	—
5		0.500	0.800	0.900	1.000	1.000	—	—	—	—
6		0.371	0.657	0.829	0.886	0.943	1.000	1.000	—	—
7		0.321	0.571	0.714	0.786	0.893	0.929	0.964	1.000	1.000
8		0.310	0.524	0.643	0.738	0.833	0.881	0.905	0.952	0.976
9		0.267	0.483	0.600	0.700	0.783	0.833	0.867	0.917	0.933
10		0.248	0.455	0.564	0.648	0.745	0.794	0.830	0.879	0.903
11		0.236	0.427	0.536	0.618	0.709	0.755	0.800	0.845	0.873
12		0.217	0.406	0.503	0.587	0.678	0.727	0.769	0.818	0.846
13		0.209	0.385	0.484	0.560	0.648	0.703	0.747	0.791	0.824
14		0.200	0.367	0.464	0.538	0.626	0.679	0.723	0.771	0.802
15		0.189	0.354	0.446	0.521	0.604	0.654	0.700	0.750	0.779
16		0.182	0.341	0.429	0.503	0.582	0.635	0.679	0.729	0.762
17		0.176	0.328	0.414	0.485	0.566	0.615	0.662	0.713	0.748
18		0.170	0.317	0.401	0.472	0.550	0.600	0.643	0.695	0.728
19		0.165	0.309	0.391	0.460	0.535	0.584	0.628	0.677	0.712
20		0.161	0.299	0.380	0.447	0.520	0.570	0.612	0.662	0.696
21		0.156	0.292	0.370	0.435	0.508	0.556	0.599	0.648	0.681
22		0.152	0.284	0.361	0.425	0.496	0.544	0.586	0.634	0.667
23		0.148	0.278	0.353	0.415	0.486	0.532	0.573	0.622	0.654
24		0.144	0.271	0.344	0.406	0.476	0.521	0.562	0.610	0.642
25		0.142	0.265	0.337	0.398	0.466	0.511	0.551	0.598	0.630
26		0.138	0.259	0.331	0.390	0.457	0.501	0.541	0.587	0.619

Continued

n		0.25	0.10	0.05	0.025	0.01	0.005	0.0025	0.001	0.0005
	One-tailed	0.25	0.10	0.05	0.025	0.01	0.005	0.0025	0.001	0.0005
	Two-tailed	0.50	0.20	0.10	0.05	0.02	0.01	0.005	0.002	0.001
27		0.136	0.255	0.324	0.382	0.448	0.491	0.531	0.577	0.608
28		0.133	0.250	0.317	0.375	0.440	0.483	0.522	0.567	0.598
29		0.130	0.245	0.312	0.368	0.433	0.475	0.513	0.558	0.589
30		0.128	0.240	0.306	0.362	0.425	0.467	0.504	0.549	0.580
31		0.126	0.236	0.301	0.356	0.418	0.459	0.496	0.541	0.571
32		0.124	0.232	0.296	0.350	0.412	0.452	0.489	0.533	0.563
33		0.121	0.229	0.291	0.345	0.405	0.446	0.482	0.525	0.554
34		0.120	0.225	0.287	0.340	0.399	0.439	0.475	0.517	0.547
35		0.118	0.222	0.283	0.335	0.394	0.433	0.468	0.510	0.539
36		0.116	0.219	0.279	0.330	0.388	0.427	0.462	0.504	0.533
37		0.114	0.216	0.275	0.325	0.382	0.421	0.456	0.497	0.526
38		0.113	0.212	0.271	0.321	0.378	0.415	0.450	0.491	0.519
39		0.111	0.210	0.267	0.317	0.373	0.410	0.444	0.485	0.513
40		0.110	0.207	0.264	0.313	0.368	0.405	0.439	0.479	0.507
41		0.108	0.204	0.261	0.309	0.364	0.400	0.433	0.473	0.501
42		0.107	0.202	0.257	0.305	0.359	0.395	0.428	0.468	0.495
43		0.105	0.199	0.254	0.301	0.355	0.391	0.423	0.463	0.490
44		0.104	0.197	0.251	0.298	0.351	0.386	0.419	0.458	0.484
45		0.103	0.194	0.248	0.294	0.347	0.382	0.414	0.453	0.479
46		0.102	0.192	0.246	0.291	0.343	0.378	0.410	0.448	0.474
47		0.101	0.190	0.243	0.288	0.340	0.374	0.405	0.443	0.469
48		0.100	0.188	0.240	0.285	0.336	0.370	0.401	0.439	0.465
49		0.098	0.186	0.238	0.282	0.333	0.366	0.397	0.434	0.460
50		0.097	0.184	0.235	0.279	0.329	0.363	0.393	0.430	0.456

Probability (P)

Appendixes • 375 •

Appendix 8

Random Number Table

ID	1—10	11—20	21—30	31—40	41—50
1	88 69 22 93 86	34 87 52 64 67	85 29 90 06 61	39 00 68 69 23	82 05 45 29 18
2	37 96 71 27 39	38 18 07 31 33	95 66 33 65 76	78 61 05 59 93	01 86 01 65 56
3	39 50 41 65 95	02 02 75 18 06	28 77 31 87 37	63 95 22 59 54	75 42 23 99 69
4	44 61 61 04 61	45 05 67 02 96	13 89 39 65 59	88 52 12 85 06	94 30 76 13 09
5	35 52 42 71 12	02 94 23 59 81	19 41 24 83 74	92 34 41 08 61	6 15 12 16 00
6	35 19 33 29 64	84 15 27 27 99	84 18 68 46 13	41 86 65 37 20	97 10 25 23 95
7	40 07 33 74 07	56 84 60 82 46	20 34 70 39 29	21 38 52 39 38	25 56 19 69 29
8	16 50 08 32 88	00 48 34 47 73	05 81 52 56 16	42 17 39 50 53	00 05 74 25 50
9	04 23 41 25 70	09 53 50 72 17	09 04 86 65 46	48 98 53 04 37	23 09 65 88 33
10	39 03 86 03 69	79 78 09 55 84	51 48 82 38 88	47 09 02 77 78	36 97 78 68 92
11	20 97 61 38 82	00 79 54 59 42	86 89 36 81 80	41 36 23 21 41	04 70 12 41 66
12	00 21 45 44 37	80 85 61 07 94	98 65 41 55 83	01 18 39 14 38	47 16 64 53 25
13	92 47 80 25 30	75 30 35 43 65	38 73 27 99 20	98 94 36 88 48	85 78 26 90 08
14	41 97 55 77 12	21 70 47 75 94	29 95 56 39 87	92 56 56 16 50	33 92 39 70 56
15	09 67 70 42 77	87 07 01 07 27	68 36 27 55 63	42 04 15 44 57	07 09 29 33 77
16	24 36 37 95 29	02 72 27 39 27	17 65 96 55 67	67 27 42 57 18	09 35 27 60 34
17	72 88 99 63 42	10 48 10 08 83	59 10 30 21 74	04 71 83 88 28	42 62 02 58 04
18	48 97 89 54 53	53 54 20 99 09	56 45 49 26 21	88 73 89 93 53	67 52 65 52 03
19	51 16 11 09 24	89 07 72 74 51	33 13 00 94 84	81 92 02 48 92	53 29 93 06 53
20	75 67 53 15 79	79 73 43 38 75	92 54 80 72 91	82 07 58 05 66	36 41 60 29 53
21	45 64 16 79 62	83 03 74 43 82	26 74 85 68 91	53 59 45 45 28	63 99 42 29 97
22	66 91 82 85 42	11 78 95 18 69	38 77 70 71 91	87 06 94 69 54	22 63 40 94 67
23	72 83 61 98 37	97 89 54 56 27	41 30 79 28 87	75 81 39 21 77	94 41 34 52 37
24	03 50 92 81 20	92 72 87 22 30	38 30 88 33 64	28 34 65 60 30	86 91 97 94 54
25	99 52 61 47 98	43 52 67 36 05	91 56 46 35 83	46 95 41 08 11	26 17 70 88 25

Continued

ID	1—10	11—20	21—30	31—40	41—50
26	74 94 92 22 30	14 04 63 87 13	87 89 74 39 89	03 98 70 21 56	64 80 59 23 26
27	32 98 72 70 22	66 98 76 70 59	32 94 81 58 43	64 39 57 45 35	84 28 30 83 11
28	39 10 95 09 83	90 49 94 58 13	81 18 18 67 77	82 72 56 20 74	36 85 94 06 94
29	23 79 88 40 92	91 63 73 79 37	19 37 52 72 71	78 22 38 61 52	20 61 72 01 62
30	91 67 82 72 10	88 51 63 69 46	56 66 58 21 91	90 82 26 84 91	52 27 37 01 86
31	29 82 41 79 19	53 18 04 38 49	88 41 12 04 32	20 88 70 21 24	73 92 03 78 19
32	63 95 60 38 71	96 42 47 71 48	23 05 01 72 07	13 25 92 42 35	15 89 79 83 56
33	55 89 21 83 51	06 83 19 78 32	01 19 99 99 48	54 60 31 59 33	10 31 30 92 99
34	51 22 66 68 24	72 32 64 47 78	59 12 53 96 94	50 43 56 34 36	28 80 82 3 82
35	38 26 96 14 31	17 38 69 63 65	63 16 95 25 83	48 12 91 69 77	69 33 39 25 83
36	24 04 51 07 44	21 58 47 02 59	65 11 86 41 80	33 41 63 95 78	53 36 61 59 60
37	21 36 55 87 64	80 41 28 84 58	73 69 97 96 37	80 05 88 50 75	08 81 88 12 23
38	92 00 95 46 70	36 92 21 65 40	58 21 23 55 89	68 61 60 47 71	52 83 22 37 31
39	27 09 02 96 73	52 82 60 25 18	57 74 39 81 79	88 19 99 56 15	89 91 26 74 34
40	52 94 64 60 62	92 16 76 14 55	43 41 88 86 87	03 08 02 24 71	33 70 88 98 75
41	49 95 47 75 75	45 50 75 87 20	29 11 29 52 30	96 30 66 27 57	95 92 57 35 90
42	29 67 86 51 76	34 07 57 64 71	02 81 26 00 97	00 74 63 87 88	53 93 69 55 35
43	27 55 02 92 10	16 36 11 08 16	58 25 63 15 84	91 53 34 39 98	09 51 45 23 55
44	62 79 06 85 40	85 01 97 47 43	64 39 58 24 77	19 07 89 98 20	82 00 85 54 09
45	90 68 20 46 68	39 77 57 86 97	18 76 19 20 17	61 70 39 18 70	89 86 88 12 84
46	94 71 25 51 24	38 01 94 19 91	32 87 73 19 43	69 18 82 83 47	71 87 22 21 80
47	04 84 08 54 85	19 59 46 33 95	77 91 26 61 94	75 16 82 88 96	59 41 26 94 53
48	84 79 41 24 48	02 30 30 84 66	34 61 15 44 76	50 66 72 89 26	29 63 61 86 02
49	73 68 33 46 81	37 83 92 02 73	05 11 69 17 65	37 84 70 17 68	28 41 76 92 30
50	09 98 42 09 49	19 20 43 72 64	97 97 74 78 65	11 14 83 53 76	98 75 65 83 85

Appendix 9

Random Permutation Table ($n=20$)

ID	1	2	3	4	5	6	7	8	9	10	11	12	13	14	15	16	17	18	19	20	r_s
1	1	15	19	13	17	5	4	7	9	14	12	18	10	16	11	20	3	6	2	8	−0.1519
2	13	19	15	11	4	10	17	9	5	7	12	14	1	18	8	2	3	16	20	6	−0.1850
3	13	12	20	3	9	6	14	17	1	16	19	18	7	4	10	2	5	11	15	8	−0.1955
4	2	12	7	11	5	8	15	10	6	17	20	18	9	16	1	19	14	4	3	13	0.1368
5	4	7	20	13	6	19	2	14	16	5	18	3	17	1	11	9	15	10	8	12	−0.0090
6	15	4	1	12	17	19	13	8	7	14	18	9	10	16	11	2	3	6	5	20	−0.0947
7	10	11	1	18	5	12	14	20	19	8	3	17	4	9	6	13	7	15	16	2	−0.0692
8	14	7	9	18	17	5	6	20	11	12	2	4	13	10	15	3	16	8	1	19	−0.1128
9	3	16	6	14	13	10	5	1	9	12	19	11	20	15	18	7	8	17	4	2	0.0361
10	4	13	1	19	10	11	6	17	15	2	7	12	3	18	14	9	16	8	20	5	0.1729
11	13	5	20	3	8	15	4	19	7	6	12	17	14	2	11	1	18	10	16	9	0.0301
12	2	16	9	18	13	8	11	19	1	10	15	7	20	5	12	6	3	17	14	4	−0.0947
13	7	15	5	9	11	10	13	6	17	14	16	1	19	4	8	3	20	18	12	2	0.0316
14	14	13	15	1	17	12	5	3	16	4	8	20	10	11	18	19	6	2	7	9	−0.1188
15	8	7	6	4	5	14	10	16	12	17	11	20	19	15	13	3	9	18	1	2	0.0496
16	1	2	18	19	11	12	17	9	8	7	5	13	16	4	6	15	20	3	14	10	0.0827
17	6	18	7	19	8	10	20	9	17	16	1	5	3	14	4	11	13	12	2	15	−0.1865
18	19	14	15	1	4	3	13	18	9	11	16	5	2	12	7	10	20	8	6	17	−0.0181
19	13	3	14	11	20	5	17	16	1	8	9	12	2	18	15	6	4	10	19	7	−0.0647
20	9	17	12	7	8	6	15	10	2	20	13	5	11	1	3	16	19	18	4	14	0.0677
21	7	13	10	11	20	5	4	14	15	16	9	19	18	8	1	2	17	3	12	6	−0.1835
22	17	9	11	4	6	15	16	8	14	2	12	10	20	1	18	13	3	5	19	7	−0.0496
23	11	8	4	10	19	3	17	15	16	7	1	18	20	2	6	9	12	13	14	5	−0.0105
24	8	11	10	13	17	18	15	19	2	5	6	16	9	4	7	3	14	1	20	12	−0.1729
25	1	10	15	19	6	9	20	7	14	12	16	4	8	2	18	11	5	3	17	13	−0.0195
26	6	18	3	10	19	1	14	5	20	11	16	2	17	7	4	12	9	8	15	13	0.0421
27	20	1	16	3	14	12	19	4	15	7	10	18	13	5	8	2	6	9	11	17	−0.1218
28	14	10	16	9	5	3	20	2	4	11	12	18	13	1	7	15	19	17	8	6	0.0526
29	11	16	5	4	15	17	13	6	18	2	14	19	1	9	3	8	12	7	10	20	−0.0286
30	15	9	18	4	5	7	3	17	12	1	10	16	14	20	19	2	13	8	6	11	0.0301